AF443476

Oral Cancer:
Clinical and Pathological Considerations

Editors

Bruce A. Wright, D.D.S., M.D.
Assistant Professor
Division of Oral and Maxillofacial Surgery
Dalhousie University
Halifax, Nova Scotia, Canada

John M. Wright, D.D.S., M.S.
Professor
Department of Pathology
Baylor College of Dentistry
Dallas, Texas

William H. Binnie, D.D.S., M.S.D., F.R.C. Path.
Professor and Chairman
Department of Pathology
Baylor College of Dentistry
Dallas, Texas

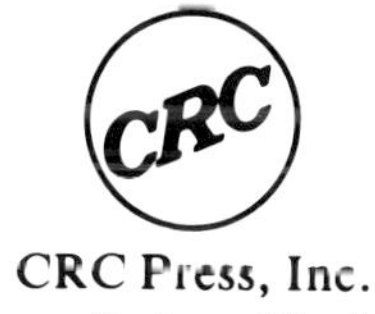

CRC Press, Inc.
Boca Raton, Florida

Library of Congress Cataloging-in-Publication Data

Oral cancer.

Includes bibliographies and index.
1. Mouth--Cancer.   I. Wright, Bruce A.   II. Wright, John M., 1948-   .   III. Binnie, William H.
[DNLM: 1. Mouth Neoplasms.   WU 280 0628]
RC280.M6068   1988   616.99′492   87-23892
ISBN 0-8493-6774-3

This book represents information obtained from authentic and highly regarded sources. Reprinted material is quoted with permission, and sources are indicated. A wide variety of references are listed. Every reasonable effort has been made to give reliable data and information, but the author and the publisher cannot assume responsibility for the validity of all materials or for the consequences of their use.

Direct all inquiries to CRC Press, Inc., 2000 Corporate Blvd., N.W., Boca Raton, Florida, 33431.

International Standard Book Number 0-8493-6774-3

Library of Congress Card Number 87-23892
Printed in the United States

FOREWORD

Between the inception and completion of this book, at least four other texts on oral cancer have appeared. All have a different approach to the subject. *Oral Cancer: Clinical and Pathological Considerations* focuses exclusively on squamous cell carcinoma of the oral cavity, not neoplasia of the head and neck.

This monograph is concerned with the scope of the problem, its cause, pathogenesis, presentation, and management. We have also added our thoughts on future trends and research, some of which no doubt will have been overtaken by the time of publication.

Oral cancer is a complex problem which requires a team of many different specialists for its management. It is important that each member of that team understands the problems of the other members. The purpose of this book is to help in the promotion of that understanding.

ACKNOWLEDGMENTS

We are indebted to many for their help and tolerance. The contributors worked hard to meet the deadline we set. Our families and institutions have allowed us time from various committments. Special thanks are due to Joanell Rawlins for typing the manuscript, Linda Ford for carrying the extra load of departmental secretarial duties, and the Department of Media Resources for producing the illustrations.

Our interest in this subject is due mainly to the influence of three men. Our thanks to William G. Shafer, Roderick A. Cawson, and Jens J. Pindborg for the stimulus they have provided.

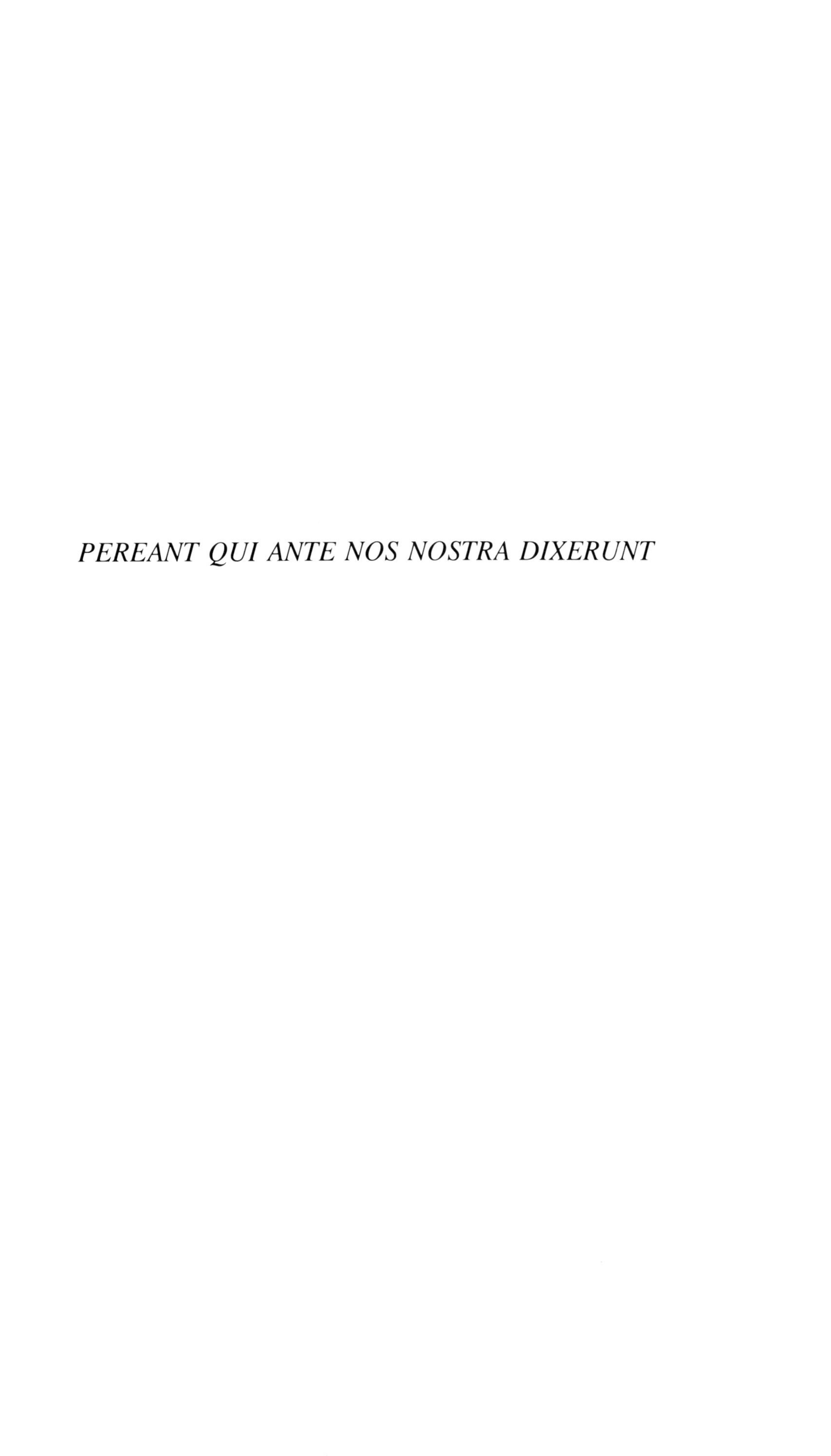

PEREANT QUI ANTE NOS NOSTRA DIXERUNT

THE EDITORS

Bruce A. Wright is an Assistant Professor in the Department of Oral Surgery at Dalhousie University, Halifax, Nova Scotia, Canada, and is presently engaged in a residency in General Pathology at the Victorial General Hospital in Halifax.

He received his Bachelor in Dental Surgery from Guy's Hospital, London; a doctorate in Dental Surgery from Dalhousie University; a Masters of Science in Oral Pathology from Indiana University School of Dentistry; and his M.D. from Dalhousie University.

Dr. Wright is a Diplomate of the American Board of Oral Pathology as well as a Junior Member of the College of American Pathology.

Dr. Wright's major research interests include oral cancer and premalignancy and the role which chronic fungal infections play in the genesis and natural history of these entities.

John M. Wright is Professor of Pathology at Baylor College of Dentistry, Associate Attending in the Department of Pathology at Baylor University Medical Center, and a consultant to the Veterans Administration Hospital in Dallas, Texas.

Dr. Wright received his D.D.S. from West Virginia University School of Dentistry in 1973, and an M.S. in Oral Pathology from Indiana University School of Dentistry in 1977. He held a Clinical Fellowship from the American Cancer Society from 1976 to 1977 and was Assistant Professor in the Department of Oral Pathology at Indiana University School of Dentistry from 1977 to 1980. In 1980, Dr. Wright was appointed Associate Professor of Pathology at Baylor College of Dentistry.

Dr. Wright is a member of the American Dental Association, the Texas Dental Association, the Dallas County Dental Association, the International Association of Oral Pathologists, the Dallas section of the International Association for Dental Research, and the American Association of Dental Schools. He is a Fellow of the American Academy of Oral Pathology and a member of its governing Council. Dr. Wright is certified by both the American Board of Oral Pathology and the American Board of Oral Medicine.

Dr. Wright has published numerous scientific articles in the field of oral pathology. His major research interests are oral mucosal diseases, with a particular interest in premalignancy.

William H. Binnie is Professor and Chairman of Pathology at Baylor College of Dentistry in Dallas, Texas. He is on the attending staff at Baylor University Medical Center and a consultant oral pathologist at Methodist and Veterans Administration Hospitals in Dallas.

He obtained his Bachelor of Dental Surgery degree from the University of Glasgow in 1963; a doctorate in Dental Surgery in 1965 from McGill University, Montreal; and the Master of Science in Dentistry from the University of Indiana in 1967. He was appointed lecturer in Oral Medicine and Pathology at Guy's Hospital Medical School in 1967 and later senior lecturer and honorary consultant in 1975. He obtained his Fellowship in Dental Surgery from the Royal College of Physicians and Surgeons of Glasgow in 1972 and his Membership in the Royal College of Pathologists in 1975. He moved to Baylor in 1979 and is a naturalized U.S. citizen.

Dr. Binnie is a diplomate of the American Board of Oral Medicine and Secretary/Treasurer of the International Association of Oral Pathologists. He is a member of the American Academy of Oral Pathology, the British Society for Oral Pathology, the American Association of Dental Schools, the International Association for Dental Research, the American Academy of Oral Medicine, the American Dental Association, and is a Fellow of the American College of Dentists.

Dr. Binnie is the author or co-author of more than 50 scientific publications in oral pathology. His main interest is in epidemiology and etiological aspects of oral cancer.

Fritz E. Barton, M. D.
Attending, Plastic and Reconstructive
 Surgery
Attending, Oncology
Baylor University Medical Center
Chief, Division of Plastic Surgery
University of Texas Health Science
 Center
Dallas, Texas

John S. Bradfield, M.D.
Attending, Radiology
Attending, Oncology
Baylor University Medical Center
Dallas, Texas

D. Lamar Byrd, D.D.S., M.S.D.
Sammons Cancer Center
Baylor University Medical Center
Dallas, Texas

Eugene W. Dahl, D.D.S.
Assistant Professor, Prosthodontics
Baylor College of Dentistry
Dallas, Texas

Robin E. Howell, D.D.S.
Assistant Professor
Department of Oral Biology
Dalhousie University
Halifax, Nova Scotia, Canada

Zelig H. Lieberman, M.D.
Attending, Surgery
Attending, Oncology
Baylor University Medical Center
Dallas, Texas

Robert G. Mennel, M.D.
Associate Attending, Internal Medicine
Associate Attending, Oncology
Baylor University Medical Center
Dallas, Texas

John C. O'Brien, Jr., M.D.
Attending, Surgery
Attending, Oncology
Baylor University Medical Center
Dallas, Texas

Kathleen Vendrell Rankin, D.D.S.
Research Associate
Department of Pathology
Baylor College of Dentistry
Dallas, Texas

TABLE OF CONTENTS

Chapter 1

EPIDEMIOLOGY OF ORAL CANCER

William H. Binnie and Kathleen Vendrell Rankin

TABLE OF CONTENTS

I. INTRODUCTION

It has been stated[1] that it is a fundamental principle of epidemiology that disease does not occur randomly, and it is the province of epidemiology to identify the characteristics of these nonrandom occurrences. The epidemiology of cancer, specifically oral cancer, is unique in its long latent period and relatively low incidence which renders a direct cause and effect relationship more difficult to identify, particularly if one accepts the premise of multifactorial etiology. However, a high fatality rate and a high degree of diagnostic reliability generate case numbers with reliable population data, particularly with regard to death registrations. The descriptive study of this data on incidence, mortality, and survival is the foundation for analytic and experimental study of oral cancer.

II. DESCRIPTIVE STUDY

A. Incidence

Incidence and prevalence rates are two of the more commonly used indexes for describing epidemiologic patterns. Incidence may be defined as the number of new cases in a specific time period (usually 1 year) for a specified population conventionally expressed as cases per 100,000. This is in contrast to period prevalence which is the proportion of the population that has the disease at a given point in time and which is usually expressed as a percentage.

In the U.S., malignant neoplasia of the oral cavity is a small problem in numerical terms, comprising only 2 to 4% of total malignant tumors (a total which does not include non-melanotic skin cancer).[2] A similar incidence of 2% was reported by Binnie et al.[3] for neoplasms in the buccal cavity and oral mesopharynx in England and Wales, and, in fact, a range of 2 to 6% applies to most western countries.[4] Internationally, however, there are tremendous variations in incidence. A figure approaching 50% has been reported for parts of India[5] and over 40% in Sri Lanka.[6]

On a global basis oral cancer ranks fourth for men and sixth for women in incidence rank for all cancers.[7] Volume 4 of *Cancer Incidence in Five Continents* lists the four highest male incidence rates for cancer of the buccal cavity and pharynx as those from Hong Kong, Bas-Rhin (France), Bombay (India), and Newfoundland (Canada). High incidence areas have also been identified in the U.S.S.R. where the rate for males was reported to be 17.1/100,000.[8] Contrastingly low incidence (6.3/100,000) was reported from the German Democratic Republic (Table 1).

Although these figures may serve to identify areas of elevated oral cancer incidence one must exercise caution in interpretation. It is not an infrequent occurrence that figures are reported for International Classification of Diseases (ICD eighth revision) numbers 140 to 148 referred to as buccal cavity and pharynx. This grouping includes carcinoma of the lip (140), salivary gland (142), and nasopharynx (147), which have a very different epidemiologic profile when contrasted with carcinoma of the tongue (141), mouth (143 to 145), and oro- (146) and hypopharynx (148). This is clearly demonstrated in Table 1. In the case of cancer of the lip, the highest global incidence is reported in Newfoundland. However, the same geographic area is 49th in rank when isolated for carcinoma of the tongue. Similarly, cancer of the nasopharynx was responsible for approximately 75% of the incidence rate in Hong Kong and less than 3% of the rates reported for Bas-Rhin, France, and Bombay.

It should be remembered that in late stage disease it may be virtually impossible to identify a primary site. Furthermore, the method of diagnosis, classification completeness, and accuracy of reporting may vary considerably from registry to registry.

In order to make international and regional comparisons it is vital to have annual age-adjusted incidence rates. Unfortunately, these are unavailable for the U.S. as a whole on an annual basis, and so accurate studies of trends in incidence are not possible. For instance,

Table 1

AGE-ADJUSTED INCIDENCE RATES PER 100,000 MALES FOR CANCER OF BUCCAL CAVITY AND PHARYNX AROUND 1975 FOR SELECTED GEOGRAPHIC AREAS[7]

Site (ICD -)	Registry						
	Hong Kong	Bas-Rhin	Bombay	Newfoundland	Utah	Connecticut	GDR
Buccal cavity & pharynx (140—148)	41.3	40.5	30.0	27.7	16.4	10.39	6.3
Lip (140)	0.3	0.2	0.3	22.8	10.3	1.6	2.9
Tongue (141)	2.4	7.4	10.2	1.5	1.6	3.3	0.7
Mouth (142—145)	2.7	9.6	5.8	0.7	1.7	4.9	0.9
Oropharynx (146)	1.0	11.6	4.7	0.8	0.9	2.1	0.7
Nasopharynx (147)	32.9	0.5	0.7	0.8	0.6	1.6	0.3
Hypopharynx (148)	1.3	10.2	0.8	0.7	0.3	0.5	0.4

the Texas Cancer Control Act providing for the establishment of a statewide cancer registry was implemented only as recently as 1979. However, the Bureau of Epidemiology, a newly created branch of the Texas Department of Health, lists only 2 of the 12 health service areas of the state with 100% reporting to the state tumor registry.[9]

1. Site

In the white male population of the U.S.[2] and the U.K.[3] the lower lip is the most common oral site for squamous cell carcinoma to develop, and this is followed by the tongue (lateral and ventral surfaces), floor of mouth, alveolar ridge, and buccal mucosa. The hard palate and upper lip are rarely involved, and neoplasms of these sites usually originate from minor mucous glands and not from surface epithelium. Exceptions to this pattern have been identified as with the elevated incidence of oral cancer in females in the southeastern U.S.,[10] the comparatively high incidence of palatal cancer in Indian populations with the indigenous reverse smoking habit,[11] and an incidence approaching zero for lip cancer in black populations.[7] Variations in this pattern globally and locally within the U.S. give rise to many etiologic hypotheses.[1]

2. Age

Like most epithelial malignant neoplasms, oral squamous cell carcinoma is very much an age-related disease. In their study in England and Wales in 1972, Binnie et al.[3] showed that 98% of cases occurred in persons over the age of 40. The peak incidence for individual sites occurs in the 60- to 70-year age group, but age-specific incidence is progressive with age. Males 75 years of age and over have an incidence of approximately 1 in 1100 (Figures 1 and 2).

3. Sex

Oral cancer is more common in males than females. In the U.S. the total incidence is 17.4/100,000 males and 6.2/100,000 females,[12] and this 3:1 ratio represents an average ratio for most parts of the world. Ratios vary with site. In England and Wales lip cancer is eight times more common in men, whereas intraoral cancer is only twice as high.[3] In the U.S. in roughly the same time period (1969 to 1971) the ratio for lip cancer in whites was 13:1 and 2.1 for intraoral cancer[13] (Table 2).

4. Trends

Two reports[13,14] allow comparison to be made between the incidence of the disease in

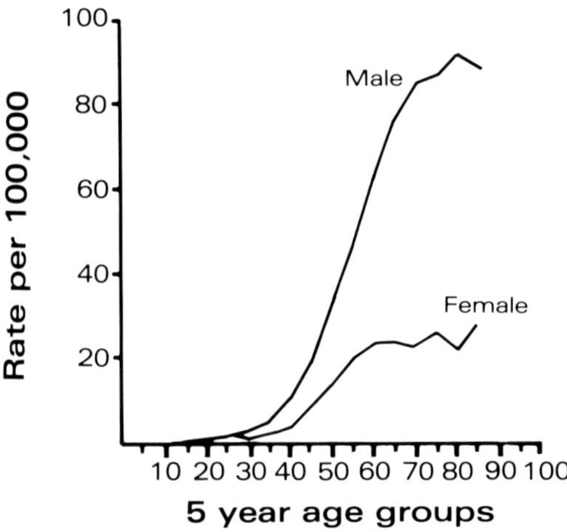

FIGURE 1.   Average annual incidence rates of cancer of the buccal cavity and pharynx by age and sex. U.S., 1973—1977.[12]

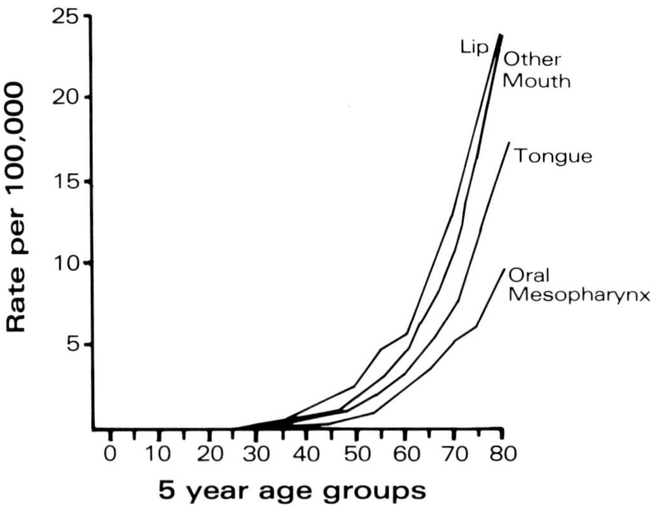

FIGURE 2.   Average annual incidence rates of oral cancer by site and age, males. England and Wales, 1962 to 1967.[3]

1947 and the average of the years 1969 to 1971 (Table 2). In this period it can be seen that lip and intraoral cancer decreased considerably in the white male population of the U.S., but intraoral cancer in both black males and females increased. The overall incidence of the disease probably remained static or slightly decreased during this period. The significant decrease in incidence in white males is similar to that reported by Binnie et al.[3] in England and Wales. No explanation for this decrease has been forthcoming. This static or downward trend must be borne in mind when considering environmental agents as etiological factors.

Comparison of incidence figures in the four volumes of *Cancer Incidence in Five Continents*[7] helps to illuminate interesting global trends for a 15- to 20-year time span. Lip cancer has decreased in nearly every population reported. Tongue cancer is rising, particularly in U.S. Alameda blacks, New York State, the German Democratic Republic, Israeli Jews, and Slovenian and Hungarian males while falling slowly or remaining static in over one half of

Table 2
ORAL CANCER IN THE U.S.
COMPARISON OF AGE-
ADJUSTED INCIDENCE RATES
PER 100,000 POPULATION, 1947
AND 1969—1971 (AVERAGE) BY
SEX AND RACE[13,14]

Lip cancer

White		Nonwhite	
Male	Female	Male	Female
5.8	0.8	0.4	0.2
4.1	0.3	0.3	0.1

Tongue cancer

White		Nonwhite	
Male	Female	Male	Female
4.2	1.2	2.7	1.1
3.1	1.1	3.5	1.3

Other mouth

White		Nonwhite	
Male	Female	Male	Female
4.6	1.5	2.0	0.5
3.9	1.9	3.9	1.6

the 32 population groups reported. Cancer of the mouth (ICD 143 to 145) rose noticeably in all four U.S. and both Polish populations as well as in the German Democratic Republic with a slightly higher increase in females. Incidence of cancers of the oro- and hypopharynx remained static.

B. Mortality

Mortality may be defined as the number of deaths from a particular disease for a given time period for a specified population conventionally expressed as deaths per 100,000. In contrast, fatality rate is deaths per year in a population with the disease. If the disease has a high fatality rate and short survival time, the mortality and incidence should be similar as is frequently the case with cancer of the esophagus.

As with incidence, mortality rates for oral cancer vary geographically as well as by sex, site, and race. It is worth mentioning that reliable mortality figures based on death certificates tend to be more readily available than incidence figures. In the U.S. (excluding Puerto Rico) the Surveillance, Epidemiology, and End Results program by the National Cancer Institute, Bethesda, Md., reports an overall mortality rate of 3.8/100,000 for cancer of the buccal cavity (including lip, tongue, salivary gland, and gum) for the years 1973 to 1977.[12] Mortality rates nearly parallel incidence rates except in the case of white females where salivary gland is the most fatal site and in black females where pharynx and buccal cavity are most fatal. Death rates are elevated in U.S. urban males and females in the rural South.[10]

Table 3 demonstrates the global variation in mortality from oral cancer. Hong Kong and

Table 3
**AGE-ADJUSTED DEATH RATES PER 100,000 POPULATION FOR
CANCER OF THE ORAL CAVITY AND PHARYNX IN MALES
AND FEMALES[2]**

Rank	Registry	Males	Rank	Registry	Females
1	Hong Kong	21.2	1	Hong Kong	7.1
2	Singapore	18.9	2	Singapore	6.3
3	France	18.5	3	Philippines	4.5
4	Malta & Gozo	9.5	4	Venezuela	3.1
5	Uruguay	8.3	5	Greece	3.0
6	Switzerland	8.0	6	Ireland	2.7
7	Hungary	7.6	7	U.S.	2.0
8	U.S.	5.8	8	Malta & Gozo	2.0
9	Poland	5.8	9	Scotland	1.9
10	Philippines	5.7	10	Iceland	1.8
11	Australia	5.3	11	Costa Rica	1.7
12	Canada	5.3	12	England & Wales	1.7
13	Ireland	5.3	13	New Zealand	1.7
14	Austria	5.2	14	Canada	1.6
15	Spain	4.8	15	Northern Ireland	1.6
16	Yugoslavia	4.5	16	Australia	1.5
17	Argentina	4.4	17	Denmark	1.5
18	Romania	4.4	18	France	1.5
19	Scotland	4.4	19	Israel	1.5
20	New Zealand	4.3	20	Hungary	1.4
21	Norway	4.3	21	Sweden	1.4
22	Paraguay	4.0	22	Poland	1.3
23	Costa Rica	3.9	23	Switzerland	1.3
24	England & Wales	3.7	24	Thailand	1.3

Singapore rank first in deaths for both males and females, followed by France in males and the Philippines in females. The same source[2] ranks Honduras and Nicaragua lowest for oral cancer mortality in both sexes. As is the case with incidence figures, mortality ranking is skewed by the inclusion of pharyngeal, lip, and salivary gland carcinomas with cancer of the buccal cavity and tongue.

Improvements in diagnosis of cancer, more accurate death certification, the possibility of improved survival as well as possible exposure to risk factors make variations over time in mortality figures difficult to explain. A number of these factors may be operational in mortality figures from cancer of the lip and tongue in England and Wales from 1868 to 1961[3] (Figure 3). Rates for cancer of the lip in both sexes and cancer of the tongue in males rose in the latter part of the 19th century and early part of the 20th century with a subsequent fall. In contrast, the rate for cancer of the tongue in females has declined gradually throughout the 100-year period.

Age-adjusted death rates for the U.S. are available which compare the 25-year period between the early 1950s and middle 1970s, and these show that there has been very little change.[15] In 1950 the age-adjusted death rate for oral cancer in males was 6.1/100,000 and females 1.5, and in 1975 the corresponding rates were 5.9 and 2.0. However, the accuracy of these figures is questionable because the same publication (citing the *World Health Statistics Annual)* shows the age-adjusted mortality rates in the U.S. for 1974 to 1975 were 4.7 and 1.6, respectively.

C. Survival
A crude method of determining the lethality of a neoplasm is to compare deaths with annual registrations. It was estimated that there would be 27,100 new cases of oral cancer

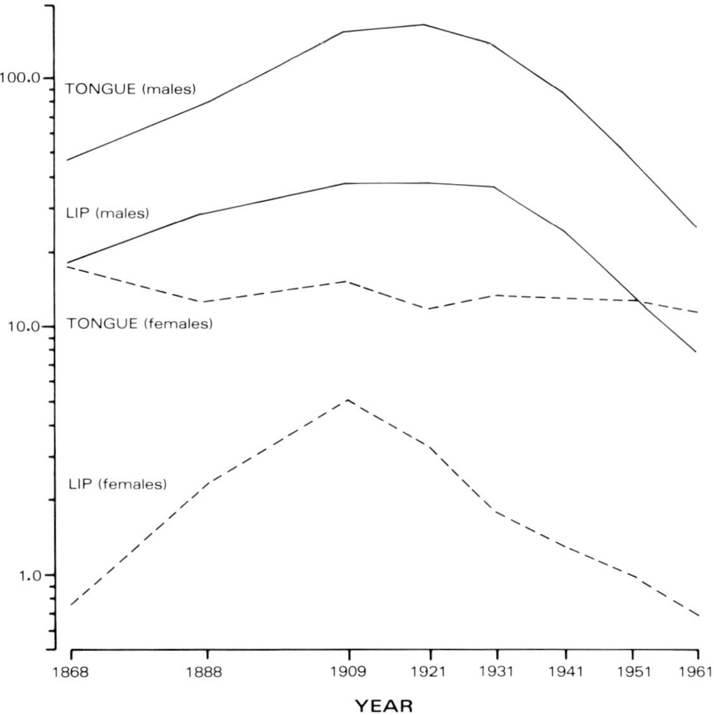

FIGURE 3.   Death rates per million from cancer of the lip and tongue. England and Wales, 1868 to 1961.[3]

Table 4
DEATH TO REGISTRATION RATIOS 1983[2]

	Total deaths (estimated)	Total new cases (estimated)	D/R
Lip	175	4000	0.04
Tongue	2000	4900	0.41
Oral pharynx	4200	7800	0.54

(including lip, salivary gland, and oral pharynx) in the U.S. in 1983 and 9150 deaths in the same year from neoplasia in these sites.[2] If this technique is applied to these figures, the death to registration ratio (D/R) would be 0.34 (Table 4). It is misleading, however, to apply this ratio (0.34) to individual oral sites as can be seen in Table 4. Carcinoma of the lip has an excellent prognosis (D/R = 0.04) compared with tongue (D/R = 0.41) and oral pharynx (D/R = 0.54). Tongue cancer then can be considered to be ten times as lethal as lip cancer. For comparison purposes, if the same technique is applied to malignant melanoma, traditionally considered a highly lethal neoplasm, the D/R is 0.35, less lethal than carcinoma of the tongue or oral pharynx.

A U.S. Department of Health Education and Welfare (DHEW) publication[16] has provided data on survival for cancers of the buccal cavity and pharynx. The report covers the period 1950 to 1973 and contains data for all newly diagnosed cancer patients seen in the entire state of Connecticut, approximately one fifth of the patients in California, and all patients seen at Charity Hospital in New Orleans and the University of Iowa Hospital. It is not possible to determine how representative this data is of the U.S. as a whole, but it is the most valid information available of a large-scale population. Table 5 shows the 5-year relative

Table 5
5-YEAR RELATIVE SURVIVAL
RATES FOR WHITE PATIENTS
BY STAGE, SEX, AND SITE:
1965—1969[18]

	All stages (%)	Localized (%)
Lip		
Male	84	87
Female	85	89
Tongue		
Male	32	55
Female	44	61
Floor of mouth		
Male	42	56
Female	47	75
Other mouth		
Male	39	56
Female	47	69
Pharynx		
Male	21	35
Female	30	47

survival rates for white patients by stage, sex, and site from registrations accumulated between 1965 and 1969. The data in Table 5 demonstrate again the importance of separating information from the different oral sites and the confusion that can arise by classifying intraoral, pharyngeal, and lip lesions in one all-inclusive category. Survival from lip cancer is far superior to intraoral cancer, which is in turn more favorable than survival from pharyngeal cancer. It is interesting to note the close correlation between the figures presented in this table and those published by Binnie et al.[3] in a national study of oral cancer in England and Wales (Figure 4). It is also intersting to note that 5-year survival rates are better in females than males, and this better prognosis for women was demonstrated previously in a survey of oral cancer patients at the Christie Hospital in Manchester, England.[17] This improved prognosis for females is almost certainly related to the fact that women have a higher percentage of localized lesions than do the males.

In fact, as will be discussed in more depth in Chapter 5, the stage at which the disease is treated is the single most important factor affecting survival. Figure 5 shows graphically the difference in survival of patients with early and late stage lip and intraoral carcinomas. The most important thing to note from the DHEW report[16] is that there has been essentially no change in the 5-year relative survival rate since 1950 for cancer of the lip, tongue, and floor of the mouth.

Equipped, then, with the available morbidity and mortality data on oral cancer it would seem appropriate to question whether these figures are alterable. The influence of changes in treatment methods of diagnosed disease requires time before adequate conclusions can be drawn. A recent review of etiological factors[18] shows that there is still no specific causative factor which if removed from the environment would significantly reduce the incidence of the disease. Even those who believe that 75 to 80% of lesions are avoidable[19] would be naive to imagine that confirmed consumers of alcohol and tobacco will abandon these habits because of the risk of developing cancer. It would seem, therefore, at the present time the emphasis should be on reducing mortality and the degree of morbidity, by improving diagnostic methods in order to institute treatment earlier or even intercept invasive disease.

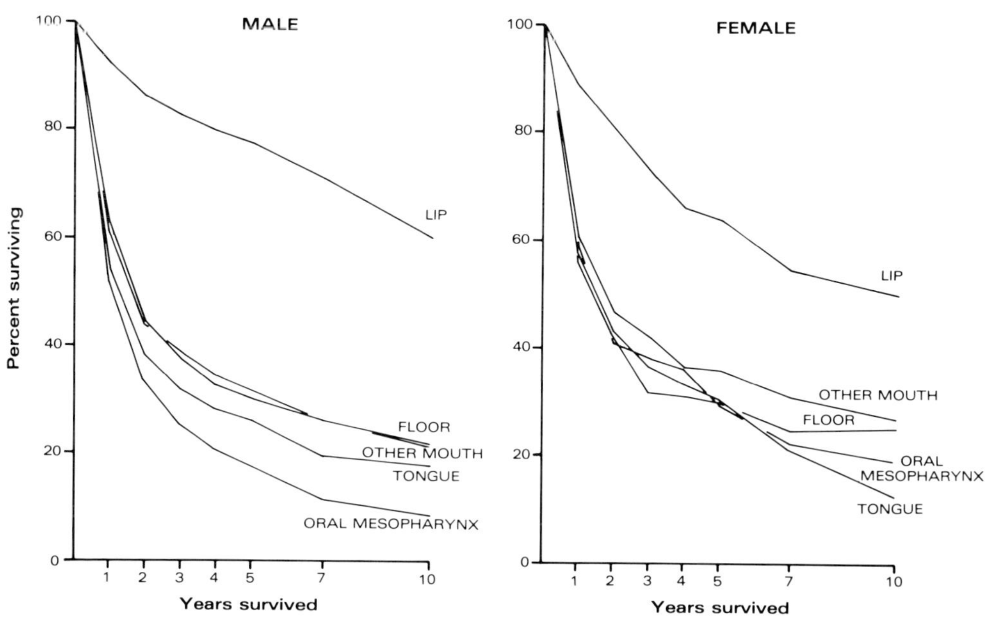

FIGURE 4. Corrected survival rates from oral cancer of different sites. England and Wales registrations, 1954 to 1960.[3]

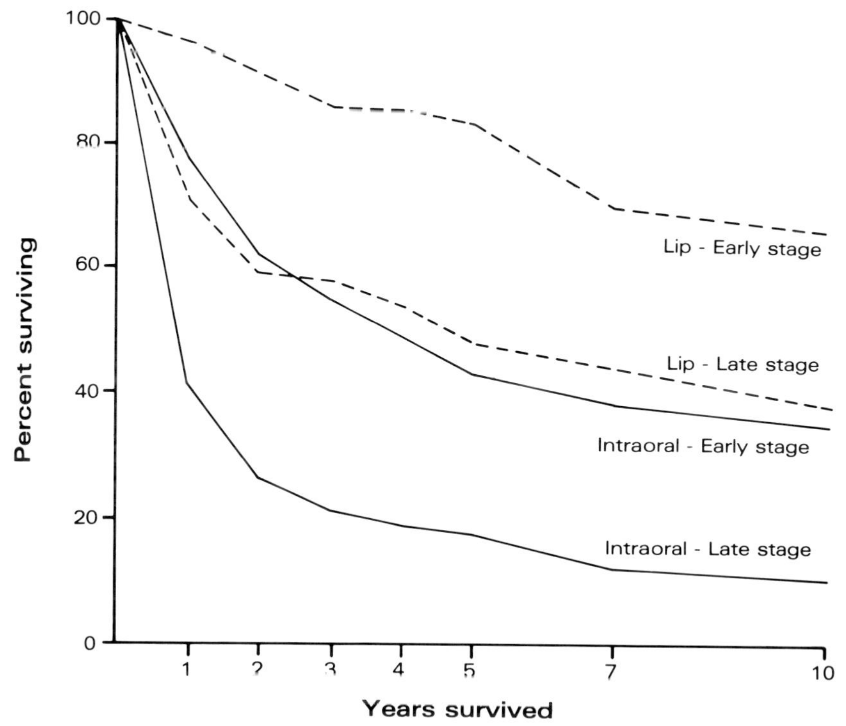

FIGURE 5. Corrected survival from lip and intraoral cancer by stage of disease. England and Wales registrations, 1954 to 1960.[3]

III. ANALYTIC STUDY

If the result of epidemiologic or descriptive study of oral cancer is the formulation of hypotheses on the causation of the disease, it is a natural progression to analytic study and manipulation within these populations to identify possible etiologic factors. Two measures of the association between possible etiologic factors and the risk of disease are relative risk (RR) and attributable risk (AR). RR is expressed as a ratio between the incidence or mortality in a population exposed to the factor and the rate in an unexposed population expressed relative to a risk of 1.0 for persons not exposed.

$$RR = \frac{\text{rate in exposed population}}{\text{rate in unexposed population}}$$

AR is calculated by subtracting the rate of disease (incidence of mortality) in an unexposed group from the rate in an exposed group: AR = rate in exposed population − rate in unexposed population. This measure assumes all other factors aside from the one being measured to be zero or to affect both populations equally.

These analytical methods are the basis for assessing the various etiological or risk factors which are discussed in the next chapter.

REFERENCES

1. **Hutchison, G. B.**, The epidemiologic method, *Cancer Epidemiology and Prevention,* Schottenfeld, D. and Fraumeni, J. F., Eds., W. B. Saunders, Philadelphia, 1982, chap. 1.
2. American Cancer Society, 1983 Cancer Facts and Figures, American Cancer Society, New York, 1983.
3. **Binnie, W. H., Cawson, R. A., Hill, G. B., and Soaper, A. E.**, Oral Cancer in England and Wales: A National Study of Morbidity, Mortality, Curability and Related Factors, Office of Population Censuses and Surveys: Studies on Medical and Population Subjects No. 23, Her Majesty's Stationery Office, London, 1972.
4. **Pindborg, J. J.**, Epidemiological studies of oral cancer, *Int. Dent. J.,* 27, 172, 1977.
5. **Mehta, F. S., Pindborg, J. J., Hammer, J. E., et al.**, Report on Investigations of Oral Cancer and Precancerous Condition in Indian Rural Population, 1966—1969, Basic Dental Research Unit, Tata Institute of Fundamental Research, Bombay, 1971.
6. **Lucas, R. B.**, *Pathology of Tumours of the Oral Tissues,* Churchill Livingstone, Edinburgh, 1976, 134.
7. **Waterhouse, J., Muir, C. S., Shanmugaratnam, K., and Powell, J., Eds.**, *Cancer Incidence in Five Continents,* Vol. 4, IARC Sci. Publ. No. 42, International Agency for Research on Cancer, Lyon, 1982.
8. **Dunham, L. J. and Bailar, J. C.**, World maps of cancer mortality rates and frequency ratios, *JNCI,* 41, 155, 1968.
9. *Interagency Center for Cancer Prevention and Control, Impact of Cancer in Texas,* 2nd ed., University of Texas System Cancer Center, M.D. Anderson Hospital and Tumor Institute, Houston, 1980, 110.
10. **Blot, W. J. and Fraumeni, J. F., Jr.**, Geographic patterns of oral cancer in the United States: etiologic implication, *J. Chron. Dis.,* 30, 745, 1977.
11. **Reddy, D. G. and Rao, V. K.**, Cancer of the mouth in coastal Andhra due to smoking cigars with the burning end inside the mouth, *Indian J. Med.,* 11, 791, 1957.
12. **Young, J. L., Jr., Percy, C. L., and Asire, A. J.**, Surveillance, Epidemiology, and End Results: Cancer Incidence and Mortality in the United States, 1973—1977, National Cancer Institute Monogr. No. 57, National Cancer Institute, Bethesda, Md., 1981.
13. **Cutler, S. J. and Young, J. L.**, Third National Cancer Survey: Incidence Data, National Cancer Institute Monogr. No. 41, U.S. Department of Health Education and Welfare, Bethesda, Md., 1975.
14. **Dorn, H. F. and Cutler, S. J.**, Morbidity from Cancer in the United States, Public Health Monogr. No. 56, U.S. Department of Health Education and Welfare, Washington, D.C., 1959.
15. American Cancer Society, 1981 Cancer Facts and Figures, American Cancer Society, New York, 1981.
16. **Hankey, B. F.**, Survival for cancers of the buccal cavity and pharynx, Department of Health Education and Welfare Publ. (NIH) 78-1539, Department of Health Education and Welfare, 1979.

17. **Easson, E. C. and Russell, M. H.,** *The Curability of Cancer in Various Sites,* Pitman Medical, London, 1968.
18. **Binnie, W. H., Rankin, K. V., and MacKenzie, I. C.,** Etiology of oral squamous cell carcinoma, *J. Oral Pathol.,* 12, 11, 1983.
19. **Rothman, K. J.,** Alcohol, in *Persons at High Risk of Cancer: An Approach to Cancer Etiology and Control,* Fraumeni, J. F., Jr., Ed., Academic Press, New York, 1975.

Chapter 2

ETIOLOGY

William H. Binnie and Kathleen Vendrell Rankin

TABLE OF CONTENTS

I. INTRODUCTION

Epidemiological studies attempt, by examination of such features as geographical distribution, racial prevalence, occupation, social class, diet, climate, hygiene, use of tobacco, and alcohol consumption, to elicit possible causative factors for the disease in question. This approach has been validated by the documented etiological significance of inhaled tobacco smoke in bronchogenic carcinoma. However, no single clearly recognizable causative factor has come to light with regard to oral carcinoma. To gain a perspective from which to identify productive areas of future research it is worthwhile reviewing the present status of etiological factors implicated in the development of oral squamous cell carcinoma.

There exists a traditional list of etiologic factors some of which are habits and others host factors. These include alcohol, smoking, syphilis, and oral sepsis. Reviewing cancer of the tongue in 1918 Power[1] concluded:

> "Cancer of the tongue has always existed in both men and in animals; the actual cause as yet unknown. Its rapid increase in men within historical times is the result of two causes: The first predisposing, the second exciting. The predisposing cause is the degenerative change taking place as a result of spirochaetal infection, the change being accentuated by lapse of years and indulgence in alcohol. The form in which the alcohol is taken does not seem to be important; beer, spirits, and wine are equally harmful. It is the amount consumed, not the quality which matters. The exciting cause is local irritation. The most effective irritant is tobacco although pyorrhea and carious teeth often act as minor exciting causes."

As vital as the actual factors themselves is the concept of "cocarcinogenesis". Goldhaber[2] discusses two distinct phases in the development of a malignant neoplasm of the mouth; initiation and promotion. In the initiation period, normal cells are converted to "tumor" cells (i.e., a malignant potential) by a carcinogenic agent in a relatively short time interval. Promotion takes much longer and involves the frequent exposure of latent tumor cells to an agent which is not itself a carcinogen, but is referred to as a cocarcinogen. Wynder et al.[3] applied the terms "intrinsic" and "extrinsic" to group factors which act together to produce malignant transformation. Intrinsic factors infer generalized defects from such things as malnutrition from alcoholism, vitamin deficiencies, sideropenia, and syphilis. Extrinsic factors are exogenous and have local effects, i.e., tobacco and sunlight in the case of cancer of the lip.

This historical list of possible etiologic factors has been expanded to include iron deficiency, chronic candidosis, and viral infection. Current studies of these factors, both traditional and provisional, continue to examine the multifactorial nature of the etiology of oral cancer. The possible mechanisms by which these factors may interrelate to produce a malignant neoplasm are as vital as the study of the individual factors themselves. However, it is worthwhile reviewing these factors individually and assessing their associations with oral cancer.

II. HABITS

A. Tobacco

The vast majority of the literature regarding the implications of the use of tobacco offers support for the historical contention that tobacco is, in fact, one of the primary factors in the etiology of oral cancer.

1. Smoking

Evidence accumulated over the past 200 years linking smoking habits with oral cancer was comprehensively reviewed by Clemmesen.[4] Rothman[5] states categorically that tobacco has been well established as a risk factor in cancer of the mouth and pharynx. This assumption, based primarily on the epidemiological association of tobacco usage with increased incidence of oral cancer, should not, however, obscure the as yet unresolved questions regarding the significance of the manner in which tobacco is smoked and the nature of the relationship established by combining smoking with other environmental variables.

Although of minor significance in the U.S., there is evidence from some parts of the world that the habit of smoking cigarettes and cigars with the burning end inside the mouth is responsible for a high incidence of oral cancer. In the state of Andhra Pradesh in India, reverse smoking is related to cancer of the palate, one of the rarest sites for squamous cell carcinoma to develop in the western world.[6-10] Reddy et al.[11] reported a relative risk of the reverse-smoking female to be 47 times that of the nonsmoking female. Gupta et al.[12] clarified that the palatal changes observed in smokers in western populations, referred to as nicotinic stomatitis, are not considered to be precancerous or analogous to palatal lesions discussed in relation to reverse smoking.

Traditionally, there has been an assumed causal relationship between pipe smoking and cancer of the lip. From evidence reviewed by Clemmesen[4] this would appear to be justified. However, he did note that earlier studies considered the additional effects of heat and condition of the pipe stem to be of significance. Levin et al.[13] and Wynder et al.[3] continued to support the association of pipe smoking and cancer of the lip. Spitzer et al.,[14] in an evaluation of etiologic variables of lip cancer in fishermen, reported that although the use of tobacco in general (cigarette, pipe, and chewing tobacco) was not an important risk factor, the risk ratio for pipe smoking taken alone was 1.50 (p <0.05; Mantel-Hanenszel χ^2 = 3.934).

There is contradictory evidence regarding the relative risk of cigarette vs. pipe/cigar as a method of tobacco consumption in the etiology of intraoral cancer. Frequently lip cancer is included in studies designed to assess the relative risk of cigarette vs. pipe/cigar usage, and it is doubtful that factors operating in lip carcinoma and intraoral carcinoma are analogous. Much of the confusion has also undoubtedly been spawned by the misrepresentation of data published by Doll and Hill.[15] Inaccurate interpretation of their data has led to the assumption that increased risk of cigarette smoking over pipe/cigar smoking in lung cancer implies an analogous situation in the oral cavity. However, they stated "...unlike lung cancer, the association is less characteristic of cigarette smoking and indeed in several studies the relationship is equally close, or closer with the smoking of pipes and cigars".

The confusion is unaided by conflicting statements from the same author. Wynder and Stellman[16] state: "Cigar and pipe smokers have a risk similar to cigarette smokers for cancer of the oral cavity." However, Wynder et al.[17] state: "Cigar and pipe smoking have also been implicated in the etiology of oral cavity and esophagus cancer, but to a lesser extent than cigarette smoking."

The method of smoking notwithstanding, there is ample evidence to support the premise of tobacco consumption as a dose/time-related entity in the etiology of intraoral cancer. Dorn and Cutler[18] combined deaths from cancers of the mouth, pharynx, and esophagus to show an increased risk for cigarette smokers with a gradient by amount smoked. Kahn[19] further analyzing Dorn and Cutler's data, examined sites individually, and showed increased risk with strong positive gradients related to the number of cigarettes smoked. Mashberg et al.[20] reported, "The relative risk for smokers adjusted for drinking rose from 3.2 to 4.5 to 5.0 for smokers of 10—19, 20—30, 40 or more cigarettes a day respectively." Wynder et al.[17] concluded, "The chance of developing a second primary is dependent principally on the intensity (i.e., quantity and duration) of the smoking and drinking habit prior to the onset of the first neoplasm."

Polycyclic aromatic hydrocarbons (PAH), regarded as the main precarcinogens in tobacco smoke, are activated to ultimate carcinogens in cells by microsomal complex enzymes commonly referred to as aryl hydrocarbon hydroxylases (AHH). Trell et al.[21] measured AHH inducibility in Swedish oral cancer patients and controls and showed high inducibility was more common and low inducibility less common in cancer cases than in the controls (p = <0.0001). Incidentally, this was found to be regardless of dental status.

The accumulated data on smoking and oral cancer are voluminous, and one of the most surprising aspects is how contradictory and inconclusive the findings are, particularly with regard to cigarette smoking. Despite many studies which have shown strong association between cigarette smoking and oral cancer, there are others in which no correlation could be found. It must be remembered that although there has been a continuous increase in cigarette consumption for most of the century, this has not produced an increase in incidence of the disease — unlike lung cancer. Perhaps much of the information has been considered in too simplistic a fashion. In some very positive studies tobacco products may have been carcinogenic, but it is becoming more apparent that many factors, both initiators and promoters, are interrelated. Smoking (and alcohol) reduce cell-mediated and humoral immunity, and it has been suggested that there is an interaction between herpes simplex virus (type 1) and tobacco smoke and tumor development.[22]

2. Smokeless Tobacco

Numerous epidemiological studies conducted on various Indian populations with peculiar indigenous tobacco habits have indicated that topical tobacco is a vital consideration in the evaluation of tobacco as a risk in oral cancer.[23] The tobacco is blended in various forms, often with lime and rolled in a betel leaf to form a quid which users may hold in the mouth as long as 24 hr/day. A papilliferous, ulcerated neoplasm at the site where the quid is habitually placed has been observed to develop after many years of leukoplakia. Mahboubi,[24] discussing the etiological implications of areas of highest oral cancer incidence in the world, states, ''Ceylon and Bombay have the highest incidence rates, as do certain areas in India and in Hong Kong. In these areas, the environmental factor responsible is the cultural habit of chewing tobacco.''

There remains, however, some disagreement as to whether it is, in fact, the tobacco component of the quid which imparts its observed carcinogenic capacity. In reviewing the literature, Khadim[25] noted that the addition of tobacco to the betel quid known as ''pan'' increased the risk from 4 without tobacco to as much as 29 with its addition. Atkinson et al.,[26] however, suggested that the possible etiological agent involved may be the lime. This possibility is supported by observation of elevated oral cancer incidence related to endemic chewing habits in Malaysia[27] and Papua, New Guinea[28] where it is customary to use the betel nut with lime but without tobacco. The incidence is contrastingly low in Afghanistan and Nigeria where tobacco is chewed without lime.[29] This issue is admittedly complicated by the combination of various smoking habits in chewers.

A mixture of tobacco, ash, cotton oil, and lime referred to as ''nass'' is the smokeless tobacco equivalent in the U.S.S.R. An elevated incidence of oral carcinomas has been reported from several geographic areas of the U.S.S.R. where this habit is known to be a common practice.[30] The variability in individual nass preparation makes conclusions on its carcinogenic potential difficult. There is agreement that there is elevated incidence, and the lesions appear to be site related. However, animal studies have failed to produce malignancy or severe dysplasia, and case-control studies have not supported the geographic incidence reports. The habit may be a promoter, but the influence of smoking and nutritional deficiencies in habitues may be more important.[31]

In the U.S. an association between the use of topical tobacco and the development of oral squamous cell carcinoma has been known for some time. Ackerman[32] reported the

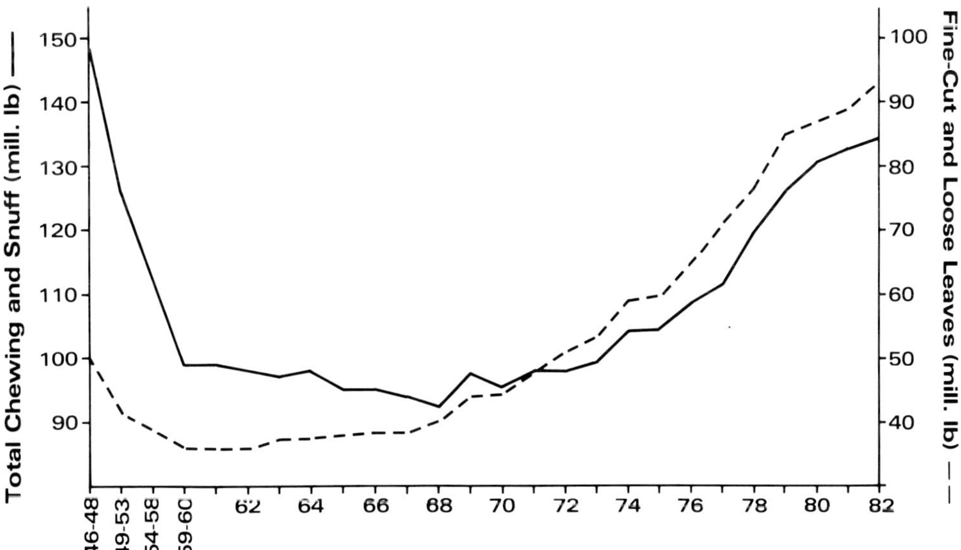

FIGURE 1.   Topical (unburned) tobacco production in the U.S. 1946—1982. (Annual Reports on Tobacco Statistics AMS-USDA. With permission.)

etiological association in his description of verrucous carcinoma. Although tobacco is not essential for the development of the lesion, most series of cases contain a high percentage of users.[33] In regions such as the southeastern U.S., where topical tobacco use is particularly prevalent, the carcinoma is so distinctive in its site distribution, appearance, and unusual female:male ratio that the lesion is referred to as "snuff dippers' cancer".[34]

Graphic demonstration for the need for continued evaluation of topical tobacco habits in the U.S. was supplied by Mason[35] and Mason et al.[36] in an atlas of cancer mortality. He identified increased oral cancer mortality in females in the southeastern U.S. which is characteristically a textile area where topical tobacco habits are known to be common among the workers. In an analysis of demographic variables characteristic of females in this area of elevated oral cancer mortality, Blot and Fraumeni[37] elaborated on the correlation between snuff use by women in the textile industry and the elevated oral cancer mortality.

More recently, in response to the dramatic increase in total production of smokeless tobacco in the U.S., Winn et al.[38] reported a 4-fold increase in the risk of oral and pharyngeal cancer and a 50-fold increase for carcinomas of the gingiva and buccal mucosa in long-term users in a similarly exclusive female population of the southeastern U.S. In the light of the increasing consumption of topical tobacco in the U.S. (particularly fine-cut and loose leaf forms) and the conscientious replacement of the cigarette with supposedly less harmful forms of tobacco consumption, this becomes an increasingly relevant issue (Figure 1).

Sundstrom et al.[39] studied 23 Swedish males with carcinomas of the anterior oral vestibule who were chronic "snuff dippers". Most of the lesions were verrucous carcinomas or exophytic verruciform squamous cell carcinomas. It is interesting to note that 11 of 19 available for histologic study showed candidal invasion (see Section IV.B).

There is no evidence from animal studies to show a cause and effect relationship between topical tobacco and oral cancer. While no animal models have been developed that exactly duplicate the human habit with smokeless tobacco, the animal studies that have been done have been negative. In the only study in which a tumor occurred,[40] a surgically created canal was used to expose the rats to snuff. These animals were known to develop squamous cell carcinomas spontaneously. Moreover, it is not known whether the one tumor that developed after 8½ months did so at the site of exposure.

Three types of chemical carcinogens have been identified in smokeless tobacco.[41] A polynuclear aromatic hydrocarbon, benzo(a)pyrene, has been detected, indicating that the tobacco has been contaminated with thermal degradation products in the curing process.[42] Varying amounts of an α-particle-emitting metal, polonium 210, originating from a specific phosphate fertilizer used in the cultivation of tobacco, have also been demonstrated as well as several of the over 300 known carcinogenic nitrosamines.[42] N'-nitrosonornicotine (NNN) was the first organic carcinogen to be isolated from unburned tobacco and is found in highest concentration in fermented snuff and fine-cut chewing tobacco. NNN is produced by bacterial and enzymatic nitrosation of nicotine and can be found by reaction of salivary nitrates with nornicotine. NNN levels increased 44% when tobacco was mixed with saliva, and it is important to realize NNN extracted from fine-cut chewing tobacco with saliva is approximately 1000 times that found in the mainstream smoke of a typical American nonfilter cigarette.[43]

The nicotine-derived N-nitrosamines and their relationship to tobacco-related cancer have recently been reviewed by Hoffman and Hecht.[44] It is interesting that although more than 300 nitrosamines have been shown to be carcinogenic in one or more of 40 animal species, no cancers have occurred in the oral cavity. It seems odd that proven powerful carcinogens, which can be shown to be in high concentrations in fermented tobacco mixed with saliva, cannot to date produce carcinomas in buccal mucosa of laboratory animals.

The current concern in the U.S. about the possible increase in buccal mucosal/gingival carcinoma due to increase in the consumption of smokeless tobacco by young people has resulted in simplistic assumptions. The facts at present show that the one study showing increased risk was in a specific population and significant risk was in very long-term users and little was known of nutritional status.[38] Increased risk does not prove cause and effect.

Finally, it should be remembered that although the U.S. population has increased significantly in the last 40 years, smokeless tobacco production is just beginning to return to the amount produced in the late 1940s (Figure 1).

B. Alcohol

The role of alcohol consumption in the etiology of oral cancer is complicated by several factors. The most commonly cited reason for the lack of definitive evidence on the carcinogenic capacity of alcohol is the difficulty in isolating heavy alcohol consumption from smoking. Wynder et al.[3] in a landmark study on the etiological implications of the combined use of alcohol and tobacco specifically addressed this as a relevant concern. Schwartz et al.,[45] however, in an analysis of the association between alcohol consumption and cancer of the tongue, hypopharynx, larynx, esophagus, buccal cavity, and oropharynx in 3937 French males excluded the possible overlapping influence of smoking and showed a definite relationship. In a review of the literature, Rothman[46] cited figures for the maximum effect of alcohol consumption in risk ratio terms controlled for amount smoked, ranging from a 2-fold increase reported by Keller and Terris,[47] a 7-fold increase reported by Wynder et al.,[3] and a 20-fold increase reported by Vincent and Marchetta.[48] Mashberg et al.[20] published impressive data controlled for smoking from which they concluded, "Drinkers of six or more whiskey equivalents a day may be at greater risk than smokers of forty or more cigarettes a day."

In their Irish study, Herity et al.[49] showed an increased tongue cancer risk of 4.6 for light drinkers and a 9-fold risk for heavy drinkers. They also made the point that there was a significant excess of alcohol-related occupations (e.g., bartenders) among the cases.

Support, by contrast, for the possible implications of alcohol consumption is derived from evaluation of cancer mortality in populations abstaining from both alcohol and tobacco. In an effort to elucidate the etiologic implication of a cancer incidence 20% below the national average in Utah, Lyon et al.[50] suggested the lower incidence was due in part to the adherence to Mormon doctrine by the majority of the population of the state. Similar findings have been reported for abstaining Seventh Day Adventists.[51]

Reviewing four follow-up studies of alcoholics[52-55] for evidence of increased risk of head and neck cancer, Rothman[46] found these studies demonstrated an association between alcohol consumption and cancer of the head and neck. He is, however, quick to point out that this does not imply that this association is due directly to ethanol. Other possible risk factors are described as possible carcinogens in the form of contaminants or congeners in the ethanol beverage and the associated health risks of smoking and poor nutrition.

Study of the prevalence and consumption of illegally produced spirits indigenous to certain parts of the world serves to comment on the possible significance of carcinogenic congeners or contaminants. Massé[56] demonstrated that by far the highest incidence of esophageal cancer in France is found in the apple-growing areas of Brittany and Normandy whose populations traditionally consume a crude home-distilled "calvados". The influence of alcohol on esophageal cancer in rural France has been further demonstrated by Tuyns and co-workers[57] and Tuyns.[58] It is possible that a similar geographic pattern applies to oral cancer. Contrasting oral cancer incidence in Puerto Rico with the mainland U.S., Fischman and Martinez[59] suggested the prevalence of home-processed rum might in part account for the higher incidence reported in Puerto Rico.

With regard to governmentally controlled alcohol products, Rothman[46] suggested that studies contrasting the effect of vodka, which is essentially pure ethanol and water, with Bourbon or Scotch whiskey, both of which contain congeners, might be a fruitful avenue in this regard. Mashberg et al.[20] surprisingly reported a greater relative risk for beer and wine drinkers than for whiskey drinkers.

In addition to the possible existence of carcinogenic contaminants and congeners, it has been suggested that the mechanism by which alcohol might promote carcinogenesis is a localized solvent action. Wynder et al.[17] state that alcohol per se is not carcinogenic, but would be more appropriately classified as a promoter. Rothman[46] suggests that one hypothesis worth pursuing to explain the synergism of alcohol and tobacco is examination of the consequence of tobacco carcinogens dissolving in alcohol which permits more intimate contact with susceptible tissues.

McCoy[60] admits the possibility that alcohol facilitates the entry of carcinogens into exposed cells but suggests, "The effect of alcohol may be more readily explained by alterations in metabolism in the oral cavity and esophageal epithelium." Elaborating on the possibility of localized alcohol effects McCoy[60] further proposes, "The oxidation of ethanol by the epithelial cells of the target tissues could alter intracellular metabolism, creating a more favorable environment for metabolic activation of procarcinogens."

The systemic impact of alcohol, the link between a high level of alcohol consumption, liver cirrhosis, and oral cancer, has been documented by several authors.[48,61-65] In an effort to explain the possible connection McCoy[60] suggests the possibility that the alcohol-compromised liver could have a decreased ability to detoxify potential carcinogens. Nutritional deficiencies also known to occur in alcoholics probably further potentiate the systemic effects of alcohol in the etiology of oral cancer. Support of the role of nutritional deficiencies in the etiology of oral cancer is derived from the observed elevated incidence of head and neck cancers in association with Paterson Kelly (Plummer-Vinson) syndrome.[66,67] Animal studies indicate that riboflavin-deficient mice tend to develop tumors more rapidly than a control group.[68]

Before one can assume recent evidence already cited showing an increased risk in alcohol consumers to be absolute, one must first reconcile the decreasing or static incidence of the disease in the U.S. and the U.K. with the vast increase in alcohol consumption per capita over the same time span. As Binnie[69] pointed out, intraoral cancer in England and Wales has been decreasing in incidence over 3 or 4 decades while alcohol consumption has been increasing rapidly (Figure 2).

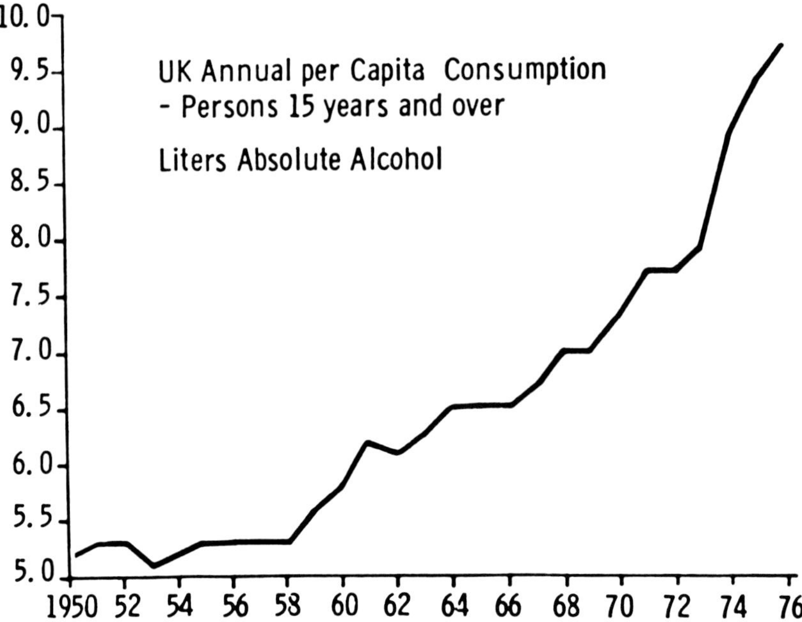

FIGURE 2.   Alcohol consumption in the U.K. 1950—1976. (H.M. Customs and Excise Annual Reports, Her Majesty's Stationery Office, London. With permission.)

Further support for the lack of definitive evidence for correlation of smoking and alcohol and oral cancer arises from a case-controlled retrospective study of oral cancer patients in the U.K. No difference was found between alcohol and cigarette consumption in cancer patients and that of controls.[70]

Much of the current literature examines the relative risk attributable to tobacco usage in concert with other possible carcinogenic agents. The predominant concern is the concurrent use of alcohol and burnt tobacco. Wynder and Stellman[16] reported a combined relative risk of 3.4 for smokers of 40 or more cigarettes per day who also consumed 7 oz or more of alcohol per day. With the addition of poor dentition to alcohol and tobacco habits, Graham et al.[71] reported a synergistic relationship increasing the risk of oral cancer 7.7 times for men possessing all three traits. The study did not, however, support the concept of synergy of alcohol and tobacco with the exclusion of dental factors. Rothman[46] offers support for a synergistic effect, concluding that joint exposure results in risk ratios 2.5 times that expected if the risk was merely additive (Table 1). Herity et al.[49] in a case-control study of head and neck cancer in the Republic of Ireland showed a similar synergistic effect. The relative risk in heavy smokers was 4.0 for cancers of the oral cavity and oropharynx and 4.8 for cancer of the tongue (for both $p < 0.01$). The relative risk of tongue cancer for heavy smokers who were also heavy drinkers was 6.0 with an index of synergy of 2.6.

III. HOST FACTORS

A. Dental Disease

Chronic neglect of the teeth and periodontal tissues has often been considered an important predisposing or exciting factor in the development of oral cancer.[72] The oral soft tissues are exposed to many chronic irritants of dental origin, both microbiological and mechanical, but the relationship between these factors and oral cancer is very difficult to assess on a scientific basis. Browne et al.[73] reported a higher incidence of poor oral hygiene and ill-fitting dentures in an examination of etiologic factors related to an increased incidence of

Table 1
RISK RATIO OF ORAL CANCER
ACCORDING TO LEVEL OF
EXPOSURE TO ALCOHOL AND
TOBACCO SMOKING (CIGARETTE
EQUIVALENTS/DAY)

Alcohol (oz/day)	0	1—19	20—39	40+
0	1.00	1.52	1.43	2.43
0.1—0.4	1.40	1.67	3.18	3.25
0.4—1.5	1.60	4.36	4.46	8.21
1.6+	2.33	4.13	9.59	15.5

Note: Risks are expressed relative to a risk of 1.00 for persons who neither smoked nor drank. 1 cigar = 4 cigarettes and 1 pipeful = 2 cigarettes.

From Rothman, K. J. and Keller, A. Z., *J. Chron. Dis.,* 25, 711, 1972. With permission.

oral cancer in Stoke-on-Trent, England. Thumfart et al.[74] observed a topographic coincidence of tumor development and chronic mechanical trauma from dental prostheses in 44% of cases of oral cancer examined. In a study of the multifactorial nature of the etiology of oral cancer, Graham et al.[71] reported, "Inadequate dentition, either posterior or anterior and upper or lower, carried a risk three times that of adequate dentition, when we controlled for heavy smoking and drinking." In contrast to these studies, however, Trell et al.[21] found dental status to be of minor importance.

Unfortunately, none of those studies provide evidence of past standards of dentition or oral hygiene, and this would be difficult to estimate with any degree of accuracy retrospectively.

Despite lack of definite evidence, it is a commonly held belief among cancer therapists in the U.K. that the decrease in oral cancer incidence is due to improved dental health. They may be right, and certain dental factors may potentiate the development of oral cancer, but at the present time there is little evidence to link the two. On the other hand, it must be stated there is no evidence which disproves an association either.

B. Iron Deficiency

Iron metabolism is important in maintaining the health of the oral mucosa, and many disease states, including carcinoma, are associated with iron depletion.[75] Iron deficiency may be the most common deficiency disease in the world, affecting both affluent and underdeveloped countries.

In 1919 Paterson[76] and Kelly[77] independently described the symptom complex of chronic dysphagia and atrophy of the mucosa of the upper GI tract in middle-aged women who were chronically anemic. Paterson was also aware at that time of the "not infrequent supervention in such cases of malignant disease of the mouth and gullet." It was not until 1939, however, that Waldenström and Kjellberg[78] pointed out the significance of diminished body iron stores associated with low serum iron levels and the absence of stainable bone marrow iron and introduced the term "sideropenic dysphagia" to describe the disease complex known as Paterson Kelly syndrome, or more commonly in the U.S., Plummer-Vinson syndrome. Further epidemiological evidence was provided by Ahlbom[66,67] in Scandinavia. This study, apart from confirming the importance of the syndrome in the development of carcinoma of the meso and hypopharynx, showed that this also applied to the buccal mucosa, tongue, and all levels of the esophagus. Other series have been reported of patients with Paterson-Kelly syndrome who have developed single or multiple oral cancers.[79-81]

Rennie and MacDonald and co-workers[82-84] in the U.K. have recently shown that in human iron deficiency anemia and in experimental iron deficiency in hamsters quantitative histological changes in the oral epithelium are demonstrable. The epithelium is atrophic with a reduced maturation compartment, but an increased keratinized compartment. Cell kinetic studies have shown an increased cell production, indicating that despite the atrophy the epithelium is turning over more rapidly. From this it is suggested that there may be an increased susceptibility to chemical carcinogens because there is an increased susceptible population of dividing cells and also the epithelium may be more permeable. Recent studies using a rat palate model painted with 4-nitroquinoline-*N*-oxide have shown that animals with iron deficiency anemia, induced by venesection and a low iron diet, develop carcinomas after a mean of 183 days as opposed to a mean of 229 days in control animals.[85] Furthermore, the early tumors are on the tongue and not the palate.

There is no doubt that iron is essential for overall integrity and health of epithelia of the upper GI tract, and its importance may lie in its contribution to normal enzyme systems. However, Joynson et al.[86] have demonstrated an impairment of cell-mediated immunity in iron deficient patients, and in their words, "This condition carries important implications with regard to the pathogenesis of malignant disease and chronic infections such as candidiasis."

Despite strong epidemiological and experimental evidence there is a surprising lack of data concerning iron status in patients who develop carcinoma of the upper aerodigestive tract. Changes in the oral mucosa can occur before significant alterations in red cell morphology or hemoglobin level are noted,[75] and in order to provide meaningful data serum iron, total iron binding capacity, or serum ferritin must be assessed. A case-control study would be interesting, but prospective information would be of more value.

At this time no cause and effect relationship exists between chronic sideropenia and malignant transformation in epithelium. There appears little doubt that there is a relationship, but whether this is passive or active remains to be seen.

C. Other Nutritional Factors

Although the most interest has been shown in iron studies, other nutritional factors may be equally or more important. The effects of iron on epithelium may, in fact, be secondary to pyridoxine deficiency.[87] Similarly, the role of folic acid[88,89] and vitamin B_{12}[90] in the etiology of tissue disturbance confuses the true effect of iron deficiency.

There has been increasing interest recently in the possible protective effects of various nutrients. Peto et al.[91] reviewed the role of β-carotene and retinol in cancer and showed that blood retinol and dietary β-carotene are inversely proportional to cancer risk. They noted that blood retinol levels are not necessarily related to dietary intake. In India, 76.2% of patients with oral and oropharyngeal carcinoma were found to have subnormal levels of serum vitamin A.[92] A Pakistani study revealed plasma vitamin A and β-carotene levels to be significantly lower in oral cancer patients than in controls.[93] In these geographic areas where smokeless tobacco and oral cancer are prevalent, it would seen important, therefore, to investigate the nutritional status of the population before laying all the blame on tobacco. A study in the U.S.S.R. designed to correlate nass consumption with the high incidence of oral and esophageal cancer, the results of which were inconclusive, revealed, however, that the surveyed population had low serum levels of riboflavin, vitamin A, and carotenoids.[31]

It should be noted that poor intake may not be the only problem. The dietary requirement for mucosal health may be compromised by alcohol consumption.[94]

D. Immunological Aspects

Since Burnet[95] introduced the concept of immunologic surveillance in 1971, the influence of immunological mechanisms on head and neck cancer has been investigated with increasing interest. A review of current knowledge was provided by Scully[96] to which little can be added, at least with regard to pathogenic mechanisms.

The immune system may influence the development of a malignancy, but it is not clearly understood whether a neoplasm develops because of lack of recognition mechanisms or because of failure in immune response.[97]

Oral cancer is an age-related disease,[98] and since aging is associated with reduced cell-mediated immune reactivity it is tempting to suggest that the increasing incidence of oral cancer with age is due to an impaired immune response.

Several factors already discussed as ''causative'' have been shown to reduce cell-mediated reactivity, i.e., smoking,[99] alcohol,[100,101] and iron deficiency.[86]

Patients with a primary immunodeficiency have an incidence rate of malignant disease over 100 times that of the general population,[102,103] but there is no evidence of increased risk of oral squamous carcinoma. However, patients with a severe primary immunodeficiency die at a young age, and information about minor immunodeficiency in oral cancer patients has not been sufficiently explored.

Patients who are iatrogenically immunosuppressed to inhibit graft rejection have an increased risk of developing a malignancy about 80 times that of the matched controls.[104] Most neoplasms are lymphoid, but there is an increase in lip and skin cancer.[105-107] Although no increased incidence of oral cancer was found in 16,290 renal transplant patients,[108] longer follow-up would be needed before an association could be excluded.

Radiation therapy also decreases immune reactivity, and this may be of primary importance in explaining the development of second primary carcinomas or the increased incidence of primary carcinomas in radiated patients.[109]

A recent review by Silverman et al.[110] of oral findings in 375 homosexual males, many of whom had acquired immune deficiency syndrome (AIDS) or AIDS-related complex (ARC), reported seven cases of oral squamous cell carcinoma. This is much more prevalent than in the general population, especially when compared to the 20- to 40-year age group. None of these carcinomas were associated with the oral hairy leukoplakia described by Greenspan et al.[111]

IV. INFECTIONS

A. Syphilis

There has been a long established relationship in the last century between syphilis and oral cancer, particularly cancer of the tongue, and this has been reviewed by Clemmesen.[4] Fry[112] compared the incidence of positive Wassermann (WR) in patients with and without oral cancer. The relative risk of cancer of the tongue in patients with a positive WR was found to be 3.1. A similar figure of 2.6 was reported by Wynder et al.[3] who also managed to eliminate the possibility of other factors, i.e., alcohol and smoking, confusing the issue. Levin et al.[113] compared registrations of syphilis with registrations of cancer of many sites in white males in New York state. Despite a low overall incidence of syphilitic infection, there was serological and clinical evidence five times greater in patients with lingual cancer than in those with other forms of malignant neoplasms. Moreover, the expected number of cases of lingual cancer was exceeded fourfold by the actual number found among the registered syphilitics. Further evidence of a specific association between the two diseases is suggested by the fact that syphilitic-linked leukoplakia or carcinoma occurs predominantly on the dorsum of the anterior two thirds of the tongue, which is nowadays an unusual cancer site. The vast majority of tongue cancers occur on the lateral border, ventral surface, or posterior third.

Despite the fact that the evidence favors a strong association between the two diseases, it by no means infers proof of syphilis being a causative factor in lingual cancer. It may well be, for instance, that substances used in the treatment of syphilis before the use of antibiotics, i.e., various preparations of arsenicals and heavy metals, were more influential as carcinogenic agents than the infection itself. However, there has been no positive evidence that the widespread introduction of penicillin has been responsible for a sharp decrease in oral cancer. The possibility of an immunological mechanism relating the two diseases is unlikely since the leukoplakia and carcinoma associated with syphilis occurs in the late tertiary stages, and it has been shown that cell-mediated immune responses at that stage are intact.[114]

Although there has been an increase in incidence of syphilis in recent years, mortality and the incidence of late syphilitic disease have been steadily falling. With modern methods of treatment it is highly unlikely that late stage syphilis will ever be prevalent, and it is therefore unlikely that more conclusive epidemiological evidence concerning the association of the two diseases will emerge.

B. Chronic Candidosis*

Traditionally it has been assumed that candidal hyphae found on the surface layers of dysplastic oral epithelium have represented a superimposed infection, but this concept has recently been challenged by Cawson and Binnie.[115] Their evidence for a relationship between chronic candidosis and squamous cell carcinoma is based on the following findings:

1. Chronic hyperplastic candidosis itself is the cause of leukoplakic lesions and as such must be regarded as having premalignant potential.
2. Clinically, *Candida* leukoplakias are frequently speckled in character and these lesions have been shown to be especially likely to show epithelial dysplasia or carcinoma.[116]
3. The development of malignancy in candidal leukoplakias is more frequent than in many other types of leukoplakia.
4. Unlike other types of leukoplakia, a possible mechanism can be demonstrated as to how chronic *Candida* infection might disturb epithelial cellular activity in a way that could lead to neoplastic change in that: (a) chick embryo ectoderm undergoes squamous metaplasia and proliferative activity which produces hyperplastic plaques when infected with *Candida albicans*; (b) ultrastructural investigation shows that *Candida albicans* is an intracellular parasite of epithelial cells, causing changes in organelle structure which might affect the behavior of epithelia.
5. Iron deficiency has long been known to have profound effects on the oral mucosa and also to have associations with both oral and pharyngeal cancer (Paterson-Kelly syndrome), and with chronic candidosis.[117] In this context further reference is made to the findings of Joynson et al.[86] where they showed an impairment of cell-mediated immunity in iron deficient patients.

It would be quite unjustifiable from present evidence to state categorically that chronic candidosis per se is a precancerous condition. The evidence at best is circumstantial. However, it is simplistic to hold to the traditional view that the candidal invasion is purely a superimposed infection. This concept requires that evidence be found of preexistence of an earlier lesion which then becomes infected by *Candida*. No such evidence has ever been reported.

C. Herpes Simplex Virus

Since 1968 when Rawles et al.[118] reported that women with cervical cancer have high

---

* Candidosis is used throughout because we are discussing a mycosis. We are aware that the term ''candidiasis'' is used equally commonly.

antibody titers to herpes simplex virus type 2 (HSV-2) there have been several dozen publications from around the world confirming this finding.[119,120] It is now accepted that at least in the early stage of cervical cancer the cells carry a fragment of the HSV-2 genome[121] and express some, but not all, HSV-2 antigens.[122] Both HSV-1 and -2 can cause malignant transformation of cells in vitro, and the transformed cells continue to express some HSV antigens.[123] Because of these findings which have been emerging over the last 10 years, some attention has been directed toward the possibility that HSV-1 might be associated with oral cancer.

Lehner et al.[124] reported a significantly higher lymphocyte response to HSV-1 in patients with oral leukoplakia and epithelial atypia than in patients without atypia. In fact, the lymphocyte level rises similarly in active primary and recurrent herpetic infection. Silverman et al.[125] correlated tumor burden with in vitro lymphocyte reactivity and antibodies to herpesvirus tumor-associated antigens (HSV-TAA) in head and neck cancer patients. They concluded that clinical tumor burden impaired lymphocyte reactivity to phytohemaglutinin and was associated with a high incidence of antibodies to HSV-TAA in patients with squamous cell carcinoma of the head and neck region. They further showed a correlation between the immune defects in clinically cured patients and tumor extent prior to treatment. Smith et al.[126] demonstrated a change in humoral immunity in a high risk group of the population who are likely to develop squamous cell carcinomas of the head and neck region. They showed that cigarette smoking and the use of alcoholic beverages were associated with heightened humoral immunity to HSV-induced antigens, particularly IgA. Further evidence has been reported recently by Shillitoe et al.[22] who studied the relationship between neutralizing antibody to HSV-1 in the serum of patients with oral cancer, patients with oral leukoplakia, and in smoking and nonsmoking control subjects. Significantly higher titers to HSV-1 were found in smoking controls than in nonsmoking controls. Patients with untreated oral cancer have HSV-1 neutralizing titers similar to those of the smoking controls, but those with later stage tumors had higher titers than those with earlier stage tumors. In patients who were tumor free after treatment for oral cancer, higher antibody titers to HSV-1 were associated with longer survival times. The conclusions were that the data were consistent with role for HSV-1 in the pathogenesis of oral cancer and suggested that the tumor results from interactions between the virus and tobacco smoke.

D. Human Papilloma Virus (HPV)

HPV play a role in a range of diseases, particularly various types of wart, and they are increasingly being implicated in the etiology of carcinomata including oral squamous cell carcinoma. An excellent review of their role in oral diseases has been prepared by Scully et al.[127]

The possible role of HPV in oral squamous cell carcinoma was suggested by studies associating the virus with carcinoma of the genital tract, bronchus, larynx, and esophagus.[128-131] Syrjanen et al.[132] studied 40 biopsies of oral squamous cell carcinomas and found that 16 showed histological features suggestive of HPV. Immunostaining showed HPV in eight, four were negative, and four were untested. No immunostaining was performed on the specimens that showed no histological features of HPV. Light microscopic findings suggestive of HPV infection were recently reported in 15 of 17 cases of verrucous carcinoma of the oral cavity.[133] Again, no immunostaining was performed.

A nodular leukoplakia demonstrating HPV viral antigens progressed to squamous cell carcinoma.[134] However, HPV viral antigens have not been found in oral verrucous carcinoma by immunostaining, although they have been in verrucous carcinoma of other mucosae.[135]

Further studies are necessary on larger samples before data on prevalence and HPV type can be established. The important question, however, is whether the presence of HPV in oral epithelial proliferation or neoplasms is causative.

V. SUMMARY OF ETIOLOGICAL FACTORS

A. Tobacco

1. Smoking is an important risk factor in the etiology of oral cancer. Cigars and pipes are strongly associated, but the effect of cigarettes is still questionable.
2. The mechanism by which smoking leads to oral cancer is probably associated with many carcinogenic chemicals produced by burning tobacco. However, interactions with other etiological factors probably occur.
3. There is an increased risk of developing mouth cancer in long-term users of smokeless tobacco.

B. Alcohol

1. Studies show consumption of alcoholic beverages to be a risk factor in oral cancer, but a negative correlation is found when trends in incidence are compared with alcohol consumption nationally.
2. There is a synergistic effect between smoking and drinking. The risk is highest in heavy drinkers who also smoke.
3. The mechanism by which drinking leads to cancer development is not known. It may be local, systemic, or both. Congeners of other agents or other alcohols may be more important than ethanol.

C. Iron Deficiency
There is strong evidence that chronic sideropenia is associated with an increase in oral cancer development.

D. Chronic Candidosis

1. *Candida albicans* infection is associated with some precancerous lesions and might lead to malignant change.
2. The mechanism by which *Candida* infection could lead to cancer is unknown, but evidence of primary involvement is stronger than the assumption that the organism has only a passive role to play.

E. HSV

1. HSV had been associated with oral cancer.
2. The mechanism by which HSV could lead to oral cancer has been investigated in depth. HSV can cause cancer in animals. Interaction with other factors could be important.

F. HPV
HPV has been found in human carcinomas (including oral squamous cell carcinoma). They have also been found in verrucous carcinomas, although not as yet by immunostaining in the oral verrucous carcinomas.

G. Concluding Remarks
Traditionally etiological factors implicated in oral cancer have been examined in isolation. In fact, many studies have gone to great lengths to standardize their results in order to separate possible conflicting influences — the classic example is the overlap of smoking and alcohol consumption in case-control studies.

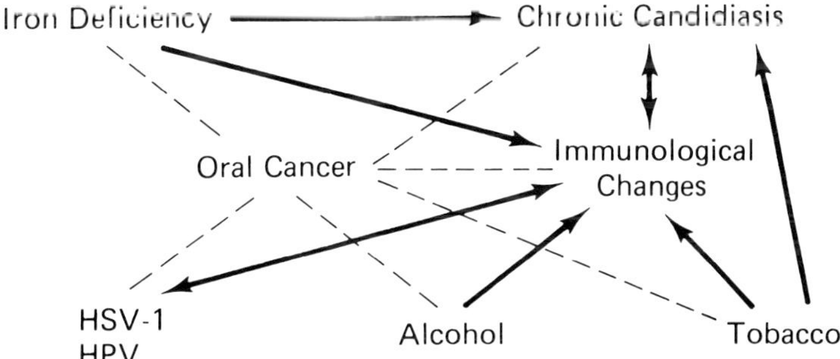

FIGURE 3.   Diagram showing interrelationships of factors associated with oral cancer.

Despite the importance of determining the influence of individual factors as carcinogens, promoters, or initiators, the combination and interrelationships of these factors may prove to be more informative about populations at risk. For instance, the realization that the combined effect of alcohol and tobacco consumption is synergistic and not merely additive is a significant contribution. A more complex challenge is posed by the question of how some or all of these etiological factors associated with oral cancer — smoking, alcohol, HSV and HPV, immunodeficiency, iron deficiency, and *Candida* infection — all have an association with at least one other factor in the list (Figure 3). It would seem, therefore, that although more information needs to be acquired about individual factors, equal priority must be given to studying the interrelationships of these factors (multifactorial influences) possibly by regression analyses.

It is unlikely that much more meaningful information will be gathered by further retrospective case-control studies, and an attempt should be made to mount a prospective study. However, this is a disease which is much less common than, for instance, lung cancer, and so the project becomes expensive and time-consuming. It does, however, allow for monitoring habits such as smoking and alcohol and also allows these to be integrated with changes in host factors. A prospective study avoids the problem of controls and would provide important information on the time and sequence of various factors in relation to the disease. Cause and effect relationships would be more easily established.

REFERENCES

1. **Power, D.,** On cancer of the tongue. The Bradshaw lecture, *Br. J. Surg.,* 6, 336, 1918.
2. **Goldhaber, P.,** The role of saliva and other environmental factors in oral carcinogenesis, *J. Am. Dent. Assoc.,* 54, 517, 1957.
3. **Wynder, E. L., Bross, I. J., and Feldman, R. M.,** A study of the etiological factors in cancer of the mouth, *Cancer,* 10, 1300, 1957.
4. **Clemmesen, J. C.,** *Statistical Studies in the Aetiology of Malignant Neoplasms,* Vol. 1, Munksgaard, Copenhagen, 1965.
5. **Rothman, K. J.,** Epidemiology of head and neck cancer, *Laryngoscope,* 88, 435, 1978.
6. **Kini, M. G. and Rao, K. V. S.,** The problem of cancer, *Indian Med. Gaz.,* 72, 677, 1937.
7. **Khanolkar, V. R. and Suryabai, B.,** Cancer in relation to usages. Three new types in India, *Arch. Pathol. Lab. Med.,* 40, 351, 1945.
8. **Reddy, D. G. and Rao, V. K.,** Cancer of the mouth in coastal Andhra due to smoking cigars with the burning end inside the mouth, *Indian J. Med.,* 11, 791, 1957.
9. **Pindborg, J. J., Mehta, F. S., Gupta, P. C., Daftary, D. K., and Smith, C. J.,** Reverse smoking in Andhra Pradesh, India. A study of palatal lesions among 10,169 villagers, *Br. J. Cancer,* 25, 10, 1971.

10. **Mehta, F. S., Pindborg, J. J., and Hammer, J. E.,** *Oral Cancer and Precancerous Conditions in India,* Munksgaard, Copenhagen, 1971.

11. **Reddy, C. R. R. M., Phranlad, D., and Ramulu, C.,** Incidence of oral cancer with particular reference to hard palate cancer in 1 million population in the district of Visakhapatnam, *Indian J. Cancer,* 12, 72, 1975.

12. **Gupta, P. C., Mehta, F. S., Daftary, D. K., Pindborg, J. J., Bhonsle, R. B., Jalnawall, P. N., Sinor, P. N., Pitkar, V. K., Murta, P. R., Irani, R. R., Shah, H. T., Kadam, P. M., Iyer, K. S. S., Iyer, H. M., Hedge, A. K., Chandrashekar, G. K., Shroff, B. C., Sahir, B. E., and Mehta, M. N.,** Incidence rates of oral cancer and natural history of oral precancerous lesions in a 10-year follow-up study of Indian villagers, *Community Dent. Oral Epidemiol.,* 8, 287, 1980.

13. **Levin, M. L., Goldstein, H., and Gerhardt, P. R.,** Cancer and tobacco smoking, *JAMA,* 143, 336, 1950.

14. **Spitzer, W. O., Hill, G. B., Chambers, L. W., Helliwell, B. F., and Murphy, H. B.,** The occupation of fishing as a risk factor in cancer of the lip, *N. Engl. J. Med.,* 293, 419, 1975.

15. **Doll, R. and Hill, A. B.,** Mortality in relation to smoking: ten years' observation of British doctors, *Br. Med. J.,* 1, 1399, 1964.

16. **Wynder, E. L. and Stellman, S. D.,** Comparative epidemiology of tobacco-related cancers, *Cancer Res.,* 37, 4608, 1977.

17. **Wynder, E. L., Mushinski, M. H., and Spirak, J. C.,** Tobacco and alcohol consumption in relation to the development of multiple primary cancers, *Cancer,* 40, 1872, 1977.

18. **Dorn, H. F. and Cutler, S. J.,** Morbidity from Cancer in the United States, Public Health Monogr. No. 56, U.S. Dept. of Health Education and Welfare, Washington, D.C., 1959.

19. **Kahn, H. A.,** The Dorn study of smoking and mortality among U.S. veterans: report on eight and one-half years of observation, *Natl. Cancer,* 19, 1, 1966.

20. **Mashberg, A., Garfinkel, L., Harris, S.,** Alcohol as a primary risk factor in oral squamous carcinoma, *CA,* 31, 146, 1981.

21. **Trell, E., Bjorlin, G., Andreasson, L., Korsgaard, R., and Mattiason, I.,** Carcinoma of the oral cavity in relation to aryl hydrocarbon hydroxylase inducibility, smoking and dental status, *Int. J. Oral Surg.,* 10, 93, 1981.

22. **Shillitoe, E. J., Greenspan, J. S., and Silverman, S., Jr.,** Neutralizing antibody to herpes simplex virus type 1 in patients with oral cancer, *Cancer,* 49, 2315, 1982.

23. **Jafarey, N. A., Mahmood, Z., and Zaidi, S. H. M.,** Habits and dietary pattern of cases of carcinoma of the oral cavity and oropharynx, *JPMA,* 27, 340, 1977.

24. **Mahboubi, E.,** The epidemiology of oral cavity, pharyngeal and esophageal cancer outside of North America and Western Europe, *Cancer,* 40, 1879, 1977.

25. **Khadim, M. I.,** The effect of pan and its ingredients on oral mucosa, *JPMA,* 27, 353, 1977.

26. **Atkinson, L., Chester, I. C., Smyth, F. G., and Ten Seldom, R. E. J.,** Oral cancer in New Guinea: a study in demography and aetiology, *Cancer,* 17, 1289, 1964.

27. **Ramanathan, K., Ganesan, T. J., and Raghavan, K. V.,** Carcinoma of the tongue in Malaysians, *Mod. Med. Asia,* 14, 56, 1978.

28. **Henderson, B. E. and Aiken, G. H.,** Cancer in Papua New Guinea, *Natl. Cancer Inst. Monogr.,* 53, 67, 1979.

29. **Hirayama, T.,** An epidemiological study of oral and pharyngeal cancer in Central and Southeast Asia, *Bull. WHO,* 34, 41, 1966.

30. **Paches, A. I. and Milievskaya, I. L.,** An epidemiologic study of carcinoma of the mucous membrane of the oral cavity in the USSR, in *Cancer Epidemiology in the USA and USSR,* NIH Publ. 80-2044, Levin, D. L., Ed., National Cancer Institute, Bethesda, Md., 1980, chap. 7B.

31. **Zaridze, D. G., Blettner, M., Trapeznikov, N. N., Kuvshinov, J. P., Matiakin, E. G., Poljakov, B. P., Poddubni, B. K., Parshikova, S. M., Rottenberg, V. I., Chamrakulov, F. S., Chodjaeva, M. C., Stich, H. F., Rosin, M. P., Thurnham, D. I., Hoffmann, D., and Brunnemann, K. D.,** Survey of a population with a high incidence of oral and oesophageal cancer, *Int. J. Cancer,* 36, 153, 1985.

32. **Ackerman, L. V.,** Verrucous carcinoma of the oral cavity, *Surgery,* 23, 670, 1948.

33. **McCoy, J. M. and Waldron, C. A.,** Verrucous carcinoma of the oral cavity, *Oral Surg.,* 52, 623, 1981.

34. **Brown, R. L, Shu, J. M., Scarborough, J. E., Wilkins, S. A., and Smith, R. R.,** Snuff dippers' intraoral cancer: clinical characteristics and response to therapy, *Cancer,* 18, 2, 1965.

35. **Mason, T. J.,** Statistics point to high-cancer localities, *Occup. Health Saf.,* 46, 44, 1977.

36. **Mason, T. J., McKay, F. W., Hoover, R., Blot, W. J., and Fraumeni, J. R.,** Atlas of Cancer Mortality for U.S. Counties 1950—69, Dept. of Health Education and Welfare, No. (NIH) 75, Washington, D.C., 1977.

37. **Blot, W. J. and Fraumeni, J. F., Jr.,** Geographic patterns of oral cancer in the United States: etiologic implications, *J. Chronic Dis.,* 30, 745, 1977.

38. **Winn, D. M., Blot, W. J., Shy, C. M., Pickle, L. W., Toledo, A., and Fraumeni, J. F., Jr.,** Snuff dipping and oral cancer among women in the southern United States, *N. Engl. J. Med.*, 304, 745, 1981.

39. **Sundstrom, B., Mornstad, H., and Axell, T.,** Oral carcinoma associated with snuff dipping, *J. Oral Pathol.*, 11, 245, 1982.

40. **Hirsch, J. M. and Johansson, S. L.,** Effect of long-term application of snuff on the oral mucosa: an experimental study in the rat, *J. Oral Pathol.*, 10, 342, 1981.

41. **Hoffman, D., Harley, N. H., Fisenne, I., Adams, J. D., and Brunnemann, K. D.,** Carcinogenic agents in snuff, *JNCI*, 76, 435, 1986.

42. **Hoffman, D.,** Snuff found to contain high concentrations of carcinogens, *Oncol. Times*, 8, 5, 1986.

43. **Hecht, S. S., Ornaf, R. M., and Hoffmann, D.,** Chemical studies on tobacco smoke. XXXIII. N' nitrosonornicotine in tobacco: analysis of possible contributing factors and biologic implications, *J. Natl. Cancer Inst.*, 54, 1237, 1974.

44. **Hoffmann, D. and Hecht, S. S.,** Nicotine-derived N-nitrosamines and tobacco related cancer: current status and future directions, *Cancer Res.*, 45, 935, 1985.

45. **Schwartz, D., Lellouch, J., Flamant, R., and Denoix, P. F.,** Alcool et cancer. Resultats d'un enquete retrospective, *Rev. Fr. Etud. Clin. Biol.*, 7, 590, 1962.

46. **Rothman, K. J.,** The effect of alcohol consumption on risk of cancer of the head and neck, *Laryngoscope*, 88 (Suppl. 8), 55, 1978.

47. **Keller, A. Z. and Terris, M.,** The association of alcohol and tobacco with cancer of the mouth and pharynx, *Am. J. Public Health*, 55, 1578, 1965.

48. **Vincent, R. G. and Marchetta, F. A.,** The relationship of the use of tobacco and alcohol to oral cancer, *Am. J. Surg.*, 106, 501, 1963.

49. **Herity, B., Moriarty, M., Bourke, B. J., and Daly, L.,** A case-control study of head and neck cancer in the Republic of Ireland, *Br. J. Cancer*, 43, 177, 1981.

50. **Lyon, J. L., Gardner, J. W., Klauber, M. R., and Smart, C. R.,** Low cancer incidence and mortality in Utah, *Cancer*, 39, 2608, 1977.

51. **Lemon, F. R., Walden, R. T., and Woods, R. W.,** Cancer of the lung and mouth in Seventh-day Adventists, *Cancer*, 17, 486, 1964.

52. **Schmidt, W. and DeLint, J.,** Causes of death of alcoholics, *Q. J. Stud. Alcohol*, 33, 171, 1972.

53. **Pell, S. and D'Alonzo, C. A.,** A five-year mortality study of alcoholics, *J. Occup. Med.*, 15, 120, 1973.

54. **Monson, R. R. and Lyon, J. L.,** Proportional mortality among alcoholics, *Cancer*, 36, 1077, 1975.

55. **Hakulinen, T., Lehtimaki, L., Lehtonen, M., and Teppo, L.,** Cancer morbidity among two male cohorts with increased alcohol consumption in Finland, *J. Natl. Cancer Inst.*, 52, 1711, 1974.

56. **Massé, L.,** Epidemiology of Cancer of the Oesophagus in Brittany, Typescript of special lecture in the University of London, London, 1972.

57. **Tuyns, A. J., Péquignot, G., and Jensen, O. M.,** Le cancer de l'oesophage en Ille et Vilaine en fonction des niveaux de consomation d'alcool et de tabac. Des risques que se multiplient, *Bull. Cancer*, 64, 63, 1977.

58. **Tuyns, A. J.,** Oesophageal cancer in non-smoking drinkers and in non-drinking smokers, *Int. J. Cancer*, 32, 443, 1983.

59. **Fischman, S. L. and Martinez, I.,** Oral cancer in Puerto Rico, *J. Surg. Oncol.*, 9, 163, 1977.

60. **McCoy, G. P.,** A biochemical approach to the etiology of alcohol related cancers of the head and neck, *Laryngoscope*, 88 (Suppl. 8), 59, 1978.

61. **Trieger, N., Ship, I. I., Taylor, G. W., and Weisberger, D.,** Cirrhosis and other predisposing factors in carcinoma of the tongue, *Cancer*, 11, 357, 1958.

62. **Trieger, N., Taylor, G. W., and Weisberger, D.,** The significance of liver dysfunction in mouth cancer, *Surg. Gynecol. Obstet.*, 108, 230, 1959.

63. **Keller, A. Z.,** Cirrhosis of the liver, alcoholism and heavy smoking associated with cancer of the mouth and pharynx, *Cancer*, 20, 1015, 1967.

64. **Vincent, R. G., Marchetta, F. A., and Nigogosyan, G.,** Incidence of cirrhosis in oral cancer, *N.Y. J. Med.*, 64, 2174, 1964.

65. **Martinez, I.,** Factors associated with cancer of the oesophagus, mouth and pharynx in Puerto Rico, *J. Natl. Cancer Inst.*, 42, 1069, 1969.

66. **Ahlbom, H. E.,** Simple achlorhydric anaemia, Plummer-Vinson syndrome and carcinoma of the mouth, pharynx and oesophagus in women, *Br. Med. J.*, 2, 331, 1936.

67. **Ahlbom, H. E.,** Pradisponierende faktorenfur platten epithelkarzinom in mund hals and speiserohre, *Acta Radiol. (Stockholm)*, 18, 163, 1937.

68. **Chan, P. C., Okamoto, T., and Wynder, E. L.,** Possible role of riboflavin deficiency in epithelial neoplasia, *J. Natl. Cancer Inst.*, 48, 1341, 1972.

69. **Binnie, W. H.,** Epidemiology and etiology of oral cancer in Britain, *Proc. R. Soc. Med.*, 69, 737, 1976.

70. **Cawson, R. A.,** unpublished data, 1986.

71. **Graham, S., Dayal, H., Rohrer, T., Swanson, M., Sultz, H., Shedd, D., and Fischman, S.,** Dentition, diet, tobacco and alcohol in the epidemiology of oral cancer, *J. Natl. Cancer Inst.*, 59, 1611, 1977.

72. **Raven, W.,** Carcinoma of the mouth and pharynx, *Br. Med. J.*, 2, 1408, 1969.

73. **Browne, R. M., Camsey, M. C., Waterhouse, J. A. H., and Manning, G. L.,** Etiological factors in oral squamous cell carcinoma, *Community Dent. Oral Epidemiol.*, 5, 301, 1977.

74. **Thumfart, W., Weidenbecher, M., Waller, G., and Pesch, H. J.,** Chronic mechanical trauma in the aetiology of oro-pharyngeal carcinoma, *J. Maxillofac. Surg.*, 6, 217, 1978.

75. **Rennie, J. S., McDonald, D. G., and Dagg, J. H.,** Iron and the oral epithelium, *J. R. Soc. Med.*, 77, 602, 1984.

76. **Paterson, D. R.,** A clinical type of dysphagia, *J. Laryngol.*, 34, 289, 1919.

77. **Kelly, A. B.,** Spasm at the entrance of the esophagus, *J. Laryngol.*, 34, 285, 1919.

78. **Waldenström, J. and Kjellberg, S. R.,** The roentgenological diagnosis of sideropenic dysphagia, *Acta Radiol.*, 20, 618, 1939.

79. **Wynder, E. L. and Fryer, J. H.,** Etiologic considerations of Plummer-Vinson (Paterson-Kelly) syndrome, *Ann. Inter. Med.*, 49, 1106, 1958.

80. **Shamm'a, M. H. and Benedict, E. B.,** Esophageal webs: a report of 58 cases and an attempt at classification, *N. Engl. J. Med.*, 259, 378, 1958.

81. **Watts, J. M.,** The importance of the Plummer-Vinson syndrome in the aetiology of carcinoma of the upper gastrointestinal tract, *Postgrad. Med. J.*, 37, 523, 1961.

82. **Rennie, J. S. and McDonald, D. G.,** Quantitative histological analysis of the epithelium of the ventral surface of the hamster tongue in iron deficiency, *Arch. Oral Biol.*, 27, 393, 1982.

83. **Rennie, J. S., McDonald, D. G., and Dagg, J. H.,** Quantitative analysis of human buccal epithelium in iron deficiency anemia, *J. Oral Pathol.*, 11, 39, 1982.

84. **Rennie, J. S., McDonald, D. G., and Douglas, J. A.,** Experimental iron deficiency in the Syrian hamster *(Mesocricates auratus)*, *Lab. Anim.*, 16, 14, 1982.

85. **Prime, S. S., McDonald, D. G., and Rennie, J. S.,** The effect of iron deficiency on experimental oral carcinogenesis in the rat, *Br. J. Cancer*, 47, 413, 1983.

86. **Joynson, D. H., Walker, D. M., Jacobs, A., and Dolby, A. E.,** Defect of cell-mediated immunity in patients with iron-deficiency anaemia, *Lancet*, 2, 1058, 1972.

87. **Jacobs, A. and Cavill, I.,** The oral lesions of iron deficiency anaemia: pyridoxine and riboflavin status, *Br. J. Haematol.*, 14, 291, 1968.

88. **Vitale, J. J., Briotman, S. A., Varrousek-Jakuba, F., Rodday, P. W., and Gottlieb, L. S.,** The effects of iron deficiency and the quality and quantity of fat on chemically induced cancer, *Adv. Exp. Med. Biol.*, 91, 229, 1978.

89. **Toskes, P. P., Smith, G. W., Bensinger, T. A., Giannella, R. A., and Conrad, M. E.,** Folic acid abnormalities in iron deficiency: the mechanism of decreased serum folate levels in rats, *Am. J. Clin. Nutr.*, 27, 355, 1974.

90. **Harrison, R. J.,** Vitamin B_{12} levels in erythrocytes in hypochromic anaemia, *J. Clin. Pathol.*, 24, 698, 1971.

91. **Peto, R., Doll, R., Buckley, J. D., and Sporn, M. B.,** Can dietary beta-carotene materially reduce human cancer rates, *Nature (London)*, 290, 201, 1981.

92. **Wahi, P. N., Kehar, U., and Lahiri, B.,** Factors influencing oral and oropharyngeal cancer in India, *Br. J. Cancer*, 19, 646, 1965.

93. **Ibrahim, N. A., Jafarey, N. A., and Zuberi, S. J.,** Plasma vitamin "A" and carotene levels in squamous cell carcinoma of oral cavity and oro-pharynx, *Clin. Oncol.*, 3, 203, 1977.

94. **Wynder, E. L.,** Dietary habits and cancer epidemiology, *Cancer*, 43, 1955, 1979.

95. **Burnet, F. M.,** Immunological surveillance in neoplasia, *Transplant. Rev.*, 7, 3, 1971.

96. **Scully, C.,** The immunology of cancer of the head and neck with particular reference to oral cancer, *Oral Surg.*, 53, 157, 1982.

97. **Klein, G.,** Tumour immunology: a general appraisal, in *Scientific Foundation of Oncology*, Symington, T. and Carter, R. L., Ed., W. Heinemann, London, 1976, 497.

98. **Binnie, W. H., Cawson, R. A., Hill, G. B., and Soaper, A. E.,** Oral Cancer in England and Wales: A National Study of Morbidity, Mortality, Curability and Related Factors, Office of Population Censuses and Surveys: Studies on Medical and Population Subjects No. 23, Her Majesty's Stationery Office, London, 1972.

99. **Chretien, P. B.,** The effects of smoking on immunocompetence, *Laryngoscope*, 88, 11, 1978.

100. **Berenyi, M. R., Straus, B., and Cruz, D.,** In vivo and in vitro studies of cellular immunity in alcoholic cirrhosis, *Am. J. Dig. Dis.*, 19, 199, 1974.

101. **Lundy, J., Raaf, J. H., Deakins, S., Jacobs, D. A., Tsung-Dao, L., Jacobowitz, D., Spear, C., Wanebo, H., and Old, L. J.,** The acute and chronic effects of alcohol on the human immune system, *Surg. Gynecol. Obstet.*, 141, 212, 1975.

102. **Gatti, R. A. and Good, R. A.**, Occurrence of malignancy in immune-deficiency diseases, *Cancer*, 28, 89, 1971.
103. **Kersey, J. H., Spector, B. D., and Good, R. A**, Primary immunodeficiency diseases and cancer: the immunodeficiency-cancer registry, *Int. J. Cancer*, 12, 333, 1973.
104. **Penn, I. and Starzl, T. E.**, Malignant tumors arising de novo in immunosuppressed organ transplant recipients, *Transplantation*, 14, 407, 1972.
105. **Hoover, R. and Fraumeni, J. F.**, Risk of cancer in renal transplant recipients, *Lancet*, 2, 55, 1973.
106. **Westburg, S. P., Stone, O. J., and Tex, G.**, Multiple cutaneous squamous cell carcinoma during immunosuppressive therapy, *Arch. Dermatol.*, 107, 893, 1973.
107. **Penn, I.**, Chemical immunosuppression and human cancer, *Cancer*, 34, 1474, 1974.
108. **Hoover, R.**, Effects of drugs-immunosuppression, in *Origins of Human Cancer, Cold Spring Harbor Conferences on Cell Proliferation*, Hiatt, H. H., Watson, J. D., and Winsten, J. A., Eds., Cold Spring Harbor Laboratories, Cold Spring Harbor, N.Y., 1977, 369.
109. **Papenhausen, P. R., Kukwa, A., Croft, C. B., Borowiecki, B., Silver, C., and Emeson, E. E.**, Cellular immunity in patients with epidermoid cancer of the head and neck, *Laryngoscope*, 89, 538, 1979.
110. **Silverman, S., Migliorati, C. A., Lozada-Nur, F., Greenspan, D., Conant, M. A.**, Oral findings in people with or at high risk for AIDS: a study of 375 homosexual males, *J. Am. Dent. Assoc.*, 112, 187, 1986.
111. **Greenspan, D., Greenspan, J. S., Conant, M., Peterson, V., Silverman, S., Jr., and De Souza, Y.**, Oral "hairy" leukoplakia in male homosexuals: evidence of association with both papillomavirus and a herpes-group virus, *Lancet*, 831, 1984.
112. **Fry, H. J. B.**, Syphilis and malignant disease: a serological study, *Br. J. Hyg.*, 29, 313, 1929.
113. **Levin, M. L., Kress, L. C., and Goldstein, H.**, Syphilis and cancer: reported syphilis prevalence among 7,761 cancer patients, *N.Y. State J. Med.*, 42, 1737, 1942.
114. **Lehner, T.**, Oral neoplasia, in *Immunology of Oral Diseases*, Roitt, I. M. and Lehner, T., Eds., Blackwell Scientific, Oxford, 1980, 429.
115. **Cawson, R. A. and Binnie, W. H.**, Candida leukoplakia and carcinoma: a possible relationship, in *Oral Premalignancy*, MacKenzie, I. C., Dabelsteen, E., and Squier, C. A., Eds., University of Iowa Press, Iowa City, 1980, 59.
116. **Pindborg, J. J., Renstrup, G., Poulsen, H. E., and Silverman, S., Jr.**, Studies in oral leukoplakias. V. Clinical and histologic signs of malignancy, *Acta Odontol. Scand.*, 21, 407, 1963.
117. **Higgs, J. M. and Wells, R. S.**, Chronic muco-cutaneous candidiasis associated abnormalities of iron metabolism, *Br. J. Dermatol.*, 86 (Suppl. 8), 88, 1972.
118. **Rawles, W. E., Tompkins, W. A. F., Figueroa, M. E., and Melnick, J. L.**, Herpesvirus type 2: association with carcinoma of the cervix, *Science*, 161, 1255, 1968.
119. **Melnick, J. L. and Adam, E.**, Epidemiological approaches to determining whether herpesvirus is the etiological agent of cervical cancer, *Prog. Exp. Tumor Res.*, 21, 49, 1978.
120. Editorial, genital herpes and cervical carcinoma, *Br. Med. J.*, 1, 807, 1978.
121. **McDougall, J. R., Galloway, D. A., Purifoy, D. J. M., Powell, K. L., Richart, R. M., and Fenoglio, C. M.**, Herpes simplex virus expression in latently infected ganglion cells and in cervical neoplasia, in *Cold Spring Harbor Conference on Cell Proliferation*, Cold Spring Harbor Laboratories, Cold Spring Harbor, N.Y., 1980, 101.
122. **Dreesman, G. R., Burek, J., Adam, E., Kaufman, R. H., and Melnick, J. L.**, Expression of herpesvirus-induced antigens in human cervical cancer, *Nature (London)*, 283, 591, 1980.
123. **Rapp, F.**, Transformation by herpes simplex viruses, in *Cold Spring Harbor Conference on Cell Proliferation*, Cold Spring Harbor Laboratories, Cold Spring Harbor, N.Y., 1980, 63.
124. **Lehner, T., Shillitoe, E. J., Wilton, J. M., and Ivanyi, L.**, Cell-mediated immunity to herpes virus type I in carcinoma and pre-cancerous lesions, *Br. J. Cancer*, 28, 128, 1973.
125. **Silverman, N. A., Alexander, J. C., Hollinshead, A. C., and Chretien, P. B.**, Correlation of tumor burden with in vitro lymphocyte reactivity and antibodies to herpes virus tumor-associated antigens in head and neck squamous carcinoma, *Cancer*, 37, 135, 1976.
126. **Smith, H. G., Chretien, P. B., Henson, D. E., Silverman, N. A., and Alexander, J. C.**, Viral-specific humoral immunity to herpes simplex-induced antigens in patients with squamous carcinoma of the head and neck, *Am. J. Surg.*, 132, 541, 1976.
127. **Scully, C., Prime, S., and Maitland, N.**, Papillomaviruses: their possible role in oral disease, *Oral Surg.*, 60, 166, 1985.
128. **Syrjanen, K. J. and Syrjanen, S. M.**, Histological evidence for the presence of condylomatous epithelial lesions in association with laryngeal squamous cell carcinoma, *ORL*, 43, 181, 1981.
129. **Lack, E., Vawter, G. F., Smith, H. G., Healy, G. B., Lancaster, W. D., and Jenson, A. B.**, Immunohistochemical localization of human papilloma virus in squamous papillomas of the larynx, *Lancet*, 2, 592, 1980.

130. **Syrjanen, K. J.,** Bronchial squamous cell carcinomas associated with epithelial changes identical to condylomatous lesions of the uterine cervix, *Lung,* 158, 131, 1980.
131. **Syrjanen, K. J.,** Histological changes identical to those of condylomatous lesions found in oesophageal squamous cell carcinomas, *Arch. Geschwulstforsch.,* 4, 283, 1982.
132. **Syrjanen, K. J., Pyrhonen, S., Syrjanen, S. M., and Lamberg, M. A.,** Immunohistochemical demonstration of human papilloma virus (HPV) antigens in oral squamous cell lesions, *Br. J. Oral Surg.,* 21, 147, 1983.
133. **Eisenberg, E., Rosenberg, B., and Krutchkoff, D. J.,** Verrucous carcinoma: a possible viral pathogenesis, *Oral Surg.,* 59, 52, 1985.
134. **Loning, T., Reichart, P., Staquet, M. J., Becker, J., and Thivolet, J.,** Occurrence of papillomavirus structural antigens in oral papillomas and leukoplakias, *J. Oral Pathol.,* 13, 155, 1984.
135. **Zachow, K., Ostrow, R., Okagaki, T., Twiggs, L., Clark, B., and Nivmara, M.,** Presence of HPV-DNA in human benign and malignant epithelial tumours, in *Papillomaviruses,* Broker, T. B. and Howley, P. M., Eds., Cold Spring Harbor Laboratories, Cold Spring Harbor, N.Y., 1982, 65.

Chapter 3

PREMALIGNANCY

John M. Wright and Bruce A. Wright

TABLE OF CONTENTS

I. INTRODUCTION

It is unlikely that oral squamous cell carcinoma arises from normal surface epithelium. The epithelium first goes through stages of initiation and promotion. These precursor stages produce morphologic changes in the cells which result in clinically detectable lesions. These early cellular and clinical alterations precede the development of carcinoma and form the basis for the concept of premalignancy or precancer.

Histologically, the cellular changes which the epithelium undergoes prior to becoming malignant are known as epithelial dysplasia. These cellular changes are usually expressed by mucosal alterations clinically, thereby producing precancerous lesions. A precancerous lesion is defined as a morphologically altered tissue in which cancer is more likely to occur than in its apparently normal counterpart.[1] In addition to individual precancerous lesions, there are generalized states associated with a significantly increased risk of cancer, and these states are known as precancerous conditions.[1]

Clinical changes occur as a result of cellular changes. Therefore, an understanding of the dysplastic process is essential prior to examining clinical lesions.

II. HISTOLOGIC FEATURES OF PREMALIGNANCY

A. Normal Oral Mucosa

The mouth is lined by a mucous membrane consisting of stratified squamous epithelium and a supporting fibrovascular connective tissue stroma called the lamina propria (Figure 1). In some locations, this mucosa lies directly over bone and is called mucoperiosteum. In other areas, it contains a submucosa where fat and/or accessory salivary glands are found. Intraorally, some epithelium is keratinized and some is not. Keratinization is a protective phenomenon, and its presence is determined by functional requirements. In general, masticatory mucosa (attached gingiva and palate) is keratinized. The type of keratinization can be either ortho- or parakeratin. Lining mucosa, on the other hand — that which does not overlie bone and has fewer functional requirements — is normally unkeratinized.

Oral stratified squamous epithelium normally consists of two, three, or four layers. All epithelium has a basal layer of cells known as a stratum basale. These cells are less differentiated and contain very little cytoplasm. The basal layer is where cellular reproduction occurs in order to replenish cells which are normally lost from its surface. The largest layer of epithelium is the stratum spinosum. As normal basal cells mature through this zone, they develop abundant cytoplasm and assume a polyhedral morphology. Nuclear chromatin becomes dispersed and the nucleus stains lighter. Nonkeratinized epithelium has only these two layers. Keratinized epithelium contains a stratum corneum of either ortho- or parakeratin. Orthokeratinization is a complete keratinization where the individual squames fully keratinize and the nucleus is lost. Parakeratin retains small, pyknotic nuclei. Orthokeratin is usually associated with well-developed keratohyalin granules, the stratum granulosum.

B. Pathologic Changes in Oral Mucosa

Oral epithelium is a dynamic tissue which continually undergoes replenishment and is highly reactive to external stimuli. A number of pathologic changes are seen in the epithelium that do not necessarily imply that a precancerous lesion exists. These conditions include:

1.   Hyperorthokeratosis: an increased thickness of orthokeratin on the surface of masticatory mucosa or the presence of any orthokeratin on lining mucosa
2.   Hyperparakeratosis: an increased thickness of parakeratin on the surface of masticatory mucosa or the presence of any parakeratin on lining mucosa; also called parakeratosis

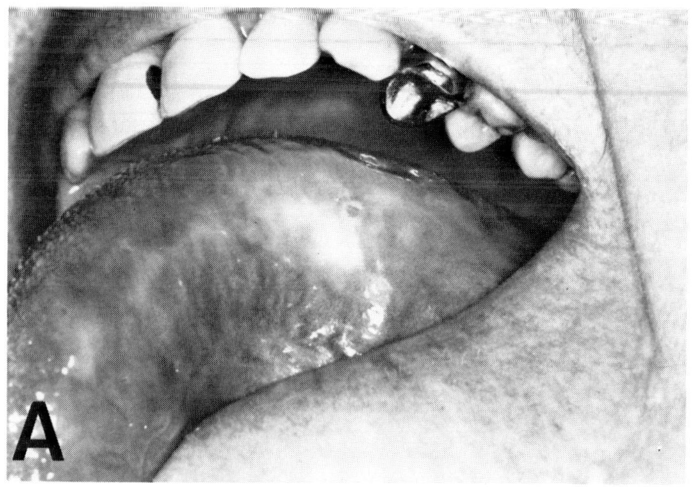

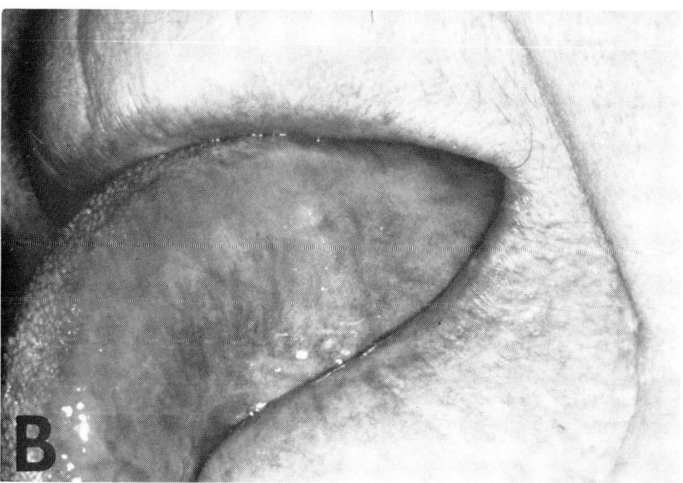

FIGURE 5. (A) Frictional keratosis on the left lateral border of the tongue which resulted from the chronic irritation from the sharp edges of a fractured lower molar. (B) Resolution of the lesion within 2 weeks following correction of the irritant.

Candida and 71% showed dysplasia. At present, the significance of finding *Candida* species in leukoplakia and its role in the subsequent development of malignancy are unknown. For those who believe that the yeast plays an etiologic role in the pathogenesis of these lesions, the name chronic hyperplastic candidosis or candidal leukoplakia has been proposed. Some of these patients are iron deficient[42] and most smoke.[1,37] Cawson and Binnie[43] followed patients with candidal leukoplakia and found that 30% developed carcinoma. However, candidal leukoplakias are most commonly speckled (red and white) lesions which show a high incidence of dysplasia and would be expected to have a higher malignant transformation rate than nondysplastic lesions. Nevertheless, we currently think that there is sufficient justification to regard candidal leukoplakia as a specific entity with malignant potential.

There remains a group of leukoplakias for which a cause is not apparent. They undoubtedly represent a heterogeneous group of lesions that will eventually be subclassified as we learn more about them. Currently, they are regarded as idiopathic leukoplakias and are considered premalignant.

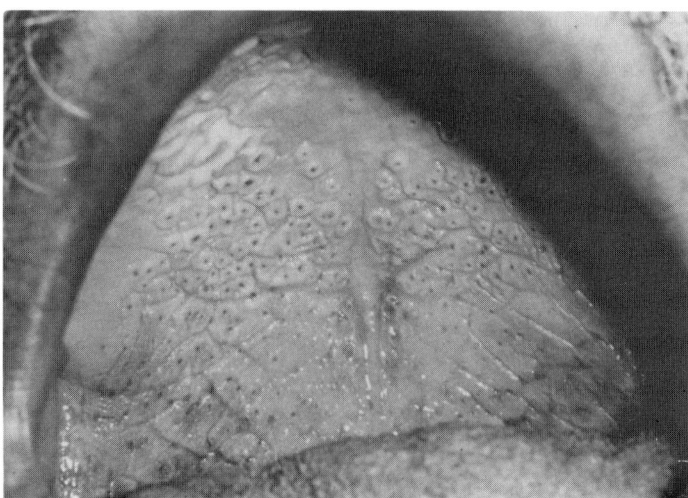

FIGURE 6.   Stomatitis nicotina.

From an etiological perspective, there are three distinct leukoplakias with malignant potential: tobacco-associated, candidal, and idiopathic.

3. Clinical Features

The prevalence of leukoplakia varies with the population studied, but Pindborg[44] recently reviewed the reported prevalences worldwide and found a range from 0.2 to 12.5%. Leukoplakia is found predominantly in the middle aged and elderly.[2,17,21,30,34,41,45] Leukoplakia was primarily a disease of men,[2,17,41,45,46] but Waldron and Shafer[30] recently reported over 3000 cases and found only a slight male predilection. This was partially explained by the increasing frequency and acceptance of tobacco use among women.

Leukoplakia occurs on all mucosal surfaces, but has a predilection for those surfaces most commonly irritated, i.e., lower alveolar mucosa and buccal mucosa.[3,21,30] In some reports, the commissures are commonly involved, particularly by the speckled type of leukoplakia.[2,39] Depending on the size of the lesion, it is not uncommon for more than one anatomic site to be contiguously involved, and a recent report showed 70% of patients had leukoplakias involving two or more areas.[21] In addition, patients may have more than one lesion, and a recent report documented that 15% of patients with leukoplakia in the floor of their mouths had separate lesions in other areas.[47]

Not all leukoplakias are homogeneous white plaques. There are a number of clinical variants which are recognized,[1-3,19,21,40,46,48-51] and these have formed the basis for past clinical classifications. Not all these classifications have used the same terminology. Designations such as leukoplakia simplex, leukoplakia verrucosa, leukoplakia erosiva, verrucous hyperplasia, speckled leukoplakia, speckled erythroplakia, nodular leukoplakia, and ulcerative leukoplakia have all been used.

While it may be difficult to remember the terminology, it is critically important to recognize the clinical changes which are possible in these lesions because it is these changes which connote different risks of malignant transformation (see Section III.A.4). In general, there are two basic clinical types of leukoplakia: homogeneous and nonhomogeneous.

The homogeneous leukoplakias (Figure 7) are basically plaque-like, and although their color may vary, it is a variation of the color white. The surface may be smooth or wrinkled and may occasionally contain fine cracks or fissures. Nonhomogeneous lesions may contain areas of ulceration or redness (Figure 8). If there are alternating areas of red and white the

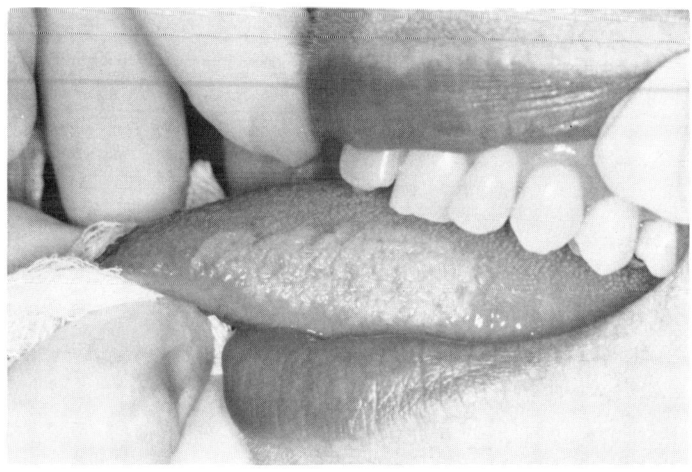

FIGURE 7. Homogeneous leukoplakia.

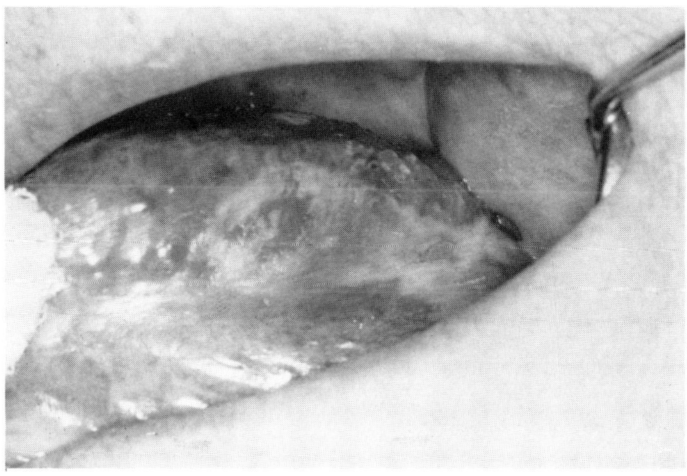

FIGURE 8. Nonhomogeneous leukoplakia with areas of redness (anterior) and ulceration (posterior) on the posterior lateral border of the tongue. Histologically, the lesion was dysplastic.

term erythroleukoplakia has been used (Figure 9). More commonly, however, there is an erythematous lesion supporting rather uniformly distributed, slightly raised, whitish nodules. This lesion has been referred to as nodular leukoplakia, speckled leukoplakia, or speckled erythroplakia (Figure 10). Some lesions are white, but contain papillary or verrucous areas entirely or in part, and this finding is suggested by the term verrucous leukoplakia (Figure 11). All types of nonhomogeneous leukoplakia have a greater malignant risk than the homogeneous form, and the magnitude of this risk is discussed later.

It is important to remember that leukoplakia is a dynamic, rather than static, process which is capable of continuous clinical and histological change.[19,21,52,53] Lesions can spontaneously regress or spread and evolve from a homogeneous to a nonhomogeneous lesion. Homogeneous leukoplakia may show only hyperkeratosis on incisional biopsy, but if untreated, may later reveal dysplastic changes histologically. Additionally, this same lesion may or may not evolve into a nonhomogeneous lesion clinically.

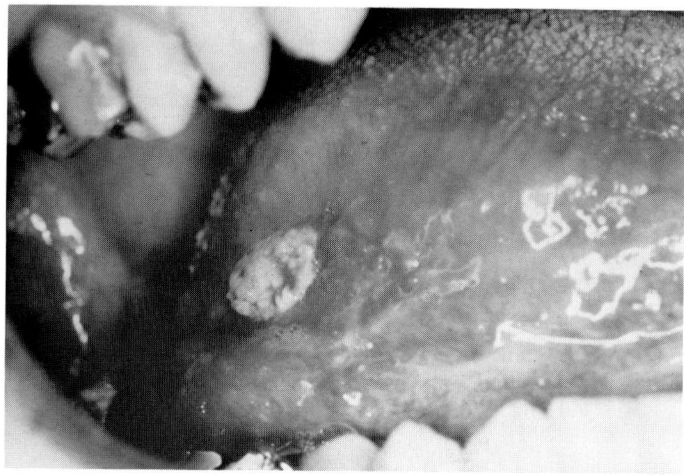

FIGURE 9.   Erythroleukoplakia of lateral posterior tongue. Anterior one half
of the lesion was red (dark). Histologically, the lesion was a superficially invasive
carcinoma.

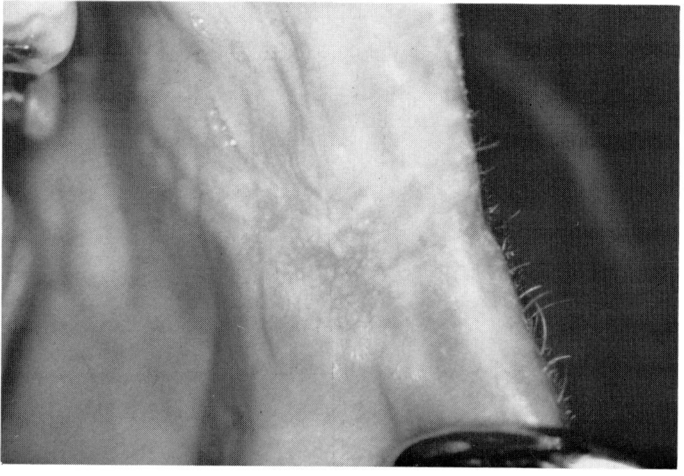

FIGURE 10.   Speckled leukoplakia at right commissure.

4. Clinicopathologic Correlation

Leukoplakia is a clinical condition only and may represent a variety of pathologic changes
microscopically. In general, it is impossible always to predict clinically which lesions will
show dysplastic changes when biopsied. Some of the most extensive and corrugated leukoplakias will show only hyperkeratosis while, on occasion, a 1-cm homogeneous leukoplakia will prove to be a superficially invasive carcinoma when biopsied. For those lesions
which persist after removal of any identifiable causative factors, biopsy is mandatory because
microscopic evaluation is the only way to assess accurately the degree of malignant risk.

Most leukoplakias, when biopsied, are characterized by varying degrees of hyperorthokeratosis, hyperparakeratosis, and acanthosis. In the largest series of leukoplakias reported,
Waldron and Shafer[30] showed that 80% of 3256 cases showed these benign and osten-
sibly reactive changes without any evidence of dysplasia. Although most leukoplakias are
benign hyperkeratoses, the reason for biopsy is to determine which lesions show dysplastic

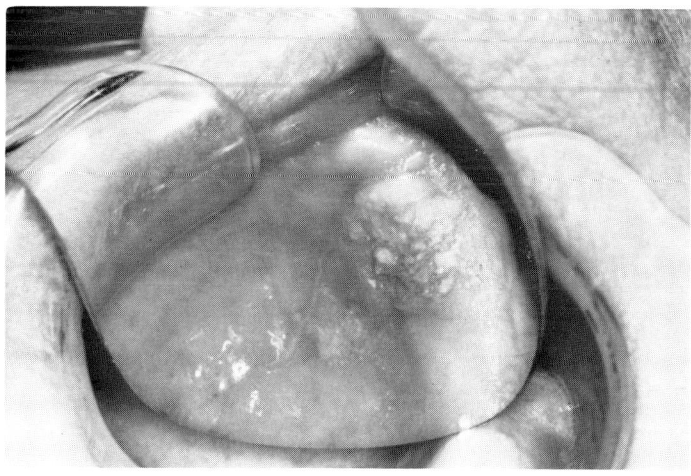

FIGURE 11.   Verrucous leukoplakia of anterior maxillary alveolar ridge. Histologically the lesion was a superficially invasive carcinoma.

or invasive epithelial changes. Most reports of large series of leukoplakias demonstrate conclusively that a significant number of lesions are premalignant (dysplastic) or malignant when first biopsied, and the figures range from approximately 10 to 25%.[2,3,17,22,25,30,41,45,54-56] In the series reported by Waldron and Shafer,[30] 12.2% of their lesions showed mild to moderate dysplasia, 4.5% showed severe dysplasia or carcinoma *in situ*, and 3.1% showed invasive squamous cell carcinoma. They reported 104 cases of squamous cell carcinoma that clinically were white plaques. Other investigators have confirmed the fact that some leukoplakias will prove to be malignant when biopsied, and the percentage in some series, 10 to 20%,[45] is alarmingly high. In a series of 153 cases, of those lesions in which the clinician suspected malignancy, roughly one third were benign hyperkeratoses; conversely, of those lesions in which the clinician suspected that the diagnosis would be hyperkeratosis, 13% were invasive carcinoma.[55] This again confirms the importance of biopsy.

Of significant clinical importance is the recent finding that the anatomic site involved by the leukoplakia alters its malignant potential. Leukoplakias involving areas where oral cancer is common have a greater chance of being precancerous when biopsied than lesions involving other areas. These "at risk" sites are the floor of the mouth, ventral and lateral border of the tongue, and lower lip.[1,18,25,47,57,58] Waldron and Shafer[30] found that 43% of 289 floor of the mouth leukoplakias were dysplastic or invasive carcinoma when first biopsied, and the corresponding figures for tongue and lower lip were approximately 25%. Kramer and colleagues[47] substantiated the high risk of malignancy in sublingual keratoses (ventral tongue and/or floor of mouth) by demonstrating that 27% of these lesions were carcinomas when first biopsied and an additional 24% developed carcinoma with follow-up.

Other reports have shown a high percentage of dysplastic lesions affecting the buccal mucosa and commissures,[2,25] and this is especially true for the nodular or speckled leukoplakias. For reasons that are unknown, these lesions are less common in the U.S.

In addition to the clinical significance of anatomic site, it is also known that clinical variants of leukoplakia impart a significant increase in the malignant potential of the lesion. Erythroleukoplakia,[2,17,21,48,59] nodular or speckled leukoplakia,[3,41,46,50,51,60] and verrucous leukoplakias[2,17,48,49,59,61,62] are significantly more likely to be dysplastic or invasive when biopsied than are homogeneous leukoplakias. Banoczy[17] has shown that 48% of erythroleukoplakias, 23% of verrucous leukoplakias, and only 6% of homogeneous leukoplakias showed

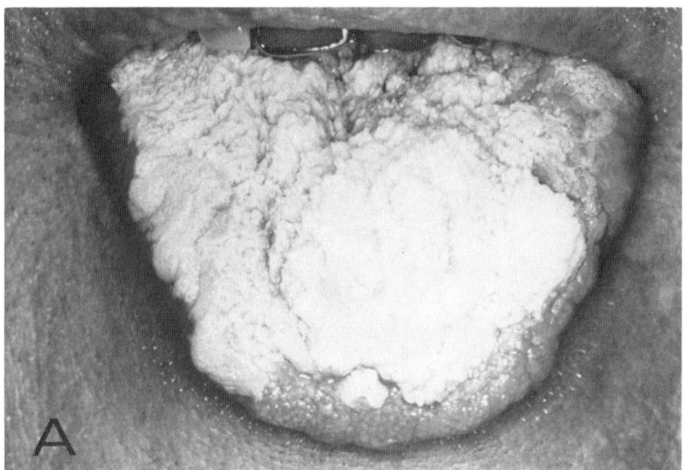

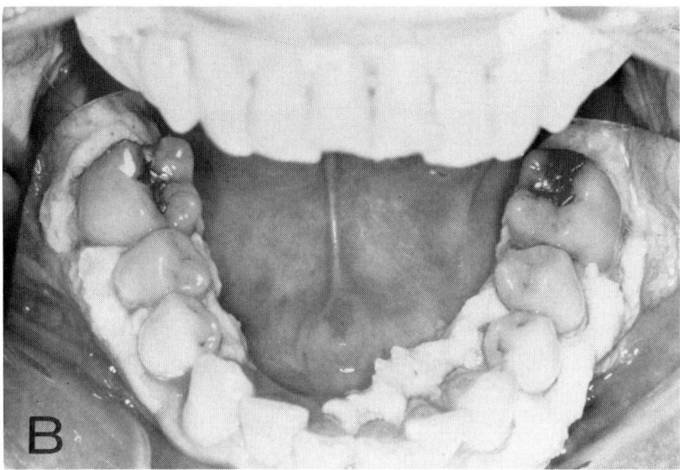

FIGURE 12.   (A and B) Proliferative verrucous leukoplakia. The lesion has progressively spread and recurred repeatedly following surgery.

histologic evidence of dysplasia while 33, 3, and 0%, respectively, showed carcinoma.[59] In a large series of nodular leukoplakias, Renstrup[41] has shown that 71% were dysplastic, while Mehta and colleagues[46] reported 59% of nodular, but only 8% of homogeneous leukoplakias, were dysplastic. Eversole and Shopper[49] have reported malignant or premalignant changes in 24% of a series of verrucous lesions. Shear and Pindborg[62] recently reported verrucous hyperplasia of the oral mucosa as a new entity, but failed to distinguish the lesion from verrucous leukoplakia. Nevertheless, clinically these white lesions were papillary or verrucous, and 66% showed epithelial dysplasia, 29% showed verrucous carcinoma, and 10% had microscopic evidence of squamous cell carcinoma. Hansen and colleagues[61] also emphasized the serious nature of verrucous lesions by reporting another new entity entitled proliferative verrucous leukoplakia (Figure 12). The condition starts as a homogeneous leukoplakia, but spreads and becomes verrucous as well as multifocal. It is slowly progressive, highly resistant to therapy, and often eventuates in carcinoma. Regardless of terminology, areas of redness or nodularity and a papillary or verrucous surface are clinical indicators of a significantly increased risk of dysplasia or malignancy.

Table 1
MALIGNANT TRANSFORMATION OF LEUKOPLAKIA

Author	Year	Country	No. of patients	Years of observation	Malignant transformation (%)
Einhorn and Wersall[20]	1967	Sweden	782	1—44	4.0
Silverman and Rozen[63]	1968	U.S.	117	5—11	6.0
Kramer[65]	1969	England	187	1—16	4.8
Roed-Petersen[64]	1971	Denmark	331	4.3 (mean)	3.6
Gangadharan and Paymaster[45]	1971	India	626	1/4—23	10.0
Malaowalla et al.[67]	1976	India (Gujarat)	4762	2	0.13
Banoczy[17]	1977	Hungary	670	1—30	6.0
Gupta et al.[22]	1980	India (Ernakulam)	410	1—10	2.2
Gupta et al.[22]	1980	India (Bhavnagar)	360	1—10	0.3
Shklar[54]	1981	U.S.	600	1—10	5.0
Silverman et al.[21]	1984	U.S.	257	7.2 (mean)	17.5

5. *Natural History*

Certain leukoplakias will progress to invasive carcinoma,[2,4,17-22,26,40,45,54,63-67] although the magnitude of this problem is unknown. The variation in malignant transformation rates as reported from around the world (Table 1) represent variations in study design, patient selection, and therapeutic intervention as much as they represent true epidemiologic differences. Despite the fact that these studies are not comparable, the generally quoted figure for malignant transformation of leukoplakia in the western world is 3 to 6%.[5,22]

In a rather alarming departure from this figure, Silverman and colleagues[21] followed 257 patients with leukoplakia for an average 7.2 years and found a malignant transformation rate of 17.5%. This high rate is most likely explained by a longer follow-up period because in their earlier report[63] they found only a 6% malignant transformation rate. Banoczy[17] also showed a higher rate with longer observation, and Einhorn and Wersall[20] reported a 2.4% rate with 10-year maximum follow-up that increased to 4% at 20 years. The highest transformation rate of Silverman et al.[21] occurred in the 2nd year of follow-up (5%), then slowly diminished to approximately 1%/year in subsequent years. These figures would seem to mandate clinical observation for the life of the lesion or the patient.

In virtually every longitudinal study employing clinicopathologic correlation, it has been shown that the risk of malignant transformation is considerably increased in those lesions showing histologic evidence of dysplasia.[2,17-22,26] Silverman et al.[21] showed a transformation rate of 36% for dysplastic lesions and 16% for those lesions originally diagnosed as hyperkeratosis, while Mincer et al.[18] reported a transformation rate of 25% in dysplastic lesions, if patients who developed carcinoma in the 1st year of observation are not omitted. Gupta et al.[22] reported a transformation rate of 7% in dysplastic lesions, but showed that the risk of malignant transformation was about 15 times greater than that of nondysplastic lesions. Although some benign hyperkeratotic lesions will progress to invasive carcinoma, it is assumed that most, if not all, of the lesions pass through a dysplastic stage. This assumption, however, has never been substantiated because of the difficulty of designing long-range, prospective studies for large groups of patients.

Of clinical significance is the fact that the nonhomogeneous leukoplakias show a significantly increased rate of malignant transformation when compared with the homogeneous lesions.[1,2,17,19,21,22,40,64] Banoczy[17] followed 670 patients and found a malignant transformation rate of 26% for leukoplakias with a red component, 5.5% for verrucous leukoplakias, and 0% for homogeneous leukoplakias. Axell et al.[1] and Silverman et al.[21] reported malignant transformation rates of 38 and 23% for erythroleukoplakias (including nodular leukoplakias) and only 3 and 6.5% rates for homogeneous lesions, respectively. As discussed earlier, the

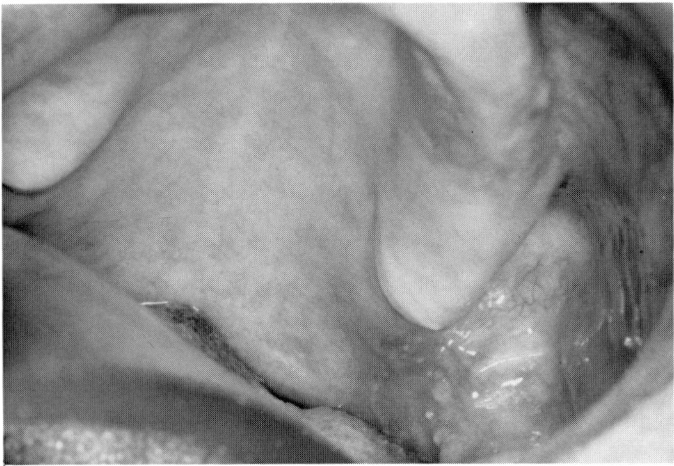

FIGURE 13.   Erythroplakia just posterior to the left maxillary tuberosity.

obvious explanation for the high rate of malignant transformation in nonhomogeneous leukoplakias is the fact that these lesions are much more likely to be dysplastic when initially biopsied. Some reports have shown a higher transformation rate for those lesions which occur in "at risk" sites, i.e., the floor of the mouth,[47,57] lower lip, and tongue.[17,20,21,64]

The effect of tobacco habits on malignant transformation rates poses an enigma. Despite the association of tobacco with leukoplakia and the development of intraoral squamous cell carcinoma, it has been shown that the idiopathic leukoplakias have a much higher risk of malignant transformation than the tobacco-associated leukoplakias.[17,20,21,64] Einhorn and Wersall[20] showed that the risk of developing carcinoma in leukoplakias from patients who did not use tobacco was about eight times that of tobacco users. The reason for this finding is not known, although Pindborg and associates[68] recently reported a chevron-type of keratinization which was found exclusively in tobacco users. This keratinization was characterized histologically by thin spires of parakeratin which extended above the surface and imparted a wavy surface appearance. Clinically it appeared as very fine "striae" described as having a pumice-like appearance. Interestingly, no dysplasia was found to be associated with chevron keratinization.

B. Erythroplakia
1. Definition
Erythroplakia is somewhat analogous to leukoplakia in that it is a clinical term which has been defined as a red, velvety plaque which cannot be characterized clinically or pathologically as being due to any other condition (Figure 13).[6]

Erythroplakia is also a diagnosis by exclusion. The most common cause of redness intraorally is inflammation. Accordingly, many infections, dermatoses, and physical and chemical injuries may cause an inflammatory reaction. Although these lesions are red, clinically they are not, by definition, erythroplakias. After all the known conditions that can produce red lesions have been eliminated, there remains a very rare, but very ominous, condition known as erythroplakia. However, unlike leukoplakia, all erythroplakias are characterized histologically by either dysplasia or invasive carcinoma.[6,69,70]

2. Clinical Features
Although the serious nature of erythroplakia is well documented, there is only a limited understanding of this condition because of its rarity. In one of the few studies on prevalence,

Lay et al.[71] reported a 0.1% prevalence for erythroplakia in a prospective study of 6000 villagers in Burma.

Like leukoplakia, erythroplakia is found most commonly in the elderly and affects the "at risk" sites for oral cancer, i.e., floor of the mouth and ventral and lateral tongue. Unlike leukoplakia, however, there is also a distinct tendency to involve the soft palate, tonsilar pilar, and retromolar trigone complex.[24,69,72,73]

The erythroplakic lesions are usually fairly well demarcated from surrounding normal mucosa and may have a smooth or rough and granular surface. Mashburg and colleagues[72] have shown that there is a greater tendency for carcinoma *in situ* and early invasive carcinoma to be rough or granular rather than smooth. In addition to the smooth or granular erythroplakias, some are interspersed with white patches or nodules.[74] The clinical distinction between speckled erythroplakia and speckled leukoplakia or erythroleukoplakia is more semantic than practical as long as one remembers that these lesions are clinically sinister and usually dysplastic or invasive when biopsied. Patients with erythroplakia can be asymptomatic or experience pain. Many patients report that the lesion burns, especially when eating hot or spicy foods.

Despite the voluminous literature on leukoplakia, less is known about erythroplakia because of its rarity. Nevertheless, the serious nature and malignant potential of erythroplakia has been unequivocally established.[5,23,24,57,69,74-76] Mashberg[77] and Mashberg et al.[72,73] have stressed the importance of erythroplakia as the most common clinical manifestation of early malignancy. Of 158 patients with early, asymptomatic oral squamous cell carcinoma, 90.5% of the lesions had a red component,[72] and another prospective study[77] showed that 86.3% of early malignancies were predominantly red. Small size does not preclude an erythroplakia from being malignant when biopsied because 42% of early malignancies detected by Mashberg and Meyers[73] were less than 1 cm. In a recent study of carcinoma *in situ*,[23] 58% of the lesions were erythroplakias, 25% were speckled erythroplakias, and 17% were leukoplakias.

3. Clinicopathologic Correlation

Most erythroplakias, when biopsied, will show microscopic evidence of dysplasia, carcinoma *in situ,* or early invasive carcinoma. Of the 65 cases reported by Shafer and Waldron,[69] 51% were invasive carcinoma, 40% were carcinoma *in situ* or severe dysplasia, and 9% were mild or moderate dysplasia. Mashberg[77] also showed that 45% of his erythroplakias were early malignancies in which he included carcinoma *in situ*.

Erythroplakias are red because the epithelium is not keratinized and is atrophic in most cases. In addition, dysplastic epithelium often induces an immune or inflammatory reaction, and the vascular changes are readily evident through the thin epithelium.

4. Clinical Diagnostic Aids

The only definitive way to determine the seriousness of persistent erythroplakic lesions is biopsy. However, not all red lesions are erythroplakias, and clinical experience, therefore, plays a significant role in patient evaluation. Toluidine blue staining of erythroplakic lesions has been shown to be a simple and relatively accurate method for distinguishing dysplastic/carcinomatous lesions from nondysplastic or inflammatory ones.[78,79] The rationale for using Toluidine blue as an intraoral supravital stain was based on its ability to detect increased nuclear activity in dysplastic or carcinomatous surface lesions. The dye has also been used as a mouth rinse to facilitate detection of lesions in high-risk patients for oral cancer.[80] If employed, the results of supravital staining should only be used as an adjunct to clinical interpretation because both false positives and false negatives have been documented.

Much has been written about the role of exfoliative cytology in the evaluation of premalignant oral lesions. The best results of cytologic examination have been reported with the erythroplakias.[59,76,81] Because the erythroplakias have no surface keratin, the likelihood of removing dysplastic or neoplastic cells by scraping is greatly increased. Banoczy and Rigo[59] reported a 72% correlation between cytologic and histologic diagnosis for erythroleukoplakias. With an occasional exception,[82] scraping leukoplakias for cytologic diagnosis simply removes keratotic cells, leaving the underlying dysplastic cells undiscovered.[83] In general, we do not feel that cytologic evaluation should play a significant role in the evaluation of premalignant oral lesions. Unlike the uterine cervix, the mouth is readily accessible and biopsy relatively easy. Furthermore, cytologic diagnosis only detects suspicious cells and cannot render a definitive diagnosis. If a cytologic smear is reported as positive, biopsy is still required.

IV. PREMALIGNANT CONDITIONS

There are several generalized conditions that are associated with an increased risk of oral cancer. With the exception of immunosuppression, the common pathological link among all these conditions is the fact that they cause atrophy of the surface oral epithelium. Presumably, this thin epithelium would then allow greater access of carcinogens to the progenitor compartment of cells within the basal epithelium.

A. Syphilis
There has been an historical association between tongue cancer, often dorsal surface, and syphilis (see Chapter 2). Unfortunately, the documentation for this association has often been anecdotal, and it is not entirely clear if the carcinomas arose as a primary result of the disease or secondarily from its treatment with arsenicals and other heavy metals.

Tertiary syphilis causes an endarteritis and interstitial glossitis. Presumably this results in atrophy of the dorsal tongue surface which is then prone to the development of leukoplakia. The association between syphilis, leukoplakia,[40,84] and tongue cancer[40,85] has been documented, but the importance of this association is conjectural since these reports do not show the prevalence of syphilis in healthy control groups.

Because of the rarity of tertiary syphilis today, its importance in the development of oral cancer has remarkably declined, and it is possible that the true relationship of syphilis to oral cancer may never be ascertained.

B. Sideropenic Dysphagia (Paterson-Kelly Syndrome, Plummer-Vinson Syndrome)
The association of iron deficiency, esophageal stricture, and dysphagia was first documented by Brown-Kelly[86] and Paterson.[87] It was subsequently shown that these patients have an increased risk of developing malignancies of their upper alimentary tracts.[88,89] It has been shown that iron deficiency results in atrophy of oral epithelium and a reduction of epithelial cell size.[90] It is interesting, however, that an increased risk of oral cancer has not been documented in iron deficient patients without sideropenic dysphagia.

Sideropenic dysphagia was found predominantly in Scandinavian women and is rare in the U.S.

C. Oral Submucous Fibrosis
Oral submucous fibrosis is a chronic disease of oropharyngeal mucosa characterized by inflammation and a progressive fibrosis of the lamina propria. The oral mucosa becomes stiff, and patients may experience trismus and dysphagia.

Oral submucous fibrosis results in epithelial atrophy, and when biopsied, it is not uncommon for the epithelium to be dysplastic.[25,91] Paymaster[92] first reported that one third of patients with submucous fibrosis developed low-grade carcinomas in their lesions. Pindborg and associates[25] subsequently reported that oral cancer was found in 10% of a group of submucous fibrosis patients at the time of diagnosis, and an additional 4.5% developed carcinomas with follow-up.

Oral submucous fibrosis occurs almost exclusively in India and has not been reported in the U.S.

D. Erosive Lichen Planus

The most controversial condition, regarding its malignant potential, is erosive lichen planus. The literature is replete with cases of malignant transformation in lichen planus. Marder and Deesen[93] reviewed the literature and found that almost 5000 patients with lichen planus had been followed, and malignant transformation rates ranged from 0.3 to 10%. In a more controlled study than the literature provided, Silverman and colleagues[94] followed 570 lichen patients for an average 5.6 years and reported malignant transformation in 1.2%. When adjusted for age and follow-up, this figure was only slightly higher than would be expected in the general population. Holmstrup and Pindborg[95] reported the concomitant occurrence of erythroplakia in approximately 1% of their 740 patients with lichen planus.

In 1977, Krutchkoff and associates[96] critically reviewed the literature and found 223 reported cases of malignancy supposedly arising from lichen planus. However, when strict clinicopathologic criteria were required for documentation, the authors concluded that only 15 cases of true malignant transformation were justified. The authors concluded that there was insufficient evidence to indict oral lichen planus as a premalignant lesion.

The controversy regarding the malignant potential of lichen planus is based on the histologic interpretation of the initial biopsy. Dysplastic epithelium is sufficiently antigenic that it often induces an immune response. This immune response takes the form of a band-like infiltrate of lymphocytes immediately beneath the epithelium, and this reaction in many ways mimics lichen planus histologically. If this dysplastic lesion is then misdiagnosed as lichen planus, the patient receives either no treatment or corticosteroids (immunosuppressants). Subsequent development of carcinoma in this lesion would not be unexpected. There is no doubt that many of the previously reported cases of malignant transformation in lichen planus are actually malignant transformation of dysplastic lesions which were misdiagnosed as lichen planus. Krutchkoff and Eisenberg[97] have recently published an excellent discussion of this dilemma and have suggested strict histological criteria to distinguish lichenoid dysplasia from lichen planus.

Lichen planus is a common oral mucosal condition, and some of these patients will develop oral cancer by chance alone. Additionally, some forms of lichen planus are clinically indistinguishable from leukoplakia, and leukoplakia and lichen planus have been reported in the same patient. There does seem to be a statistically significant association between lichen planus and the subsequent development of oral carcinoma, but the magnitude of this risk is unknown. If there is a true risk in these patients, it usually occurs in the erosive form of the disease which is characterized histologically by epithelial atrophy.

E. Chronic Immunosuppression

The association of lymphoreticular malignancies with chronic immunosuppression is widely known. As immunosuppressed patients survive longer, more epithelial malignancies are being reported. Although most epithelial malignancies are squamous carcinomas of the skin and lip,[98] intraoral carcinomas[99] have been reported. The magnitude of risk appears relatively small. Hoover and Fraumeni[98] reported the results of cancer risk in 6297 patients registered with the Human Renal Transplant Registry (National Institutes of Health) and found that lip cancer occurred approximately four times more often than expected. Whether these cancers are preceded by premalignant lesions is unknown, but Gissor[100] reported a leukoplakic lesion in association with a tongue malignancy in a 26-year-old male who had survived a renal transplant for 9 years.

Intraoral malignancy has also been documented in immunosuppressed patients with the acquired immune deficiency syndrome (AIDS). The most common intraoral malignancy is Kaposi's sarcoma,[101] but carcinomas[102] have been reported. Greenspan and colleagues[103] recently reported a new entity called hairy leukoplakia which was found principally on the lateral borders of the tongue in male homosexuals. Although none of the lesions had progressed to carcinoma, 6 of 35 lesions showed mild atypia when biopsied. Most of the lesions were associated with *Candida albicans,* human papillomavirus, and Epstein-Barr virus.[103,104] Silverman and colleagues[102] recently reported an incidence of oral cancer approximating 2% in a group of homosexual males.

V. MANAGEMENT OF PREMALIGNANCY

The most relevant, and often controversial, consideration of premalignancy is the problem of management. Einhorn and Wersall[20] reported that surgical excision of leukoplakias did not reduce the incidence of malignant transformation when compared to patients receiving no treatment. However, their decision to treat a patient was not decided randomly, and their findings obviously included a significant selection bias. Sako and colleagues[105] also reported that four patients (6.6%) developed carcinomas in their treated leukoplakias. Nevertheless, most authors suggest that therapeutic intervention actually provides some benefit to the patient.[2,17-19,106] The degree of this benefit, however, is almost impossible to determine because leukoplakia includes a heterogeneous group of lesions and the natural history of some of these is spontaneous resolution.

Chronic irritation has traditionally been the most common etiologic factor associated with leukoplakia. If a cause can be found for the lesion, its elimination usually results in clinical resolution. Some authorities today consider these frictional keratoses as specific entities and do not classify them as leukoplakias. Tobacco is the only other major etiologic factor associated with leukoplakia, and it has been shown that cessation of the tobacco habit will result in regression of the clinical lesion in some patients.[21,52,53,107,108] Pindborg[107] showed that 60% of leukoplakias disappeared within 1 year of abstinence from tobacco. Roed-Petersen[108] reported that leukoplakias regressed or disappeared within 3 months in 56% of patients who cut tobacco consumption by at least one half and in 63% of patients who abstained. Silverman and colleagues[21] reported less favorable results by showing that leukoplakias improved in 44% of smokers who stopped, but the lesions improved in 37% of smokers who continued smoking.

Some cases of candidal leukoplakia will respond to antimycotic drugs, and Pindborg[107] has shown the reversibility of dysplasia after antimycotic treatment for lesions containing *Candida.* Many of the candidal leukoplakias are clinically speckled leukoplakias. It has also been shown that many speckled candidal leukoplakias do not completely disappear after antimycotic therapy, but instead become homogeneous leukoplakias. Clinical experience has shown that some lesions do not respond at all to antimycotic therapy. The treatment of candidal leukoplakia in patients who smoke is often ineffective if the patient continues to smoke.[1]

For idiopathic leukoplakias, a cause is not apparent. Management decisions regarding these lesions are best based on biopsy and microscopic examination. An incisional biopsy should be taken from the most worrisome area of the lesion, i.e., areas of redness or surface irregularity (nodules or verrucous areas). For very large, homogeneous leukoplakias, more than one area might be sampled. From a pathologic standpoint, it is not necessary to include a margin of normal tissue in the biopsy.

Surgery is not indicated for those lesions which show reactive (reversible) histologic changes, i.e., hyperorthokeratosis, hyperparakeratosis, and/or acanthosis. It is, however, imperative to follow these patients because of the dynamic nature of leukoplakia. Should the lesions develop areas of redness or surface irregularity, rebiopsy is mandatory. Malignant transformation is well documented in these lesions, although the risk is considerably less than for dysplastic lesions.

The diagnosis of mild to moderate dysplasia is not a serious or life-threatening condition. Small lesions, particularly in "at risk" sites, can be excised easily. Other lesions can be followed without significant risk to the patient. Severe dysplasia and carcinoma *in situ* are serious, but not immediately life-threatening conditions. Surgical removal is recommended for these lesions. Carcinoma *in situ* can grow down and involve the underlying ducts of accessory salivary glands. While this is not true invasion in a biologic sense, it certainly represents "invasion" in a morphologic sense. If these lesions are superficially stripped and residual carcinoma *in situ* left in the underlying ducts, the chance for recurrence would be significantly increased.

It has been shown that the most successful method of managing premalignant lesions is surgical excision and removal of any associated etiologic factors.[17,25] While excision cures many patients, there are no reports documenting a 100% success rate. Banoczy and Csiba[2] reported that almost 70% of lesions were cured or improved after surgery. Pindborg and associates[19] and Silverman and associates[21] reported recurrence rates of 10 and 35%, respectively, for leukoplakias removed surgically. In reports dealing only with dysplastic lesions, recurrences of 30 to 35% are reported following surgical removal.[18,23]

In regard to the natural history of the lesion, it makes no difference whatsoever how ablation is accomplished. Historically, this has been done by surgical excision. Much of what is known about premalignancy was accomplished because of the advantage of studying the entire surgical specimen histologically rather than making assumptions on incisional biopsies. Recently, cryosurgery[109-112] and laser surgery[113] have been advocated for managing premalignant lesions. While these techniques are not more successful at lesion removal, they do have operative advantages and decreased postoperative morbidity. The major disadvantage to these techniques is that they destroy tissue in vivo, thereby making it impossible to determine what pathologic changes were present in the lesion.

REFERENCES

1. **Axell, T., Holmstrup, P., Kramer, I. R. H., Pindborg, J. J., and Shear, M.,** International seminar on oral leukoplakia and associated lesions related to tobacco habits, *Community Dent. Oral Epidemiol.,* 12, 145, 1984.
2. **Banoczy, J. and Csiba, A.,** Occurrence of epithelial dysplasia in oral leukoplakia, *Oral Surg.,* 42, 766, 1976.
3. **Mehta, F. S., Daftary, D. K., Shroff, B. C., and Sanghvi, L. D.,** Clinical and histologic study of oral leukoplakia in relation to habits, *Oral Surg.,* 28, 372, 1969.
4. **Pindborg, J. J., Daftary, D. K., and Mehta, F. S.,** A follow-up study of sixty-one oral dysplastic precancerous lesions in Indian villagers, *Oral Surg.,* 43, 383, 1977.
5. **Shafer, W. G., Hine, M. K., and Levy, B. M.,** *A Textbook of Oral Pathology,* W.B. Saunders, Philadelphia, 1983, 92.
6. WHO Collaborating Centre for Oral Precancerous Lesions, Definition of leukoplakia and related lesions: an aid to studies on oral precancer, *Oral Surg.,* 46, 518, 1978.
7. **Santis, H., Shklar, G., and Chauncey, H. H.,** Histochemistry of experimentally induced leukoplakia and carcinoma of the hamster buccal pouch, *Oral Surg.,* 17, 207, 1964.
8. **Shklar, G.,** Oral leukoplakia — studies in enzyme histochemistry, *J. Invest. Dermatol.,* 48, 153, 1967.
9. **Lonins, T. and Burkhardt, A.,** Dyskeratosis in human and experimental oral precancer and cancer. An immunohistochemical and ultrastructual study in men, mice and rats, *Arch. Oral Biol.,* 27, 361, 1982.
10. **Hyun, K. H., Nakai, M., Kawamura, K., and Mori, M.,** Histochemical studies of lectin binding patterns in keratinized lesions, including malignancy, *Virchows Arch.,* 402, 337, 1984.

11. **Scully, C.,** Serum beta 2 microglobulin in oral malignancy and premalignancy, *J. Oral Pathol.,* 10, 354, 1981.
12. **Scully, C.,** Immunological abnormalities in oral carcinoma and oral keratosis, *J. Maxillofac. Surg.,* 10, 113, 1982.
13. **Scully, C., Barkas, T., Boyle, P., and McGregor, I. A.,** Circulating immune complexes detected by binding of radiolabelled protein A in patients with oral cancer and oral premalignant lesions, *J. Clin. Lab. Immunol.,* 8, 113, 1982.
14. **Auclair, P. L.,** Altered H-antigen reactivity as an early indicator of malignant transformation in oral epithelium, *J. Oral Pathol.,* 13, 401, 1984.
15. **MacKenzie, I. C., Dabelsteen, E., and Zimmermann, K.,** The relationship between expression of epithelial B-like blood group antigen, cell movement and cell proliferation, *Acta Pathol. Microbiol. Scand.,* 85A, 49, 1977.
16. **Burkhardt, A.,** Advanced methods in the evaluation of premalignant lesions and carcinomas of the oral mucosa, *J. Oral Pathol.,* 14, 751, 1985.
17. **Banoczy, J.,** Follow-up studies in oral leukoplakia, *J. Maxillofac. Surg.,* 5, 69, 1977.
18. **Mincer, H. H., Coleman, S. A., and Hopkins, K. P.,** Observations on the clinical characteristics of oral lesions showing histologic epithelial dysplasia, *Oral Surg.,* 33, 389, 1972.
19. **Pindborg, J.J., Renstrup, G., Jolst, O., and Roed-Petersen, B.,** Studies in oral leukoplakia: a premalignancy report on the period prevalence of malignant transformation in leukoplakia based on a follow-up study of 248 patients, *J. Am. Dent. Assoc.,* 76, 767, 1968.
20. **Einhorn, J. and Wersall, J.,** Incidence of oral carcinoma in patients with leukoplakia of the oral mucosa, *Cancer,* 20, 2189, 1967.
21. **Silverman, S., Jr., Gorsky, M., and Lozada, F.,** Oral leukoplakia and malignant transformation. A follow-up study of 257 patients, *Cancer,* 53, 563, 1984.
22. **Gupta, P. C., Mehta, F. S., Daftary, D. K., Pindborg, J. J., Bhonsle, R. B., Jalnawalla, P. N., Sinor, P. N., Pitkar, V. K., Murti, P. R., Irani, R. R., Shah, H. T., Kadam, P. M., Iyer, K. S. S., Iyer, H. M., Hegde, A. K., Chandrashekar, G. K., Shroff, B. C., Sahiar, B. E., and Mehta, M. N.,** Incidence rates of oral cancer and natural history of oral precancerous lesions in a 10-year follow-up study of Indian villagers, *Community Dent. Oral Epidemiol.,* 8, 287, 1980.
23. **Amagasa, T., Yokoo, E., Sato, K., Tanaka, N., Shioda, S., and Takagi, M.,** A study of the clinical characteristics and treatment of oral carcinoma in situ, *Oral Surg.,* 60, 50, 1985.
24. **Shedd, D. P., Hukiu, P. B., Kligerman, M. M., and Gowen, G. F.,** A clinicopathologic study of oral carcinoma *in situ, Am. J. Surg.,* 106, 791, 1963.
25. **Pindborg, J. J., Murti, P. R., Bhonsle, R. B., Gupta, P. C., Daftary, D. K., and Mehta, F. S.,** Oral submucous fibrosis as a precancerous condition, *Scand. J. Dent. Res.,* 92, 224, 1984.
26. **Burkhardt, A.,** Der Mundhohlenkrebs und Seine Vorstadien, in *Veroffentlichungen aus der Pathologie,* Vol. 112, Bungeler, W. et al., Eds., Gustav Fischer Verlag, Stuttgart, 1980; cited by **Lonins, T. and Burkhardt, A.,** *Arch. Oral Biol.,* 27, 361, 1982.
27. **Grassel-Pietrusky, R., Deinlein, E., and Hornstein, O. P.,** DNA-ploidy rates in oral leukoplakias determined by flow-cytometry, *J. Oral Pathol.,* 11, 434, 1982.
28. **Brown, R. L., Suh, J. M., Scarborough, J. E., Wilkins, S. A., Jr., and Smith, R. R.,** Snuff dipper's intraoral cancer: clinical characteristics and response to therapy, *Cancer,* 18, 2, 1965.
29. **Smith, J. F., Mincer, H. A., Hopkins, K. P., and Bell, J.,** Snuff-dipper's lesion. A cytological and pathological study in a large population, *Arch. Otolaryngol.,* 92, 450, 1970.
30. **Waldron, C. A. and Shafer, W. G.,** Leukoplakia revisited, *Cancer,* 36, 1386, 1975.
31. **Andreasson, L., Bjorlin, G., Korssaard, R., Mattiasson, I., Trell, E., and Trell, L.,** Leukoplakia of the oral cavity, smoking and arylhydrocarbon-hydroxylase inducibility, *Postgrad. Med. J.,* 58, 138, 1982.
32. **Baric, J. M., Alman, J. E., Feldman, R. S., and Chauncey, H. H.,** Influence of cigarette, pipe and cigar smoking, removable partial dentures, and age on oral leukoplakia, *Oral Surg.,* 54, 424, 1982.
33. **Rodriguez, I., Santana, J. C., Sanabria, J., and Banoczy, J.,** Prevalence of oral leukoplakia in Havana City, Cuba, *Community Dent. Oral Epidemiol.,* 11, 379, 1983.
34. **Gupta, P. C.,** Epidemiologic study of the association between alcohol habits and oral leukoplakia, *Community Dent. Oral Epidemiol.,* 12, 47, 1984.
35. **Cawson, R. A. and Lehner, T.,** Chronic hyperplastic candidiasis — candidal leukoplakia, *Br. J. Dermatol.,* 80, 9, 1968.
36. **Roed-Petersen, B., Renstrup, G., and Pindborg, J. J.,** Candida in oral leukoplakias. A histologic and exfoliative cytologic study, *Scand. J. Dent. Res.,* 78, 323, 1970.
37. **Arendorf, T. M., Walker, D. M., Kingdom, R. J., Roll, J. R., and Newcombe, R. G.,** Tobacco smoking and denture wearing in oral candidal leukoplakia, *Br. Dent. J.,* 155, 340, 1983.
38. **Banoczy, J.,** Oral leukoplakia and other white lesions of the oral mucosa related to dermatological disorders, *J. Cutaneous Pathol.,* 10, 238, 1983.

39. **Jepsen, A. and Winther, J. E.,** Mycotic infection in oral leukoplakia, *Acta Odontol. Scand.,* 23, 239, 1965.
40. **Banoczy, J. and Sugar, L.,** Longitudinal studies in oral leukoplakias, *J. Oral Pathol.,* 1, 265, 1972.
41. **Renstrup, G.,** Occurrence of Candida in oral leukoplakias, *Acta Pathol. Microbiol. Scand.,* 78(B), 421, 1970.
42. **Jenkins, W. M. M., Macfarlane, T. W., Ferguson, M. M., and Mason, D. K.,** Nutritional deficiency in oral candidosis, *Int. J. Oral Surg.,* 6, 204, 1977.
43. **Cawson, R. A. and Binnie, W. H.,** Candida leukoplakia and carcinoma: a possible relationship, in *Oral Premalignancy,* MacKenzie, I. C., Dabelsteen, E., and Squires, C. A., Eds., University of Iowa Press, Iowa City, 1980, 59.
44. **Pindborg, J. J.,** Epidemiology and public health aspects of diseases of the oral mucosa, *J. Dent. Res.,* 56(C), 14, 1977.
45. **Gangadharan, P. and Paymaster, J. C.,** Leukoplakia — an epidemiologic study of 1504 cases observed at the Tata Memorial Hospital, Bombay, India, *Br. J. Cancer,* 25, 657, 1971.
46. **Mehta, F. S., Pindborg, J. J., Gupta, P. C., and Daftary, D. K.,** Epidemiologic and histologic study of oral cancer and leukoplakia among 50,915 villagers in India, *Cancer,* 24, 832, 1969.
47. **Kramer, I. R. H., El-Labban, N., and Lee, K. W.,** The clinical features and risk of malignant transformation in sublingual keratosis, *Br. Dent. J.,* 144, 171, 1978.
48. **Banoczy, J. and Csiba, A.,** Comparative study of the clinical picture and histopathologic structure of oral leukoplakia, *Cancer,* 29, 1230, 1972.
49. **Eversole, L. R. and Shopper, T. P.,** Oral leukoplakia: prevalence of dysplastic and carcinomatous change in verruciform and planar patterns, *Can. Dent. Assoc. J.,* 9, 45, 1981.
50. **Cawson, R. A.,** Premalignant lesions in the mouth, *Br. Med. Bull.,* 31, 164, 1975.
51. **Pindborg, J. J., Renstrup, G., Poulsen, H. E., and Silverman, S.,** Studies in oral leukoplakias. V. Clinical and histologic signs of malignancy, *Acta Odontol. Scand.,* 21, 407, 1963.
52. **Banoczy, J. and Sugar, L.,** Progressive and regressive changes in Hungarian oral leukoplakias in the course of longitudinal studies, *Community Dent. Oral Epidemiol.,* 3, 194, 1975.
53. **Mehta, F. S., Gupta, M. B., Pindborg, J. J., Bhonsle, R. B., Jalnawalla, P. N., and Sinor, P. N.,** An intervention study of oral cancer and precancer in rural Indian populations: a preliminary report, *Bull. WHO,* 60, 441, 1982.
54. **Shklar, G.,** Modern studies and concepts of leukoplakia in the mouth, *J. Dermatol. Surg. Oncol.,* 7, 996, 1981.
55. **Fischman, S. L., Ulmansky, M., Sela, J., Babi, I., and Gazit, D.,** Correlative clinico-pathological evaluation of oral premalignancy, *J. Oral Pathol.,* 11, 283, 1982.
56. **Banoczy, J.,** *Oral Leukoplakia,* Martinus Nijhoff, London, 1982, 75.
57. **Pogrel, M. A.,** Sublingual keratosis and malignant transformation, *J. Oral Pathol.,* 8, 176, 1979.
58. **Rankin, K. V., Wood, J. C., and Wright, J. M.,** Leukoplakia in Texas, *Tex. Dent. J.,* 102, 4, 1985.
59. **Banoczy, J. and Rigo, O.,** Comparative cytologic and histologic studies in oral leukoplakia, *Acta Cytol.,* 20, 308, 1976.
60. **Laskaris, G. C. and Nicolis, G. D.,** Erythroplakia of Queyrat of the oral mucosa, a report of 2 cases, *Dermatologica,* 162, 395, 1981.
61. **Hansen, L. S., Olson, J. A., and Silverman, S.,** Proliferative verrucous leukoplakia. A long term study of thirty patients, *Oral Surg.,* 60, 285, 1985.
62. **Shear, M. and Pindborg, J. J.,** Verrucous hyperplasia of the oral mucosa, *Cancer,* 46, 1855, 1980.
63. **Silverman, S. and Rozen, R. D.,** Observations on the clinical characteristics and natural history of oral leukoplakia, *J. Am. Dent. Assoc.,* 76, 772, 1968.
64. **Roed-Petersen, B.,** Cancer development in oral leukoplakia: follow-up of 331 patients, *J. Dent. Res.,* 50, 771, 1971.
65. **Kramer, I. R. H.,** Precancerous conditions of oral mucosa: a computer aided study, *Ann. R. Coll. Surg. Engl.,* 45, 340, 1969.
66. **Roch-Berry, C. S.,** Malignant changes in glossal leukoplakia, *Clin. Radiol.,* 32, 693, 1981.
67. **Malaowalla, A. M., Silverman, S., Mani, N. I., Bilimoria, K. F., and Smith, L. W.,** Oral cancer in 57,518 industrial workers of Gujarat, India, *Cancer,* 37, 1882, 1976.
68. **Pindborg, J. J., Reibel, J., Roed-Petersen, B., and Mehta, F. S.,** Tobacco induced changes in oral leukoplakic epithelium, *Cancer,* 45, 2330, 1980.
69. **Shafer, W. G. and Waldron, C. A.,** Erythroplakia of the oral cavity, *Cancer,* 36, 1021, 1975.
70. **Pindborg, J. J.,** Oral precancer, in *Surgical Pathology of the Head and Neck,* Barnes, L., Ed., Marcel Dekker, New York, 1985, 315.
71. **Lay, K. M., Sein, K., Myint, A., Ko, S. K., and Pindborg, J. J.,** Epidemiologic study of 6000 villagers of oral precancerous lesions in Bilugyun: preliminary report, *Community Dent. Oral Epidemiol.,* 10, 152, 1982.

72. **Mashberg, A., Morrissey, J. B., and Garfinkel, L.,** A study of the appearance of early asymptomatic oral squamous cell carcinoma, *Cancer,* 32, 1436, 1973.
73. **Mashberg, A. and Meyers, H.,** Anatomical site and size of 222 early asymptomatic oral squamous cell carcinomas, *Cancer,* 37, 2149, 1976.
74. **Shear, M.,** Erythroplakia of the mouth, *Int. Dent. J.,* 22, 460, 1972.
75. **Mehta, F. S., Pindborg, J. J., and Hamner, J. E.,** *Oral Cancer and Precancerous Conditions in India,* Munksgaard, Copenhagen, 1971.
76. **Frederick, K. L. and George, D. I., Jr.,** Erythroplakia and the detection of oral malignancy, *Quintessence Int.,* 12, 1023, 1981.
77. **Mashberg, A.,** Erythroplakia: the earliest sign of asymptomatic oral cancer, *J. Am. Dent. Assoc.,* 96, 615, 1978.
78. **Mashberg, A.,** Reevaluation of toluidine blue application as a diagnostic adjunct in the detection of asymptomatic oral squamous carcinoma: a continuing prospective study of oral cancer. III., *Cancer,* 46, 758, 1980.
79. **Silverman, S., Migliorati, C., and Barbosa, J.,** Toluidine blue staining in the detection of oral precancerous and malignant lesions, *Oral Surg.,* 57, 379, 1984.
80. **Mashberg, A.,** Final evaluation of tolonium chloride rinse for screening of high-risk patients with asymptomatic squamous carcinoma, *J. Am. Dent. Assoc.,* 106, 319, 1983.
81. **Craig, R. M.,** Speckled leukoplakia of the floor of the mouth, *J. Am. Dent. Assoc.,* 102, 690, 1981.
82. **King, O. H. and Coleman, S. A.,** Analysis of oral exfoliative cytologic accuracy by control biopsy technique, *Acta Cytol.,* 9, 351, 1965.
83. **Dabelsteen, E., Roed-Petersen, B., Smith, C. J., and Pindborg, J. J.,** The limitations of exfoliative cytology for the detection of epithelial atypia in oral leukoplakias, *Br. J. Cancer,* 25, 21, 1971.
84. **Hobaek, A.,** Leukoplakia oris, *Acta Ondontol. Scand.,* 2, 61, 1946.
85. **Trieger, N., Ship, I. I., Thomas, G. W., and Weisberger, D.,** Cirrhosis and other predisposing factors in carcinoma of the tongue, *Cancer,* 11, 357, 1958.
86. **Brown-Kelly, A.,** Spasm at the entrance to the esophagus, *J. Laryngol.,* 34, 285, 1919.
87. **Paterson, D. R.,** A clinical type of dysphagia, *J. Laryngol.,* 34, 289, 1919.
88. **Jacobsson, F.,** Carcinoma of the tongue. A clinical study of 277 cases treated at Radiumhemmet, 1931—1942, *Acta Radiol.,* 68(Suppl.), 1, 1948.
89. **Wynder, E. L. and Fryer, J. H.,** Etiologic considerations of Plummer-Vinson (Paterson-Kelly) syndrome, *Ann. Intern. Med.,* 49, 1106, 1958.
90. **Rennie, J. S., MacDonald, D. G., and Dagg, J. H.,** Iron and the oral epithelium: a review, *J. R. Soc. Med.,* 77, 602, 1984.
91. **Pindborg, J. J.,** Is submucous fibrosis a precancerous condition in the oral cavity?, *Int. Dent. J.,* 22, 474, 1972.
92. **Paymaster, J. C.,** Cancer of buccal mucosa. Clinical study of 650 cases in Indian patients, *Cancer,* 9, 431, 1956.
93. **Marder, M. Z. and Deesen, K. C.,** Transformation of oral lichen planus to squamous cell carcinoma: a literature review and report of case, *J. Am. Dent. Assoc.,* 105, 55, 1982.
94. **Silverman, S., Gorsky, M., and Lozada-Nur, F.,** A prospective follow-up study of 570 patients with oral lichen planus: persistence, remission and malignant association, *Oral Surg.,* 60, 30, 1985.
95. **Holmstrup, P. and Pindborg, J. J.,** Erythroplakic lesions in relation to oral lichen planus, *Acta Dermatol. Venereol.,* 59(Suppl. 85), 77, 1979.
96. **Krutchkoff, D. S., Cutler, L., and Laskowski, S.,** Oral lichen planus: the evidence regarding potential malignant transformation, *J. Oral Pathol.,* 7, 1, 1978.
97. **Krutchkoff, D. J. and Eisenberg, E.,** Lichenoid dysplasia: a distinct histopathologic entity, *Oral Surg.,* 60, 308, 1985.
98. **Hoover, R. and Fraumeni, J. F.,** Risk of cancer in renal-transplant recipients, *Lancet,* 2, 55, 1973.
99. **Lee, Y. W. and Gisser, S. D.,** Squamous cell carcinoma of the tongue in a nine year renal transplant survivor. A case report with the discussion of the risk of development of epithelial carcinomas in renal transplant survivors, *Cancer,* 41, 1, 1978.
100. **Gisser, S. D.,** Papovavirus and squamous cell carcinoma, *Human Pathol.,* 12, 190, 1981.
101. **Lozada, F., Silverman, S., Migliorati, C. A., Conant, M. A., and Volberding, P. A.,** Oral manifestations of tumor and opportunistic infections in the acquired immunodeficiency syndrome (AIDS): findings in 53 homosexual men with Kaposi's sarcoma, *Oral Surg.,* 56, 491, 1983.
102. **Silverman, S., Jr., Migliorati, C. A., Lozada-Nur, F., Greenspan, D., and Conant, M. A.,** Oral findings in people with or at high risk for AIDS: a study of 375 homosexual males, *J. Am. Dent. Assoc.,* 112, 187, 1986.
103. **Greenspan, D., Greenspan, J. S., Conant, M., Petersen, V., Silverman, S., and DeSouza, Y.,** Oral "hairy" leucoplakia in male homosexuals: evidence of association with both papillomavirus and a herpes-group virus, *Lancet,* 2, 831, 1984.

104. **Greenspan, J. S., Greenspan, D., Lennette, E. T., Abrams, D. I., Conant, M. A., Petersen, V., and Freese, V. K.,** Replication of Epstein-Barr virus within the epithelial cells of oral "hairy" leukoplakia, an AIDS-associated lesion, *N. Engl. J. Med.,* 313, 1564, 1985.
105. **Sako, K., Marchetta, F. C., and Hayes, R. L.,** Cryotherapy of intraoral leukoplakia, *Am. J. Surg.,* 124, 482, 1972.
106. **Al-Drouby, H. A.,** Oral leukoplakia and cryotherapy, *Br. Dent. J.,* 155, 124, 1983.
107. **Pindborg, J. J.,** Pathology of oral leukoplakia, *Am. J. Dermatopathol.,* 2, 277, 1980.
108. **Roed-Petersen, B.,** Effect on oral leukoplakia of reducing or ceasing tobacco smoking, *Acta Dermatol. Venereol.,* 62, 164, 1982.
109. **Malmstrom, M. and Leikomaa, H.,** Experiences with cryotherapy in the treatment of oral lesions, *Proc. Finn. Dent. Soc.,* 76, 117, 1980.
110. **Tal, H., Cohen, M. A., and Lemmer, J.,** Clinical and histological changes following cryotherapy in a case of widespread oral leukoplakia, *Int. J. Oral Surg.,* 11, 64, 1982.
111. **Gongloff, R. K. and Gase, A. A.,** Cryosurgical treatment of oral lesions: report of cases, *J. Am. Dent. Assoc.,* 106, 47, 1983.
112. **Leopard, P. J. and Poswillo, D. E.,** Practical cryosurgery for oral lesions, *Br. Dent. J.,* 136, 185, 1974.
113. **Frame, J. W., Das Gupta, A. R., Dalton, G. A., and Rhys Evans, P. H.,** Use of the carbon dioxide laser in the management of premalignant lesions of the oral mucosa, *J. Laryngol. Otol.,* 98, 1251, 1984.

Chapter 4

CLINICAL AND HISTOLOGICAL ASPECTS

Bruce A. Wright and John M. Wright

TABLE OF CONTENTS

I. INTRODUCTION

As stated in the preface, the emphasis in this book is on squamous cell carcinoma of oral mucous membranes. Other malignancies may appear in the oral cavity, e.g., adenocarcinoma of minor salivary glands, carcinomas of the maxillary antrum extending through the palate, primary intraalveolar carcinomas, metastatic carcinomas to the oral cavity, and sarcomas, including lymphomas. These are all uncommon and outside the scope of this book. Greater than 90% of all malignancies in the mouth are squamous cell carcinomas.[1]

It is sad to reflect that although the oral cavity is readily accessible to inspection and biopsy and that early, small lesions are "curable",[2] the number of people dying with oral cancer today is similar to the number dying 30 years ago.[3,4] There are numerous factors to explain this apparent failure to improve oral cancer survival. Many patients fail to report nonhealing oral lesions. Also, medical and dental practitioners may not be aware of the true nature of premalignant and malignant oral lesions.

II. DIAGNOSIS

The first emphasis for early diagnosis must be on clinical suspicion. The clinical appearance of squamous cell carcinoma can be quite varied. Once a suspicious lesion is identified perhaps the next most important step is biopsy. We believe that there is little value for exfoliative cytology in the initial diagnosis of oral cancer. This is obviously not true for other, less accessible, anatomic sites, such as cervix or bronchus. In most instances oral malignancies can be adequately biopsied under local anesthetic with little or no resultant morbidity. It is only by accurate tissue diagnosis and subsequent clinical staging of the disease that a rational approach to treatment can be adopted. Mashberg[5] has reviewed the use of tolonium chloride (toluidine blue) oral rinse as a screening method for suspicious oral lesions. He advocates the use of a solution containing acetic acid and alcohol rather than an aqueous solution. Combining the results of both toluidine blue staining with clinical suspicion he was able to reduce his false-negative (under diagnosing) rate to 1.9%. It would seem, therefore, that this is a very useful adjunct to the clinical evaluation of oral mucosal lesions and helpful in the selection of biopsy sites. A positive result with toluidine blue rinse makes biopsy mandatory.[5]

III. BIOPSY

The first question to be asked is whether a lesion should be biopsied by the referring doctor or dentist. If the lesion appears obviously malignant then it would seem that immediate referral to the clinician who will treat the carcinoma would be the most appropriate course. This will avoid unnecessary delay while awaiting biopsy results and will also allow the clinician who will provide the definitive treatment to examine the primary lesion in an untouched state. There will be times, however, when a lesion which did not appear clinically malignant will turn out to be carcinoma histologically. In this instance immediate referral of the patient along with the pathology report and a description of the type and extent of biopsy is the most prudent course. It might also be wise to leave in any sutures so that the clinician who will carry out the definitive treatment can evaluate the biopsy site in its proper context.

The technique of biopsy is important. It is essential to obtain an adequate amount of representative tissue in order to give the pathologist the best opportunity to make a diagnosis. Oral squamous cell carcinoma originates as a surface lesion and as such is amenable to an incisional or even a punch biopsy. This latter type of biopsy is preferred because it causes less disruption of the tumor bed and has the major advantage of leaving the bulk of the

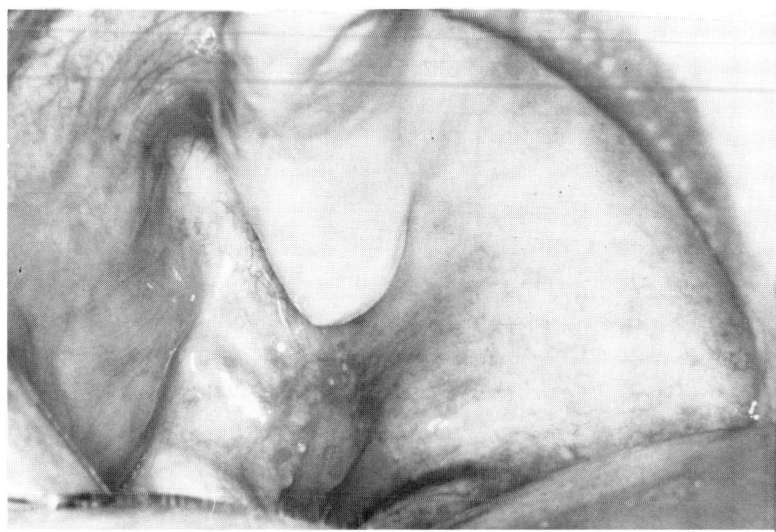

FIGURE 1.   An early asymptomatic squamous cell carcinoma of the soft palate/tonsillar pillar complex.

tumor intact so that members of the cancer team can visualize the anatomic extent of the lesion. The opportunity to examine the relatively intact anatomic extent of the tumor is of the utmost importance in clinical staging and planning adequate treatment.

Excisional biopsy should be performed only by a clinician who is prepared and has the ability to remove the entire lesion. A wide margin of normal tissue (up to 1 cm) should be taken. Also, the specimen must be submitted so that the adequacy of the resection margins may be properly assessed by the pathologist. In addition, the biopsy should be oriented anatomically by means of sutures. An excisional biopsy has several disadvantages if the tumor is not completely removed:

1.   The treatment team has no opportunity to visualize the primary tumor.
2.   The reaction from the biopsy makes accurate staging of the original lesion difficult.
3.   The tumor bed has been disturbed.
4.   The margins of any subsequent resection are more difficult to plan (and frequently excessive resection or radiation is required owing to the inability to define accurately the residual tumor boundaries).

As stated previously, if the lesion clinically appears malignant, then biopsy may be incorporated into the initial assessment visit. If one biopsy proves negative but the lesion remains clinically suspicious, then further biopsies must be obtained.

IV. CLINICAL APPEARANCE

The clinical appearance of oral squamous cell carcinoma can vary from an asymptomatic white patch (leukoplakia) or red patch (erythroplakia) to a large fungating, ulcerated, indurated lesion. Mashberg and Meyers[6] have emphasized that early asymptomatic carcinomas of the oral cavity occur predominantly in the floor of mouth, ventral and lateral tongue, and soft palate complex. These lesions were primarily erythroplakic lesions, and over 80% were 2 cm or less in size. Figure 1 illustrates one such lesion which appears relatively innocuous. Waldron and Shafer[7] pointed out that 15 out of 110 leukoplakias in the floor of the mouth were invasive squamous cell carcinoma at the time of the biopsy. From the foregoing it can

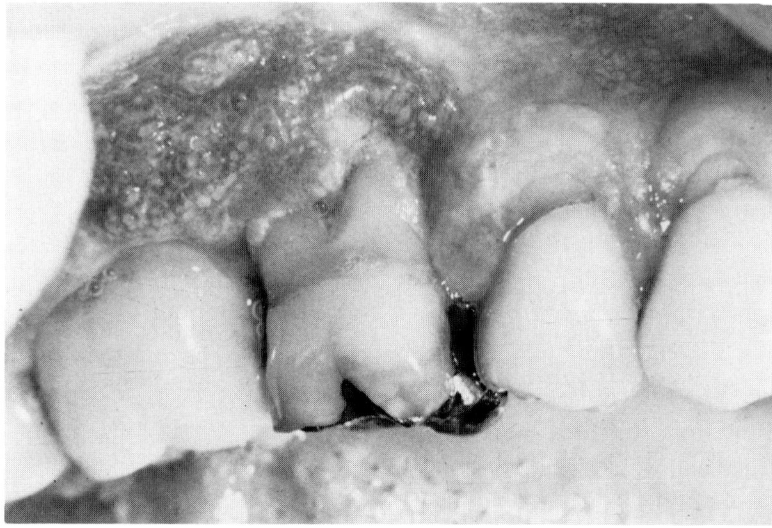

FIGURE 2.   Gingival carcinoma appearing clinically relatively innocuous.

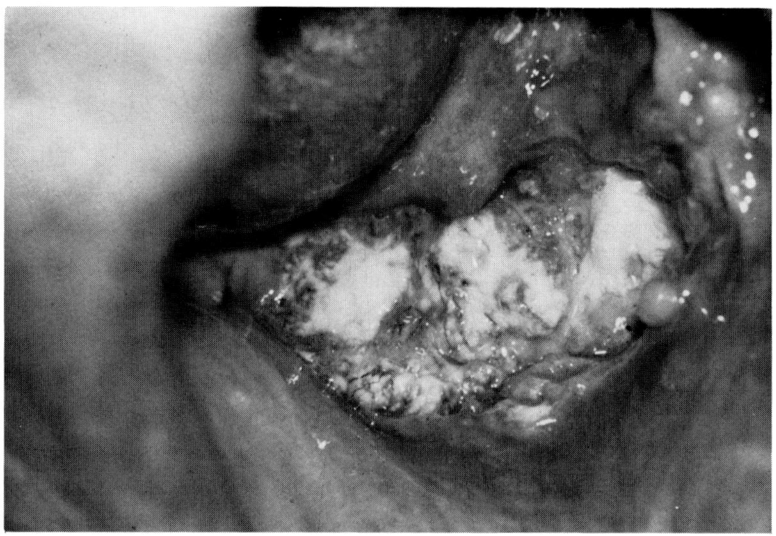

FIGURE 3.   A large, fungating squamous cell carcinoma of (and destroying) the anterior mandibular ridge.

be deduced that the clinical appearance of oral carcinomas can hide their serious nature. This is especially true for carcinomas of the gingiva which often mimic periodontal disease (Figure 2). Clinicians, therefore, must always be suspicious of any unexplained red, white, or ulcerated lesion. More advanced lesions will present as indurated, exophytic, or invasive growths which are obviously clinically malignant (Figure 3).

The practical clinical approach to any suspicious oral mucosal lesion, e.g., white patch, red patch, etc., would be a thorough search for local etiologic factors, such as tooth or denture irritation. If none is found the lesion may be biopsied as soon as is practical or the patient referred to a clinician experienced in dealing with oral cancer. If local factors are found these should be dealt with in an appropriate manner (e.g., the temporary removal of a prosthesis). If there has been no regression after an appropriate length of time, then a biopsy of the lesion is mandatory. Inflammatory lesions should resolve in 1 to 2 weeks once the inciting cause has been removed. Leukoplakia from tobacco usage may take much longer to resolve.

The clinical differential diagnosis of white and red lesions of the oral mucosa has been adequately covered in Chapter 3. When confronted with advanced lesions, clinicians will have little difficulty in arriving at a clinical diagnosis and arranging appropriate biopsy or immediate referral.

Given the markedly better prognosis for small lesions when compared with more advanced disease it behooves all clinicians to maintain a high degree of suspicion for any unusual or unexplained oral lesion. For example, Maddox[2] found that carcinomas of the tongue less than 1 cm in size had a 100% 10-year survival while those 3 to 4 cm had only a 46% survival.

V. HISTOLOGIC APPEARANCE

A. Light Microscopy

At the light microscopic level squamous cell carcinomas of the oral cavity, as of other areas of the body, can range from well differentiated to poorly or undifferentiated. Differentiation is defined according to the traditional concepts put forward by Broders,[8,9] i.e., grade I was highly differentiated with 75 to 100% of cells producing keratin while grade IV was used for those cases which were very poorly differentiated or undifferentiated carcinomas, i.e., producing no keratin and barely recognizable as epithelial malignancies. These are illustrated in Figure 4A through D. It is recognized that tumors can vary from area to area in their degree of differentiation. Nowadays most pathologists use a descriptive phrase to reflect the degree of differentiation of the tumor. Proper emphasis must also be given to the areas showing the least or poorest degree of differentiation. The degree of histologic differentiation has some bearing on prognosis especially as it relates to lymph node metastases. In Broders' original papers no grade I lip cancer metastasized while 100% of grade IV lip lesions had regional nodal involvement.[8,9] Shear et al.[10] found that poorly differentiated carcinomas were more likely to metastasize to regional lymph nodes than well-differentiated tumors. However, the correlation was not absolute. It has also been recognized that there are other features of squamous cell carcinomas which are important. Based on some initial work by Jackobsson et al.[11] other authors[12] have utilized a complex point scoring system which includes points being ascribed for the degree of differentiation of the tumor (tendency to keratinize); nuclear pleomorphism; the number of mitoses; mode of invasion; stage of invasion; and inflammatory response ("tumor cell population" — first three and "tumor-host relationship" — last three). One study has shown a correlation between point score and prognosis.[12] What has not been demonstrated convincingly is whether these factors merely correlated with the size and degree of differentiation of the primary lesion and/or reflect regional nodal metastases or whether they were genuine independent variables. Obviously this is an area where further research is needed.

The reporting pathologist should also note the presence or absence of vascular invasion. The presence of vascular invasion has been shown adversely to affect the prognosis in oral cancer.[13] However, Anneroth and Hansen[12] have discussed the problem of deciding what constitutes vascular invasion histologically. Perineural invasion has also been associated with a poor prognosis (Figure 5).[2,14,15] One caution should be mentioned in this regard. There have been numerous reports of benign nests of epithelium occurring in perioral soft tissues and jaws in a perineural location which should not be mistaken for perineural invasion by a carcinoma.[16-18]

Recently there have been reports evaluating both tumor size and depth of invasion (tumor

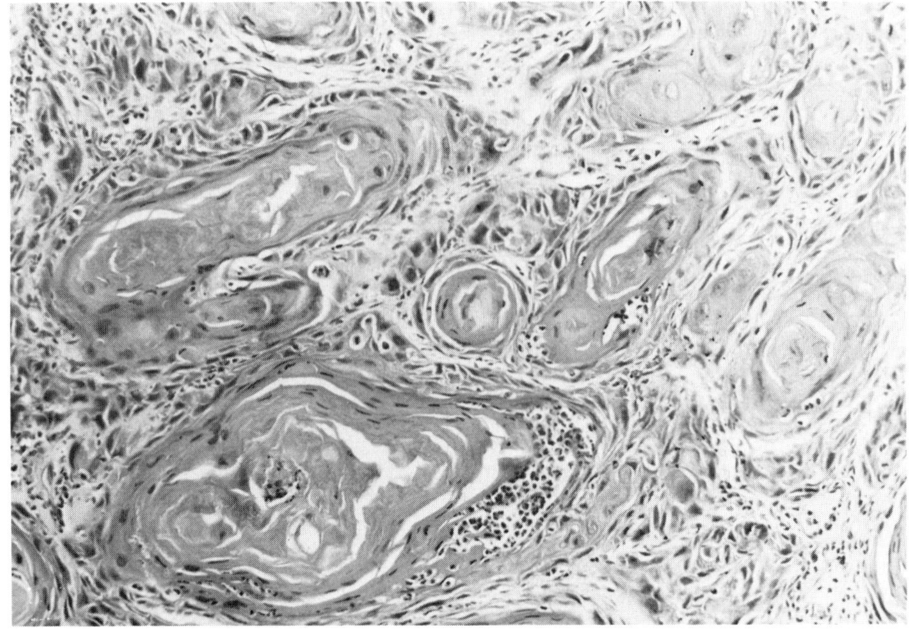

A

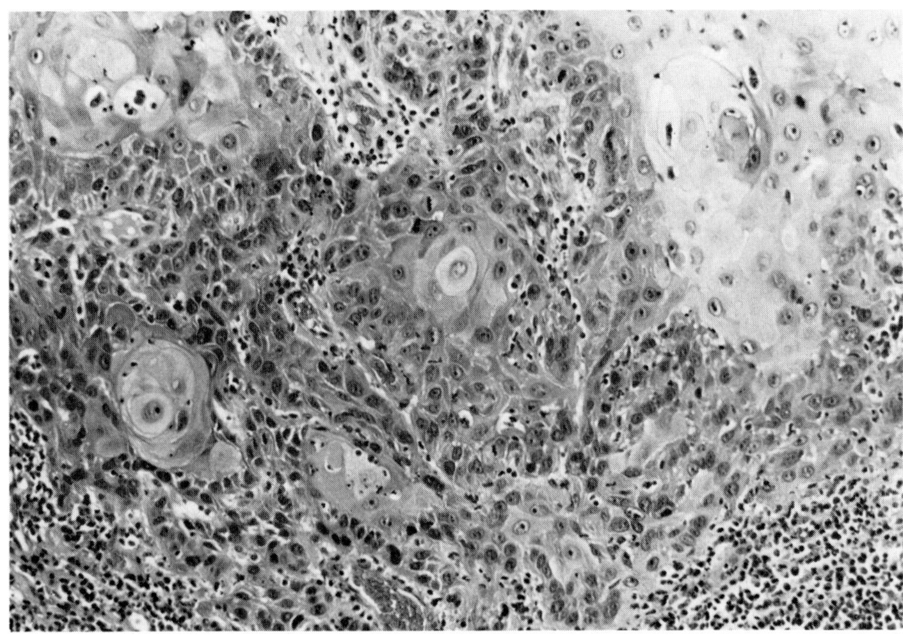

B

FIGURE 4.   (A) Photomicrograph of invasive squamous cell carcinoma greater than 75% keratinized. (H & E. Magnification × 25.) (B) Grade II invasive squamous cell carcinoma, between 50 and 75% keratinized. (H & E. Magnification × 25.) (C) Grade III invasive squamous cell carcinoma, less than 25% keratinized. (H & E. Magnification × 25.) (D) Poorly differentiated grade IV carcinoma with no evidence of keratinization. (H & E. Magnification × 25.) (It is important to note that the degree of keratinization, i.e., grade, does not necessarily correlate with cytologic atypia.)

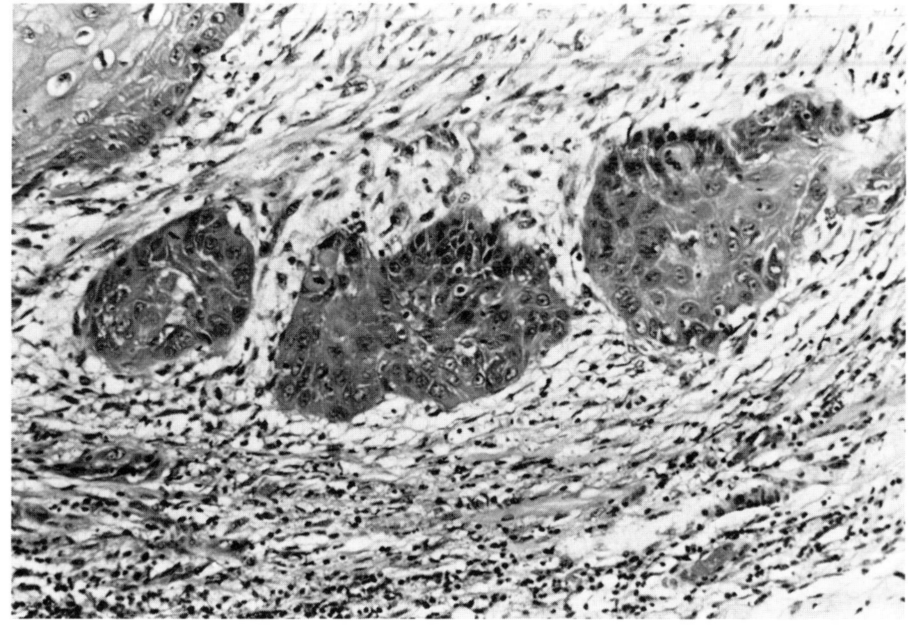

C

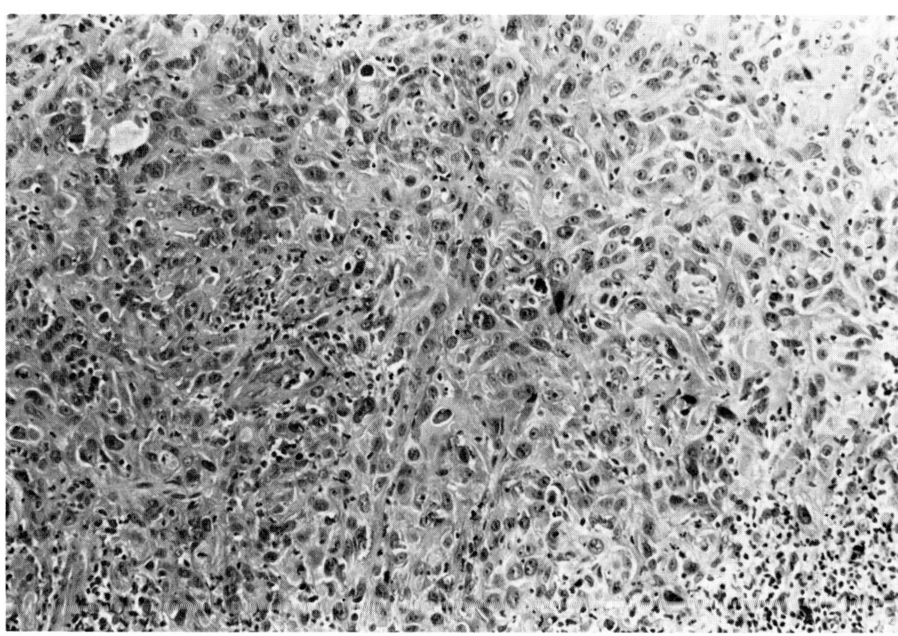

D

thickness) to prognosis.[15,19-21] Preliminary data show a very good correlation with clinical outcome. Tumors whose thickness was less than 2 mm had either a less than 2% incidence of metastases or had a 98% 2-year determinate cure rate.[20] Tumors with greater thickness had correspondingly poorer outcomes. This technique of evaluating tumor thickness or depth of invasion has been used in pathologic reporting of melanomas for many years and correlates

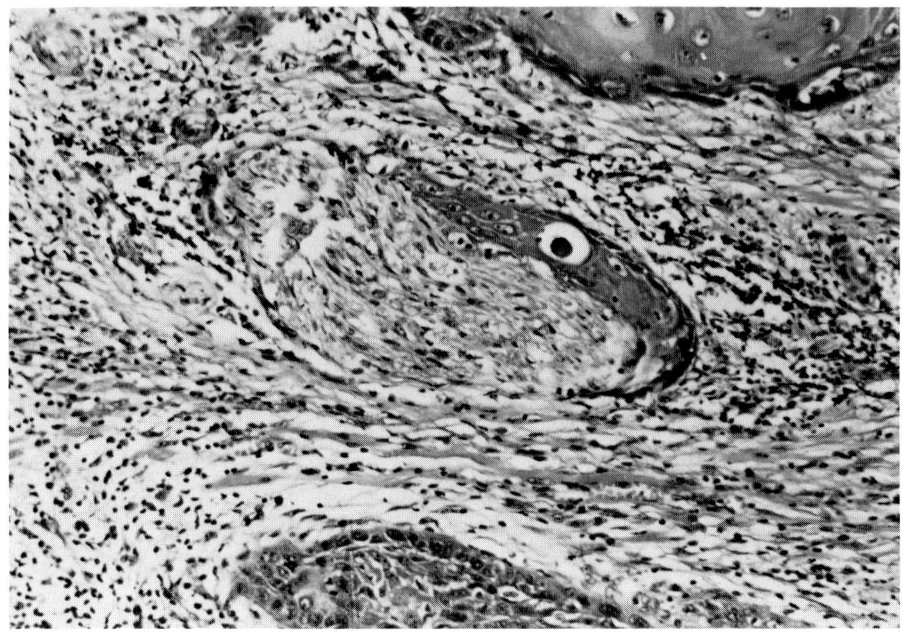

FIGURE 5.   Prominent perineural invasion in a squamous cell carcinoma of the tongue. This feature connotes a poor prognosis. (H & E. Magnification × 40. Courtesy of Dr. N. Ali Ridha.)

with clinical outcome.[22,23] What is not clear as yet is whether depth of invasion is an independent variable or related to degree of tumor differentiation, i.e., grading.

B. Special Stains

There are no specific special stains for oral squamous cell carcinoma. However, there has been a great deal of interest in recent years in intermediate filaments.[24-33] Intermediate filaments, so called because they are 10 nm in diameter and intermediate between microfilaments (6 nm) and microtubules (25 nm), are found in the cytoplasm of most cells. These intermediate filaments include (1) keratins which are found in almost all true epithelia, (2) vimentin primarily in mesenchymal cells, (3) desmin of muscle cells, (4) glial fibrillary acid protein of glial cells, and (5) neurofilaments in neurones.[24]

Further studies on human keratin intermediate filaments showed them to be a diverse subset of up to 19 different types.[28] Keratins have been subclassified into acid (AE1) and basic (AE3).[24] Once the initial isolation techniques of human keratins were described they were used with immunoperoxidase staining methods in attempts to categorize various epithelia.[29,30] Monoclonal antibodies to AE1 and AE3 keratins are now commercially available.

Antikeratin antibodies have been used in diagnostic and experimental studies on human oral epithelium in a number of ways.[30-32] One initial hope was that antikeratin antibodies would be useful in distinguishing so-called undifferentiated tumors as either epithelial or mesenchymal. One major problem encountered is that undifferentiated neoplasms often do not stain with antibodies to intermediate filaments, perhaps reflecting the "primitive" nature of the cells.

Another area of interest is the staining of premalignant epithelial lesions in an attempt to characterize these entities with regard to their malignant potential. Further work will be needed in this area before it can be used for diagnostic and prognostic purposes.[31,32]

Said et al.[33] noted that keratins are not specific for squamous epithelium since they occur in glandular as well as other epithelia. They also described involucrin, a precursor of the cross-linked envelope protein in human stratum corneum, as a marker for squamous differentiation. Whether involucrin staining will have any role in the diagnosis and study of oral cancers remains to be seen.

C. Electron Microscopic Studies

The electron microscopic appearance of oral cancer has been infrequently studied. Chen and Harwick[34] studied 16 cases of moderately differentiated oral cancer. They observed that there were many areas where the basement membrane was absent. These corresponded to psuedopodal or microvillous cytoplasmic projections of neoplastic epithelial cells. There were also foci of reduplication of basement membrane which they postulated represented the "trailing edge" of the carcinoma. Desmosomes were present but in small numbers. Their studies also revealed concentrically arranged filaments and granules as well as clustered ribosomes and many lysosomal bodies. The nuclei which were irregularly ovoid, often with a corrugated borders, were large relative to the cytoplasm. Some cells contained numerous crowded swirled bundles of tonofilaments in focal areas of the cytoplasm. None of these features is specific for squamous cell carcinoma, but may reflect the activity of the cells. Burkhardt[35] has observed that ultrastructural studies can contribute little to routine diagnostic procedures, but may give insight into the biological disturbances of malignant epithelia.

VI. HISTOLOGIC VARIANTS

A. Verrucous Carcinoma

Verrucous carcinoma, a variant of squamous cell carcinoma with an apparently distinctive biological behavior, was first recognized as a separate clinicopathological entity by Ackerman[36] in 1948. It is a slow growing, indolent neoplasm which has a deceptively benign histologic appearance with broad pushing rete ridges and little, if any, cytologic atypia. Since the original report there have been over 400 cases reported in the literature.[36-39] The most common site of occurrence of verrucous carcinoma, over 80% of all cases, is the oral cavity.[37] The larynx is probably the second most frequent location.[40] Other sites include different locations in the upper aerodigestive tract as well as penis, vagina,[37] and skin.[43] Verrucous carcinoma comprises approximately 5% (range 1 to 10%) of all cases of oral squamous cell carcinoma.[40-42,44]

Recently there have been two interesting reports attempting to elucidate further the relationship between hyperplastic verrucous oral lesions, verrucous carcinoma, and squamous cell carcinoma. The first of these, by Shear and Pindborg,[45] introduced the concept of verrucous hyperplasia in an apparent attempt to delineate those cases which did not fulfill the criteria for verrucous carcinoma. They distinguished verrucous hyperplasia from verrucous carcinoma by the proliferation of the former mainly above the surrounding normal epithelium while the latter showed an endophytic growth pattern. They reported that verrucous hyperplasia could be seen in association with verrucous carcinoma or squamous cell carcinoma. Subsequently Slootweg and Muller[46] have suggested, based on a study of age and site of occurrence, that verrucous hyperplasia is a morphologic variant of verrucous carcinoma. In 1985 Hansen et al.[47] introduced the term proliferative verrucous leukoplakia which they used to describe a particular form of epithelial change representing a spectrum and possibly a continuum from clinical leukoplakia through verrucous hyperplasia and verrucous carcinoma to papillary squamous cell carcinoma. They still used the term verrucous carcinoma in a conventional sense for patients with solitary lesions, especially when associated with tobacco use. Proliferative verrucous leukoplakia as described by them started as a simple hyperkeratosis and tended to spread, becoming multifocal with a strong tendency to develop areas of carcinoma.[47]

Clinically verrucous carcinoma usually appears as a large, exophytic, papillary or ver-

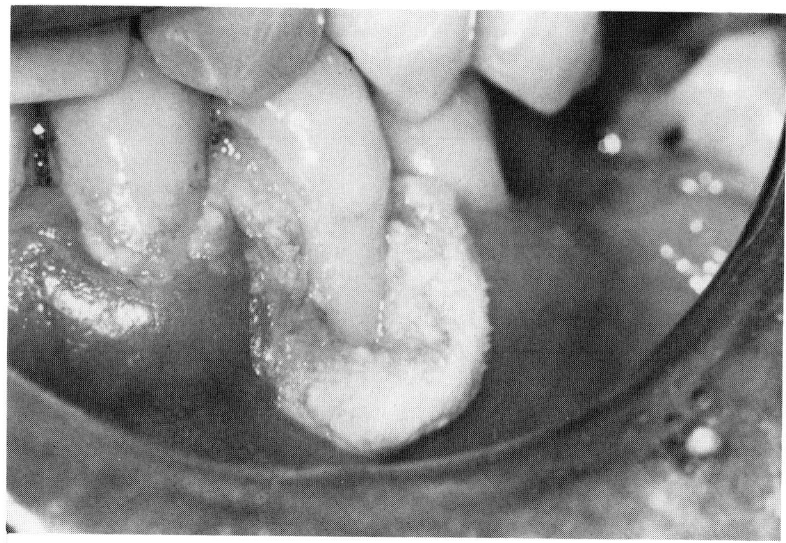

FIGURE 6.   Verrucous carcinoma of the mandibular gingiva. (Courtesy of Dr. B. Harsanyi.)

rucous lesion with a white mamillated surface (Figure 6). The usual age of occurrence is in the 6th to 8th decades of life with a male preponderance. However, series from the U.S.[48] and Norway[49] had a larger number of females than males. Many of the original series of cases showed a strong correlation with tobacco usage, although again the reports by McCoy and Waldron[48] and Tornes et al.[49] did not show such a strong correlation. The most common location, intraorally, is the buccal mucosa with over one half of all cases occurring there.[36,37,40,41,50] This is followed by the gingiva with the tongue, floor of mouth, palate, and lip being much rarer sites of occurrence.[36,37,40,41,51] Verrucous carcinoma shows virtually no tendency to metastasize to regional lymph nodes. In a review of 180 cases of oral verrucous carcinoma, Batsakis et al.[40] found only four cases of lymph node metastasis, and all of these were so-called anaplastic transformation in previously radiated verrucous carcinomas.

Microscopically the diagnosis of verrucous carcinoma is not an easy one. There is generally hyperkeratosis and papillomatosis with downward extension of broad rete ridges into the underlying connective tissue. The crypts between the papillary proliferations of epithelium are characteristically filled with parakeratin. The broad pushing margin of the downward epithelial proliferation can only be appreciated on a deep biopsy (Figure 7A).[36,38,44] This epithelium is well differentiated and lacks nuclear pleomorphism, cytologic atypia, or frequent mitoses which are all features of squamous cell carcinoma (Figure 7B). Evidence of anaplasia or of breaching of the epithelial basement membrane with invasion into the underlying connective tissue would be evidence of a coexisting squamous cell carcinoma or even, theoretically, transformation within the original verrucous carcinoma. There is frequently a moderately dense inflammatory cell infiltrate in the underlying connective tissue, which may on occasion obscure the epithelium-connective tissue interface.[44] Medina et al.[50] found the coexistence of less differentiated squamous carcinoma in 20% of their verrucous lesions of the oral cavity. These patients did not appear to differ clinically from the remainder, but since they showed a recurrence rate nearly double that of pure verrucous carcinoma, proper histologic sampling of these tumors is essential.

The lesions of oral verrucous carcinoma are often quite extensive at the time of initial treatment because they grow slowly, cause few symptoms, and have little tendency to metastasize.[40] In the past the main mode of therapy has been surgical. That this was the "treatment of choice" may have been due, in part, to the often quoted danger of "anaplastic" transformation in verrucous carcinoma subjected to radiation therapy. In an extensive review of oral verrucous carcinoma McDonald et al.[39] could only find four acceptable cases of transformation to an invasive carcinoma subsequent to radiation therapy. They also identified six cases of transformation which occurred either prior to or without previous radiation treatment. A review of treatment modalities for verrucous carcinoma still seems to favor surgical treatment with up to 82% of patients having disease control with one surgical procedure[37,50,51] and 90% controlled after more than one surgical procedure.[50] Medina et al.[50] reported over 80% control in the group initially treated with radiation and subsequent surgical salvage. Thus it would appear that while surgical treatment still affords the best opportunity for disease control, now that the fears of "anaplastic" transformation have been minimized radiation therapy offers an acceptable alternative treatment in selected cases.

As far as the etiology of verrucous carcinoma is concerned there is a correlation between the occurrence of verrucous carcinoma and tobacco usage, although McCoy and Waldron[48] noted that in 20% of patients for whom information was available there was no history of tobacco use. Tornes et al.[49] found a history of tobacco use in less than one half of their patients. More recently Eisenberg et al.[44] noted "virus-like changes" in 15 of 17 cases of verrucous carcinoma. In addition there has been recent interest in the immunohistochemical demonstration human papilloma virus antigen in oral leukoplakias and papillomas.[52] Whether the nontobacco-related cases are associated with this virus remains to be seen.

B. Adenoid Squamous Cell Carcinoma

In 1947, Lever[53] reported four cases of what he believed were adenocarcinomas of exocrine sweat glands. It is now generally held that tubular and alveolar formations seen in some squamous cell carcinomas are a result of dyskeratosis and subsequent acantholysis.[54] In a series of 155 cases of adenoid squamous cell carcinoma over 90% occurred in the head and neck, suggesting that solar damage may play a role in the genesis of the gland-like appaearance.[55] Jacoway et al.,[56] Tomich and Hutton,[57] and Weitzner[58] in their reports of cases from the lip supported the concept that these lesions arise in areas of sun-damaged skin. Histochemical studies failed to demonstrate epithelial mucins, further supporting this idea.[56] However, it is difficult to accept sun damage as a cause of the intraoral cases reported by Takagi et al.[59]

With the exception of the cases occurring intraorally,[59] the majority of lesions have been reported on the lip. They occur in older adults, with a mean age of 56 years and usually on the vermillion border.[56-58] Clinically they are described as ulcerated, hyperkeratotic, or exophytic. Microscopically, these lesions are characterized by a downward proliferation of epithelium with many of the deeper nests showing a tubular appearance lined by cuboidal cells with the lumina containing desquamated acantholytic cells.

The treatment of choice is surgical excision. These lesions have a tendency to recur, but none has been reported to metastasize. The overall prognosis is excellent.

C. Polypoid Spindle Cell Carcinoma

Polypoid usually exophytic tumors with a dimorphic histologic appearance are unusual lesions occurring mainly in the upper aerodigestive tract and have been the subject of much controversy.[60-67] In the head and neck these neoplasms seem to occur most frequently in the larynx followed by the oral cavity, esophagus, and pharynx.[61,67] Similar biphasic tumors also occur in other parts of the body.[67]

The main controversy regarding these lesions has centered on the histogenesis of the spindle cell component. This is reflected in the variety of names used, e.g., carcinosarcoma, pseudosarcoma, spindle cell or pleomorphic carcinoma, and sarcomatoid carcinoma.[62,67]

There are three main theories regarding the origin of the spindle cell component:[60,67]

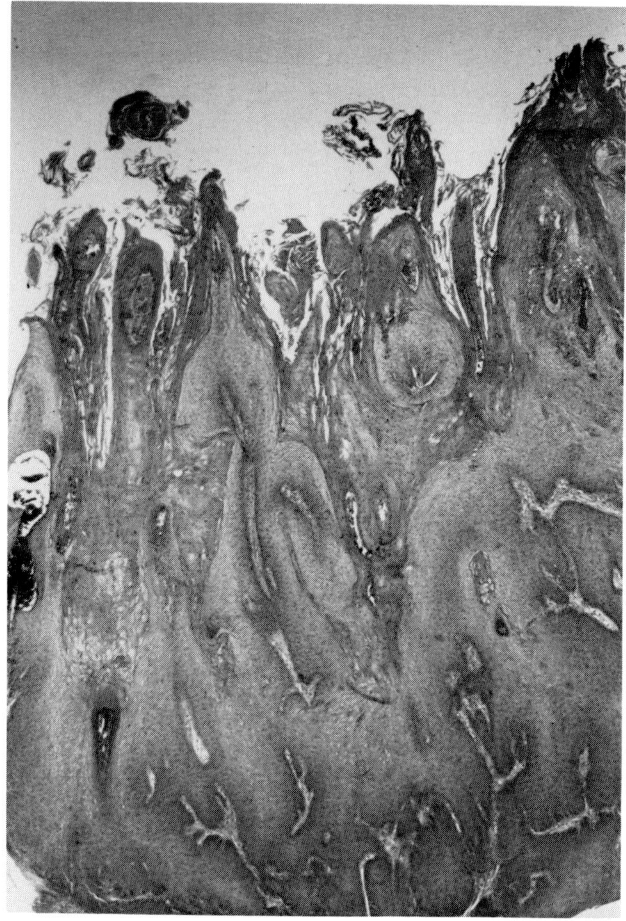

A

FIGURE 7.   (A) Low-power view of verrucous carcinoma. Note the parakeratin-filled clefts and "papillary" surface. (H & E. Magnification × 2.3.) (B) A high-power view of the deep aspect of verrucous carcinoma. Note the absence of cytologic atypia and mitoses. (H & E. Magnification × 40.)

1.   The tumor in fact represents a "collision" between a squamous cell carcinoma and a genuine soft tissue sarcoma.
2.   The spindle cell component represents an atypical but benign connective tissue reaction.
3.   The lesion represents spindle cell anaplasia in a form of squamous cell carcinoma.

Unfortunately, this controversy has not been settled by electron microscopic studies.[64,65]

Virchow is credited (cited in Lichtiger et al.[64]) with introducing the term carcinosarcoma to reflect the apparent dual origin of these lesions. Stout and Lattes[61] and Lane[60] felt that the spindle cell component was an atypical, benign reactive process. The finding of a spindle cell component in some lymph node metastases would tend to refute this theory.[65] The finding in some tumors of a "transition" from dysplastic or neoplastic epithelium to a spindle cell component, together with ultrastructural analysis, has led several authors to support the epithelial origin of the spindle cells. In a review of 59 cases of oral spindle cell carcinoma by Ellis and Corio,[62] a prerequisite for inclusion in their series was "histologic demonstration

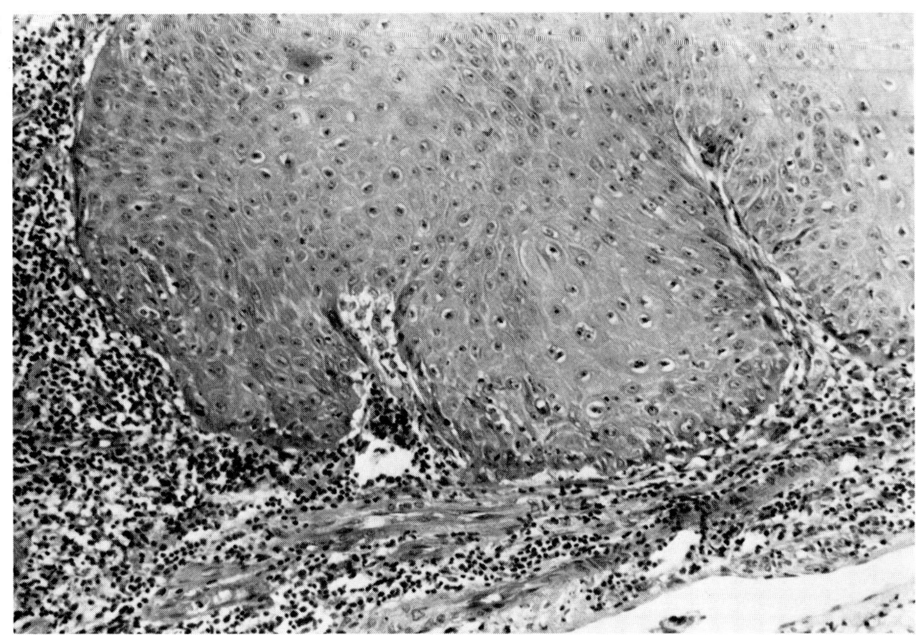

FIGURE 7B.

of epithelial changes ranging from prominent dysplasia to frank squamous cell carcinoma in conjunction with a dysplastic spindle cell element or evidence of direct transition of epithelial cells to dysplastic spindle cells''. Leventon and Evans[66] used similar selection criteria. Recognizing that in fact this may yet prove to be a heterogeneous group of neoplasms without a single unifying histogenetic origin, the term polypoid spindle cell carcinoma will be used.

In the oral cavity the most common anatomic locations for this tumor appear to be the lower lip, followed by the tongue and alveolar ridge or gingiva,[62] with other cases from the floor of the mouth being reported.[67] Clinically these tumors present with pain, as swelling or nonhealing ulcers. The mean age at presentation in the series reported by Ellis and Corio[62] was 57 years with a range from 29 to 93.

Histologically these lesions usually show extensive ulceration with an immediate subjacent layer of highly vascular tissue.[60,62] The spindle cell component is comprised of streaming cells or more myxomatous masses of cells which may be arranged in a fasciculated manner.[62,65,66] Bizarre and multinucleated giant cells as well as numerous typical and atypical mitoses are present. Epithelial dysplasia or a squamous carcinoma with or without "transition" to the underlying spindle cell tumor is usually found (Figure 8). Leventon and Evans[66] divided their cases into superficial and those showing deep invasion, i.e., into underlying muscle and salivary gland. All eight cases from the oral cavity were deeply invasive. They found a very strong correlation between growth pattern and prognosis.

There are only limited numbers of cases from which to draw inference regarding treatment modalities and survival figures. However, it would seem that surgery with or without radical neck dissection affords the best treatment with a 31% disease-free survival after a mean follow-up of 4 to 5 years.[62] This figure is slightly lower than some reports for polypoid spindle cell carcinoma. Tumor size was not found to influence survival.[62] Leventon and Evans[66] found that seven of the eight patients with invasive cases from the oral cavity died from their disease while there were no tumor-related deaths from superficial lesions outside the oral cavity. However, the obvious factors, such as regional and distant spread of the

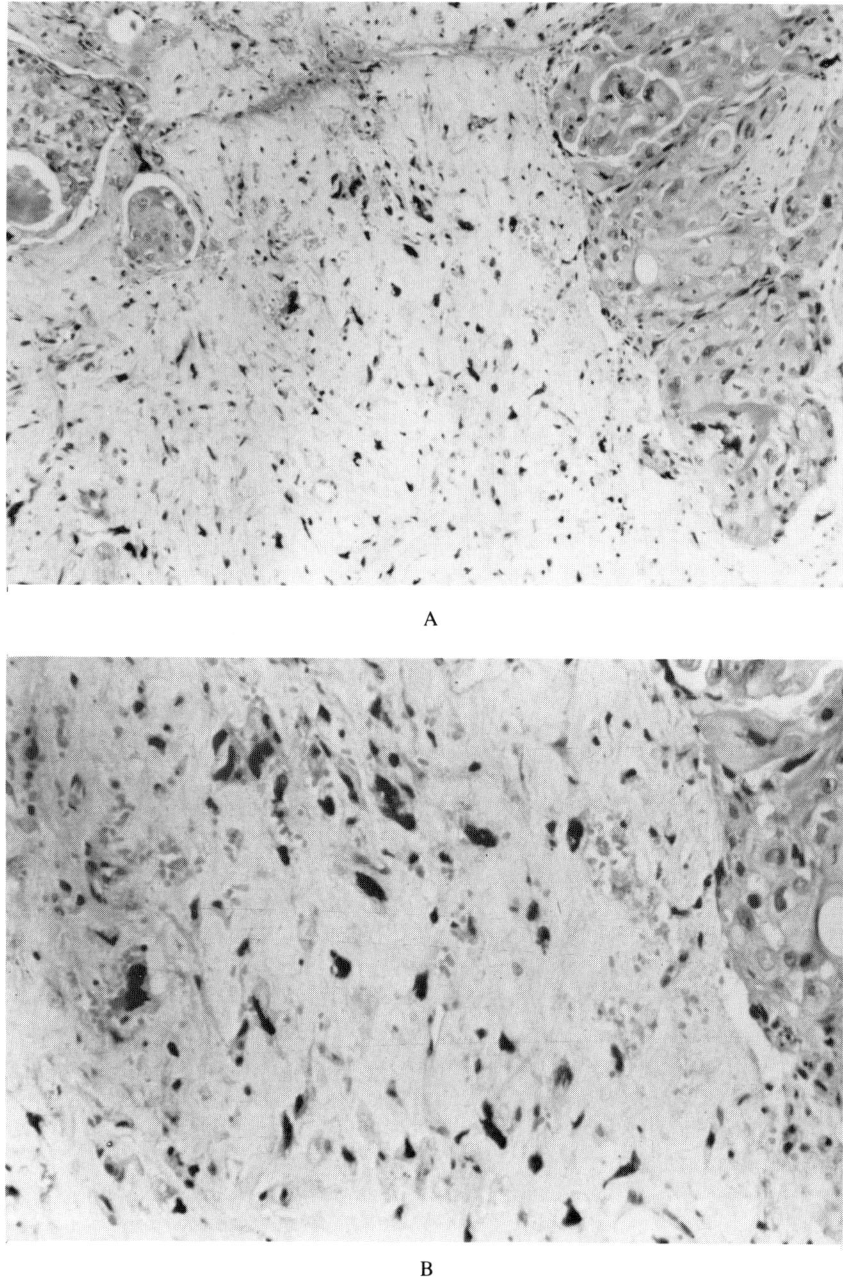

FIGURE 8.   (A, B) Low- and high-power view of polypoid spindle cell carcinoma. Note the presence of dysplastic squamous epithelium and a spindle cell component showing marked cytologic atypia. (H & E. Magnification (A) × 16; (B) × 40.)

disease, had the same disastrous effect on survival as they would for traditional squamous cell carcinoma.

Some cases of polypoid spindle cell carcinoma have been reported following treatment of squamous cell carcinoma by radiation therapy.[64-66] However, this is an inconsistent finding and cannot be implicated in the pathogenesis of most cases.

In summary, polypoid spindle cell carcinoma is a rare biphasic tumor which can occur in the oral cavity. The balance of evidence favors an epithelial origin for the spindle cell component. The prognosis with surgical intervention seems to be the same or slightly better than traditional squamous cell carcinoma.

D. Adenosquamous Carcinoma

In 1968 Gerughty et al.[68] reported ten cases of what they called adenosquamous carcinoma. They described four distinctive components, i.e., ductal carcinoma *in situ,* adenocarcinoma, squamous cell carcinoma, and a mixed carcinoma. Cases biopsied early in their development showed only ductal carcinoma *in situ* with later biopsies showing the other three elements. Histochemical studies revealed varying numbers of cells with intracytoplasmic mucin in all cases. They felt that these features separated their lesion from adenoid squamous carcinoma. Although differentiation from mucoepidermoid carcinoma may be difficult, it was argued that the histologic features together with the biological behavior (eight of their ten cases had documented metastases) were sufficient to make the distinction.

Three of the ten cases occurred on the tongue and two were from the floor of the mouth.[68] There have been sporadic case reports of adenosquamous carcinoma from other anatomic locations. The term adenosquamous carcinoma has also been used for a variant of endometrial carcinoma.[69,70] This lesion contains both malignant glandular and squamous components arising in hormonally responsive tissue. It was originally argued that this lesion from the endometrium had a worse prognosis than either adenoacanthomas or regular adenocarcinoma.[69] However, it now appears that the prognosis relates more to the grade of the glandular component than to the presence of malignant squamous elements.[70] Whether the same holds true for oral adenosquamous carcinoma remains to be seen.

VII. SPECIAL CONSIDERATIONS

A. Carcinoma in the Younger Age Group

Carcinoma of the oral cavity is generally considered a disease of older adults with the average age of occurrence being 60 years or greater. However, there is a certain percentage of cases of oral cancer which occurs in patients under the age of 40.[70-71] Some series report the incidence of all head and neck carcinomas[72-74,76] in patients under 40 while others report only oral cancers.[71,75,77-79] The incidence of oral squamous cell carcinoma in this younger age group varies, but averages between 1.8[75] and 3.6%[71] of all cases of oral cancer seen in the reporting institutions.

The most common intraoral location is the tongue[71,72,75] with three series reporting lesions from the tongue alone.[77-79] The most common symptoms are pain, a nonhealing ulcer, or a neck mass. With one exception[73] there does not appear to be a consistent association of the usual predisposing factors, i.e., a history of smoking and excessive alcohol intake. For example, in the series of McGregor et al.,[71] only 17 of 36 patients were tobacco users. Suggestions have been made that oral cancer in the younger population may be related to a genetic disorder or immunodeficiency.[72] However, this has yet to be documented.

Treatment methods have varied in different series, but usually include surgery and radiation either alone or in combination. In most instances the numbers of cases are too small to draw any firm conclusions with regard to optimum treatment regimes. This problem of treatment selection is further compounded by the widely varying survival figures. Son and Kapp[77] present a dismal picture of a 17% 3-year actuarial survival. Venables and Craft[79] found a 36% 5-year survival, while Byers,[78] a 45% survival in tongue carcinomas in patients under 30 years. This latter figure compared unfavorably to the 65% survival in patients over 30 years with tongue cancer from the same center.[78] At the other end of the spectrum, McGregor et al.[71] reported an 80% survival for the patients in their series with tongue malignancies. This compared extremely well with their institutional figure of 43% survival for older patients.

In summary, approximately 1 to 3% of all oral cancers occur in patients under 40 years, many of whom do not have the usual predisposing factors of tobacco use and alcohol abuse. Although there is speculation with regard to genetic disorders or immunodeficiencies, to date none has been documented specifically in this patient population. No one center has sufficient numbers of patients to make a definite recommendation regarding treatment. The reported survival for oral cancer in the younger population varies from a dismal 17% to an encouraging 80%.

B. Renal Transplant Patients

Over the past number of years successful renal transplantation, either living related donor or cadaveric, has been a means of prolonging relatively high quality of life (without the problems of dialysis) in patients with what would have previously been terminal renal disease. There have been a number of reports documenting an increase in the development of neoplasms in successful renal transplant recipients.[80-85] The majority of these neoplasms have been malignant lymphomas. Successful homograft patients have a 35-times greater risk of developing this neoplasm than the general population.[81] However, there is also an increase in incidence of other neoplasms. Skin and lip are sites especially at risk. Hoover and Fraumeni[81] calculated that there was a four-times greater risk of developing skin and lip cancers in successful transplant recipients than in people living in a low risk area for these cancers. Other cases of lip,[80] skin,[82,83] and even tongue[84] cancer have been reported.

Whereas the increased risk of lymphomas occurs fairly soon after successful transplantation, the risk of skin and lip cancer seems to increase with time. The reported cases, where details are available, show that the lip and tongue cancers have developed in young adults under the age of 30.[80,84]

Whether these neoplasms develop as a result of decreased immune surveillance following immunosuppression, as a result of oncogenic viral infection, or as a result of chromosomal abnormalities due to the immunosuppression which was used prior to the advent of cyclosporin has not been proven.[80] However, in this context it is interesting that Mullen[82] et al. found a markedly decreased inflammatory cellular response to the carcinomas of the transplant group when compared to nonimmunosuppressed controls.

It is of interest that Sheil et al.[85] found that not only did transplant patients have an increased risk of developing malignancies, but those on dialysis were also at risk. However, they did not find an increase in cancers of the ''buccal cavity''.

C. Acquired Immune Deficiency Syndrome (AIDS)/AIDS-Related Complex

In 1981 in the U.S. the first cases of AIDS were reported.[86] Since that time it has been shown that AIDS is caused by a retrovirus, HTLVIII/LAV*,[87,88] which produces an irreversible immune deficiency rendering the host susceptible to a variety of opportunistic infections and neoplastic disorders. These include Kaposi's sarcoma in persons under 60 years of age and opportunistic infections, i.e., pneumocystis carinii pneumonia, bronchial or pulmonary candidiasis (diagnosed by microscopy or the characteristic white plaques), and specific forms of tuberculosis. These patients must have no other cause of immune suppression and be HTLVIII/LAV antibody positive. For complete details the original case definitions and modifications should be consulted.[89,90] It has also been recognized that HTLVIII/LAV infection represents a spectrum of disease ranging from the relatively rare AIDS, through AIDS-related complex (ARC), which displays some but not all of the features of AIDS, to asymptomatic carriers. Persons at high risk for developing AIDS or ARC are homosexual males, i.v. drug abusers, and hemophiliacs.

There has been a great deal of interest in the oral manifestations of AIDS.[91-93] More recently interest centered on hairy leukoplakia as an oral manifestation of AIDS, ARC, and

---

* Since the preparation of this section on AIDS, the preferred nomenclature for the HTLVIII/LAV RNA retrovirus has been changed to HIV (human immundeficiency virus).

high risk patients.[92] It seems to be associated with both papilloma virus and a herpes-group virus.[92] Silverman and others[93] found seven cases of oral cancer in 375 homosexual males for an incidence of 1.9% in a group with a mean age of 36 years. One occurred in a full-blown case of AIDS, five cases occurred in the "high risk group" (defined as a patient with clinical signs and symptoms, laboratory abnormalities, or both, that do not meet the criteria described for ARC or AIDS as defined by the Centers for Disease Control), and the last case of oral cancer was in a sexual partner of a known AIDS case. Six of the seven cases of squamous cell carcinoma were on the tongue. It is of interest that the "high risk group" had both the highest incidence of hairy leukoplakia, with its known viral associations, and the largest numbers of oral cancer. Obviously there is a great deal of research needed in this area.

REFERENCES

1. **Batsakis, J. G.,** *Tumors of the Head and Neck,* 2nd ed., Williams & Wilkins, Baltimore, 1979, 145.
2. **Maddox, W. A.,** Vicissitudes of head and neck cancer, *Am. J. Surg.,* 148, 428, 1984.
3. **Ildstad, S. T., Bigelow, M. E., and Remensnyder, J. P.,** Squamous cell carcinoma of the tongue: a comparison of the anterior two thirds of the tongue with its base, *Am. J. Surg.,* 146, 456, 1983.
4. **Callery, C. D., Spiro, R. H., and Strong, E. W.,** Changing trends in the management of squamous carcinoma of the tongue, *Am. J. Surg.,* 148, 449, 1984.
5. **Mashberg, A.,** Final evaluation of tolonium chloride rinse for screening of high-risk patients with asymptomatic squamous carcinoma, *J. Am. Dent. Assoc.,* 106, 319, 1983.
6. **Mashberg, A. and Meyers, H.,** Anatomical site and size of 222 early asymptomatic oral squamous cell carcinomas, A continuing prospective study of oral cancer. II, *Cancer,* 37, 2149, 1976.
7. **Waldron, C. A. and Shafer, W. G.,** Leukoplakia revisited. A clinicopathologic study of 3,256 oral leukoplakias, *Cancer,* 36, 1386, 1975.
8. **Broders, A. C.,** Squamous-cell epithelium of the lip; a study of five hundred and thirty-seven cases, *JAMA,* 74, 656, 1920.
9. **Broders, A. C.,** The microscopic grading of cancer, *Surg. Clin. North Am.,* 21, 947, 1941.
10. **Shear, M., Hawkins, D. M., and Farr, H. W.,** The prediction of lymph node metastases from oral squamous carcinoma, *Cancer,* 37, 1901, 1976.
11. **Jakobsson, P. A., Eneroth, C.-M., Killander, D., Moberger, G., and Martensson, B.,** Histologic classification and grading of malignancy in carcinoma of the larynx (a pilot study), *Acta Radiol. Ther. Phys. Biol.,* 12, 1, 1973.
12. **Anneroth, G. and Hansen, L. S.,** A methodologic study of histologic classification and grading of malignancy in oral squamous cell carcinoma, *Scand. J. Dent. Res.,* 92, 448, 1984.
13. **Poleksic, S. and Kalwaic, H. J.,** Prognostic value of vascular invasion in squamous cell carcinoma of the head and neck, *Plast. Reconstr. Surg.,* 61, 234, 1978.
14. **Byers, R. M., O'Brien, J., and Waxler, J.,** The therapeutic and prognostic implications of nerve invasion in cancer of the lower lip, *Int. J. Radiat. Oncol. Biol. Phys.,* 4, 215, 1978.
15. **Frierson, H. F. and Cooper, P. H.,** Prognostic factors in squamous cell carcinoma of the lower lip, *Hum. Pathol.,* 17, 346, 1986.
16. **Wysocki, G. P. and Wright, B. A.,** Intraneural and perineural epithelial structures, *Head Neck Surg.,* 4, 69, 1981.
17. **Jensen, J. L., Wuerker, R. B., Correll, R. W., and Erickson, J O.,** Epithelial islands associated with mandibular nerves. Report of two cases in the walls of mandibular cysts, *Oral Surg. Oral Med. Oral Pathol.,* 48, 226, 1979.
18. **Danforth, R. A. and Baughman, R. A.,** Chievitz's organ: a potential pitfall in oral cancer diagnosis, *Oral Surg. Oral Med. Oral Pathol.,* 48, 231, 1979.
19. **Moore, C., Flynn, M. B., and Greenberg, R. A.,** Evaluation of size in prognosis of oral cancer, *Cancer,* 58, 158, 1986.
20. **Spiro, R. H., Huvos, A. G., Spiro, J. D., Wong, G. Y., Gnecco, C. A., and Strong, E. W.,** The predictive value of tumor thickness in patients with squamous carcinoma confined to the tongue and the floor of the mouth, in Abstracts, 32nd Annu. Meet., Society of Head and Neck Surgeons, Colorado, 1986.

21. **Mohit-Tabatabi, M. A., Sobel, H. J., Rush, B. F., Jr., and Mashberg, A.,** Relation of thickness of the primary to regional metastases in stage I and II floor of mouth cancers, in Abstracts, 32nd Annu. Meet., Society of Head and Neck Surgeons, Colorado, 1986.
22. **Breslow, A.,** Tumor thickness, level of invasion and node dissection in stage 1 cutaneous melanoma, *Ann. Surg.,* 182, 572, 1975.
23. **Breslow, A.,** Prognostic factors in the treatment of cutaneous melanoma, *J. Cut. Pathol.,* 6, 208, 1979.
24. **Cooper, D., Schermer, A., and Sun, T.-T.,** Classification of human epithelia and their neoplasms using monoclonal antibodies to keratins: strategies, applications and limitations, *Lab. Invest.,* 52, 243, 1985.
25. **Sun, T.-T. and Green, H.,** Immunofluorescent staining of keratin fibers in cultured cells, *Cell,* 14, 469, 1978.
26. **Sun, T.-T. and Green, H.,** Keratin filaments of cultured human epidermal cells: formation of intermolecular disulfide bands during terminal differentiation, *J. Biol. Chem.,* 253, 2053, 1978.
27. **Franke, W. W., Schiller, D. L., Moll, R., Winter, S., Schmid, E., Englebrecht, I., Denk, H., Krepler, R., and Platzer, B.,** Diversity of cytokeratins, *J. Mol. Biol.,* 153, 933, 1981.
28. **Moll, R., Franke, W. W., Schiller, D. L., Geiger, B., and Krepler, R.,** The catalog of human cytokeratins: patterns of expression in normal epithelia, tumors and cultured cells, *Cell,* 31, 11, 1982.
29. **Schlegel, R., Banks-Schlegel, S., and Pinkus, G. S.,** Immunohistochemical localization of keratin in normal human tissues, *Lab. Invest.,* 42, 91, 1980.
30. **Wright, B. A., Tingey, I. C., and Fleming, B.,** Antikeratin antibodies: their production and potential uses, in Abstracts, Annu. Meet. Am. Acad. Oral Pathol., Reno, 1982.
31. **Moi, M., Nakai, M., Hyum, K.-H., Noda, Y., and Kawamura, K.,** Distribution of keratin proteins in neoplastic and tumor-like lesions of squamous epithelium, *Oral Surg. Oral Med. Oral Pathol.,* 59, 63, 1985.
32. **Reibel, J., Clausen, H., and Dabelsteen, E.,** Staining patterns of humans pre-malignant oral epithelium and squamous cell carcinomas by monoclonal anti-keratin atnbidoes, *Acta Pathol. Microbiol. Immunol. Scand. (A),* 93, 323, 1985.
33. **Said, J. W., Nash, G., Sassoon, A. F., Shintaku, I, P., and Banks-Schlegel, S.,** Involucrin in lung tumors. A specific marker for squamous differentiation, *Lab. Invest.,* 49, 563, 1983.
34. **Chen, S.-Y. and Harwick, R. D.,** Ultrastructure of oral squamous-cell carcinoma, *Oral Surg. Oral Med. Oral Pathol.,* 44, 744, 1977.
35. **Burkhardt, A.,** Advanced methods in the evaluation of premalignant lesions and carcinomas of the oral mucosa, *J. Oral Pathol.,* 14, 751, 1985.
36. **Ackerman, L. V.,** Verrucous carcinoma of the oral cavity, *Surgery,* 23, 670, 1948.
37. **Kraus, F. T. and Perez-Mesa, C.,** Verrucous carcinoma. Clinical and pathologic study of 105 cases involving oral cavity, larynx and genitalia, *Cancer,* 19, 26, 1966.
38. **Shafer, W. G.,** Verrucous carcinoma, *Int. Dent. J.,* 22, 451, 1972.
39. **McDonald, J. S., Crissman, J. D., and Gluckman, J. L.,** Verrucous carcinoma of the oral cavity, *Head Neck Surg.,* 5, 22, 1982.
40. **Batsakis, J. G., Hybels, R., Crissman, J. D., and Rice, D. H.,** The pathology of head and neck tumors: verrucous carcinoma. XV., *Head Neck Surg.,* 5, 29, 1982.
41. **Goethals, P. L., Harrison, E. G., and Devine, K. D.,** Verrucous squamous carcinoma of the oral cavity, *Am. J. Surg.,* 106, 845, 1963.
42. **Jacobsen, S. and Shear, M.,** Verrucous carcinoma of the mouth, *J. Oral Pathol.,* 1, 66, 1972.
43. **Brownstein, M. H. and Shapiro, L.,** Verrucous carcinoma of skin, *Cancer,* 38, 1710, 1976.
44. **Eisenberg, E., Rosenberg, B., and Krutchkoff, D.,** Verrucous carcinoma: a possible viral pathogenesis, *Oral Surg. Oral Med. Oral Pathol.,* 59, 52, 1985.
45. **Shear, M. and Pindborg, J. J.,** Verrucous hyperplasia of the oral mucosa, *Cancer,* 46, 1855, 1980.
46. **Slootweg, P. J. and Muller, H.,** Verrucous hyperplasia or verrucous carcinoma. An analysis of 27 patients, *J. Maxillofac. Surg.,* 11, 13, 1983.
47. **Hansen, L. S., Olson, J. A., and Silverman, S., Jr.,** Proliferative verrucous leukoplakia. A long-term study of thirty patients, *Oral Surg. Oral Med. Oral Pathol.,* 60, 285, 1985.
48. **McCoy, J. M. and Waldron, C. A.,** Verrucous carcinoma of the oral cavity. A review of forty-nine cases, *Oral Surg. Oral Med. Oral Pathol.,* 52, 623, 1981.
49. **Tornes, K., Bang, G., Koppang, H. S., and Pedersen, K. N.,** Oral verrucous carcinoma, *Int. J. Oral Surg.,* 14, 485, 1985.
50. **Medina, J. E., Dichtel, W., and Luna, M. A.,** Verrucous-squamous carcinoma of the oral cavity. A clinicopathologic study of 104 cases, *Arch. Otolaryngol.,* 110, 437, 1984.
51. **Burns, H. P., van Nostrand, A. W. P., and Palmer, J. A.,** Verrucous carcinoma of the oral cavity: management by radiotherapy and surgery, *Can. J. Surg.,* 23, 19, 1980.
52. **Loning, Th., Reichart, P., Staquet, M. J., Becker, J., and Thivolet, J.,** Occurrence of papillomavirus structural antigens in oral papillomas and leukoplakias, *J. Oral Pathol.,* 13, 155, 1984.

53. **Lever, W. F.**, Adenocanthoma of sweat glands, carcinoma of sweat glands with glandular and epidermal elements: report of four cases, *Arch. Dermatol. Syph.*, 56, 157, 1947.
54. **Lever, W. F. and Schaumburg-Lever, G.**, *Histopathology of the Skin*, 6th ed., J.B. Lippincott, Philadelphia, 1983, 503.
55. **Johnson, W. C. and Helwig, E. B.**, Adenoid squamous cell carcinoma (adenoacanthoma): a clinicopathologic study of 155 patients, *Cancer*, 19, 1639, 1966.
56. **Jacoway, J. R., Nelson, J. F., and Boyers, R. C.**, Adenoid squamous cell carcinoma (adenoacanthoma) of the oral labial mucosa. A clinicopathologic study of fifteen cases, *Oral Surg. Oral Med. Oral Pathol.*, 32, 444, 1971.
57. **Tomich, C. E. and Hutton, C. E.**, Adenoid squamous cell carcinoma of the lip: report of cases, *J. Oral Surg.*, 30, 592, 1972.
58. **Weitzner, S.**, Adenoid squamous cell carcinoma of vermillion mucosa of the lower lip, *Oral Surg. Oral Med. Oral Pathol.*, 37, 589, 1974.
59. **Takagi, M., Sakota, Y., Takayama, S., and Ishikawa, G.**, Adenoid squamous cell carcinoma of the oral mucosa: report of two autopsy cases, *Cancer*, 40, 2250, 1977.
60. **Lane, N.**, Pseudosarcoma (polypoid sarcoma-like masses) associated with squamous cell carcinoma of the mouth, fauces and larynx: report of ten cases, *Cancer*, 10, 19, 1957.
61. **Stout, A. P. and Lattes, R.**, Tumors of the esophagus, in *Atlas of Tumor Pathology*, Sec. 5, Fasc. 20, Armed Forces Institute of Pathology, Washington, D.C., 1957, 95.
62. **Ellis, G. L. and Corio, R. L.**, Spindle cell carcinoma of the oral cavity: a clinicopathologic assessment of fifty-nine cases, *Oral Surg. Oral Med. Oral Pathol.*, 50, 523, 1980.
63. **Someren, A., Karcioglu, Z., and Clairmont, A. A.**, Polypoid spindle cell carcinoma (pleomorphic carcinoma), *Oral Surg. Oral Med. Oral Pathol.*, 42, 474, 1976.
64. **Lichtiger, B., MacKay, B., and Tessmer, C. F.**, Spindle cell variant of squamous carcinoma. A light and electron microscopic study of 13 cases, *Cancer*, 26, 1311, 1970.
65. **Leifer, C., Miller, A. S., Putong, P. B., and Min, B. H.**, Spindle-cell carcinoma of the oral mucosa. A light and electron microscopic study of apparent sarcomatous metastasis to cervical lymph nodes, *Cancer*, 34, 597, 1974.
66. **Leventon, G. S. and Evans, H. L.**, Sarcomatoid squamous cell carcinoma of the mucous membranes of the head and neck, *Cancer*, 48, 994, 1981.
67. **Anonsen, C., Doble, R. A., Hoekema, D., Huang, T. W., and Gown, A. M.**, Carcinosarcoma of the floor of mouth, *J. Otolaryngol.*, 14, 215, 1985.
68. **Gerughty, R. M., Hennigar, G. R., and Brown, F. M.**, Adenosquamous carcinoma of the nasal, oral and laryngeal cavities. A clinicopathologic study of ten cases, *Cancer*, 22, 1140, 1968.
69. **Ng, A. G.**, Mixed carcinoma of the endometrium, *Am. J. Obstet. Gynecol.*, 102, 506, 1968.
70. **Silverberg, S. G., Bolin, M. G., and DeGiorgi, L. S.**, Adenoacanthoma and mixed adenosquamous carcinoma of the endometrium. A clinicopathologic study, *Cancer*, 30, 1307, 1972.
71. **McGregor, G. I., Davis, N., and Robins, R. E.**, Squamous cell carcinoma of the tongue and lower oral cavity in patients under 40 years of age, *Am. J. Surg.*, 146, 88, 1983.
72. **Son, Y. H. and Kapp, D. S.**, Oral cavity and oropharyngeal cancer in a younger population, *Cancer*, 55, 441, 1985.
73. **Lipkin, A., Miller, R. H., and Woodson, G. E.**, Squamous cell carcinoma of the oral cavity, pharynx and larynx in young adults, *Laryngoscope*, 95, 790, 1985.
74. **Mendez, P., Jr., Maves, M. D., and Panje, W. R.**, Squamous cell carcinoma of the head and neck in patients under 40 years of age, *Arch. Otolaryngol.*, 111, 762, 1985.
75. **Amsterdam, J. T. and Strawitz, J. G.**, Squamous cell carcinoma of the oral cavity in young adults, *J. Surg. Oncol.*, 19, 65, 1982.
76. **Carniol, P. J. and Fried, M. P.**, Head and neck carcinoma in patients under 40 years of age, *Ann. Otol. Rhinol. Laryngol.*, 91, 152, 1982.
77. **Newman, A. N., Rice, D. H., Ossoff, R. H., and Sisson, G. A.**, Carcinoma of the tongue in persons younger than 30 years of age, *Arch. Otolaryngol.*, 109, 302, 1983.
78. **Byers, R. M.**, Squamous cell carcinoma of the oral tongue in patients less than thirty years of age, *Am. J. Surg.*, 130, 475, 1975
79. **Venables, C. W. and Craft, I. L.**, Carcinoma of the tongue in early adult life, *Br. J. Cancer*, 21, 645, 1967.
80. **Berger, H. M., Goldman, R., Gonick, H. C., and Waisman, J.**, Epidermoid carcinoma of the lip after renal transplantation. Report of two cases, *Arch. Intern. Med.*, 128, 609, 1971.
81. **Hoover, R. and Fraumeni, J. F., Jr.**, Risk of cancer in renal transplant recipients, *Lancet*, 2, 55, 1973.
82. **Mullen, D. L., Silverberg, S. G., Penn, I., and Hammond, W. S.**, Squamous cell carcinoma of the skin and lip in renal homograft recipients, *Cancer*, 37, 729, 1976.
83. **Hoxtell, E. O., Mandel, J. S., Murray, S. S., Schuman, L. M., and Goltz, R. W.**, Incidence of skin carcinoma after renal transplantation, *Arch. Dermatol.*, 113, 436, 1977.

84. **Lee, Y. W. and Gisser, S. D.,** Squamous cell carcinoma of the tongue in a nine year renal transplant survivor. A case report with a discussion of the risk of development of epithelial carcinomas in renal transplant survivors, *Cancer,* 41, 1, 1978.

85. **Sheil, A. G. R., Flavel, S., Disney, A. P. S., and Mathew, T. H.,** Cancer in dialysis and transplant patients, *Transplant. Proc.,* 17, 195, 1985.

86. **Curran, J. W.,** The epidemiology and prevention of the acquired immunodeficiency syndrome, *Ann. Intern. Med.,* 103, 657, 1985.

87. **Gallo, R. C. and Wong-Stall, F.,** A human T-lymphotrophic retrovirus (HTLVIII) as the cause of acquired immunodeficiency syndrome, *Ann. Intern. Med.,* 103, 679, 1985.

88. **Montagnier, L.,** Lymphadenopathy-associated virus: from molecular biology to pathogenicity, *Ann. Intern. Med.,* 103, 689, 1985.

89. Update: acquired immunodeficiency syndrome (AIDS) — United States, *MMWR,* B2, 688, 1984.

90. Revision of the case definition of acquired immunodeficiency syndrome for national reporting — United States, *Ann. Intern. Med.,* 103, 402, 1985.

91. **Lozada, F., Silverman, S., Jr., Migliorati, C. A., Conant, M. A., and Volberding, P. A.,** Oral manifestations of tumor and opportunistic infections in the acquired immunodeficiency syndrome (AIDS): findings in 53 homosexual males with Kaposi's sarcoma, *Oral Surg. Oral Med. Oral Pathol.,* 56, 491, 1983.

92. **Greenspan, D., Conant, M., Silverman, S., Jr., Greenspan, J. S., Petersen, V., and de Souza, Y.,** Oral "hairy" leukoplakia in male homosexuals: evidence of association with both papillovirus and herpes-group virus, *Lancet,* 2, 831, 1984.

93. **Silverman, S., Jr., Migliorati, C. A., Lozada-Nur, F., Greenspan, D., and Conant, M. A.,** Oral findings with or at high risk for AIDS: a study of 375 homosexual males, *J. Am. Dent. Assoc.,* 112, 187, 1986.

Chapter 5

ASSESSMENT OF THE ORAL CANCER PATIENT

Bruce A. Wright and John C. O'Brien

TABLE OF CONTENTS

I. INTRODUCTION

Given the complexities of the oral cavity and the fact that so many different disciplines are involved in its day-to-day management, the concept of integrated management is vital to the assessment and treatment planning for oral cancer patients.[1] In addition, each patient with oral cancer is unique and requires separate evaluation. With this in mind a tumor board is essential in the evaluation, treatment planning, and rehabilitation of oral cancer patients.

II. TUMOR BOARD (INTEGRATED MANAGEMENT)

The phrase "tumor board" is used to denote all members of the team involved in the diagnosis, clinical staging, treatment planning, definitive treatment, and rehabilitation of the oral cancer patient. Obviously, the composition of the team will vary from patient to patient depending on the complexities of the case to be treated and the availability of specialists. However, typically the tumor board should include the clinician (usually a head and neck or oral surgeon) to whom the patient is referred and who will orchestrate the patient's evaluation and treatment. If the diagnosis of oral cancer is readily apparent clinically the patient should be referred for assessment by the team which usually comprises not only the clinician, but ideally also a radiation oncologist, a specialist in chemotherapy, a plastic surgeon, an oral surgeon, a pathologist, and a dentist (often a prosthodontist with expertise in the assessment and rehabilitation of oral cancer patients). A speech therapist may be involved, and if they are deemed necessary in any individual case they should be brought in at the planning stages.

If biopsy has been deferred so that all members of the board can see the lesion in its untouched state (see Chapter 4), then it (biopsy) should be included in this initial assessment. Also at this visit the extent of disease, i.e., clinical staging,[2] will be done. The pathologist will also be involved, not only to confirm the diagnosis but to provide information about tumor thickness and vascular and perineural invasion.[3-8] Next the various treatment options should be discussed both by members of the board and the patient. Surgery, radiation, and chemotherapy are not mutually exclusive treatment modalities, but rather complementary therapeutic approaches which may be used separately or in conjunction with one another depending on the complexities of the situation and the extent of disease.[9-30] Two brief examples will serve to illustrate this. The first situation is a lip cancer less than 4 cm in greatest dimensions without any lymph node involvement. Lesions such as this can be treated equally well with either surgery or radiation therapy with little or no post-treatment morbidity,[12,14,16] except that some post-treatment fibrosis may be expected with radiation. The treatment modality used will often depend on to whom the patient is referred in the first instance. If radiation therapy is chosen as the definitive treatment then a stent may have to be constructed to protect the teeth and periodontal tissues from unnecessary radiation. However, with this exception there will really be no necessity to involve all the other members of the tumor board. The second example might be a floor of mouth carcinoma with possible mandibular bone involvement in a person who still has many teeth present. In this instance all members of the tumor board will have to be involved. The initial visit, biopsy, and assessment with clinical staging will be carried out as usual. However, in this instance dental radiographs, bone scans, or computed tomography (CT) scans may be necessary to determine bony involvement.[31-34] The dental status of the patient will have to be carefully evaluated, especially if radiation therapy is considered.[35-39] It may also be necessary to involve the speech therapist for post-treatment rehabilitation. The treatment planning and selection of therapeutic modalities with a view to control of local and regional disease as well as rehabilitation will obviously require careful deliberation by all members of the board.

Two other factors must be considered in patient evaluation. First a high percentage of oral cancer patients develop second primary neoplasms.[40,41] This matter is discussed in greater detail below, but it must be constantly borne in mind both at the initial assessment and at follow-up visits. Many oral cancer patients are elderly, sometimes in poor health, and many have been extensive users of tobacco and alcohol.[40] Therefore, a complete assessment of the patient's general health and his ability to undergo the selected treatment modalities is vital. It may be necessary to involve the various subspecialities of internal medicine, e.g., cardiology, respirology, etc., at this stage.

From the above it is obvious that there is no one individual health care professional who can provide all the expertise necessary for the complete assessment, treatment, and rehabilitation of oral cancer patients, and, therefore, the tumor board is important. Regular consultation between the board members and mutual respect for what each specialist has to offer the patient will markedly enhance patient care and increase the chances for a successful outcome. However, it is recognized that while every effort should be made to establish a tumor board or refer the patient to an existing one there will be instances when this is not possible either for logistical or financial reasons.

III. STAGING

A. Definition

A fundamental part of the initial assessment of any oral cancer patient is accurate clinical staging. The basis of clinical staging is assessment of the extent of disease in each individual patient. The use of a uniform staging system which correlates closely with prognosis will allow clinicians to give meaningful information to the patient with regard to his or her possible outcome. In addition, accurate staging will allow comparison from center to center and between one anatomic site and another for various treatment regimes. Sometimes the results are educational. For example, it was generally held that carcinoma of the tongue base had a lower survival rate than carcinoma of the mobile tongue. However, when the same clinical stages for each location were compared, Ildstad et al.[42] could find no significant differences in survival.

To be useful a clinical staging system must be straightforward to use, easily reproducible, and correlate closely with clinical outcome. The most widely used system in North America is the TNM classification.[2] The system detailed by the Union Internationale Centre le Cancer (UICC) is very similar with some minor modifications.[43] Recently Platz et al.[44] have compared AJC and UICC classifications and concluded that neither fulfilled the criteria needed by staging systems. However, they felt that the STNMP[45] (see below) may be a starting point for further work in this area.

The TNM systems are based on three parameters, i.e., the size of the primary lesion (T), the status of the regional lymph nodes (N), and the presence or absence of distant metastases (M). These are detailed in Table 1.[2] The TNM classification is subdivided into clinical stages I through IV (Table 2). There are innumerable reports showing that the overall prognosis for oral cancer correlates well with the clinical stage, with stage I having the best prognosis and stage IV the worst.[14,15,18,27,29,46]

It is recognized that the TNM system does have some limitations as a prognostic indicator, and this led Rapidis et al.[45] to propose a new staging system (STNMP) where the site (S) and pathology (P) of the lesion are also taken into consideration. Point values are assigned to each of the STNMP categories and clinical stages determined by total points (Table 3A and B). They found no significant difference between their system and the conventional TNM staging up to 5 years follow-up. However, with longer follow-up they found the STNMP system and improvement as a prognostic indicator. However, Rich and Radden[46] failed to show any advantage of the STNMP system over the conventional TNM classification.[46] With the recent emphasis on the pathologic evaluation of tumor thickness[6-8] it may

Table 1
DEFINITIONS OF T, N, AND M CATEGORIES OF ORAL CANCER

Tumor

T1	Greatest diameter of primary tumor 2 cm or less
T2	Greatest diameter of primary tumor > 2 cm, but not > 4 cm
T3	Greatest diameter of primary tumor > 4 cm
T4	Massive tumor > 4 cm in diameter, with deep invasion involving antrum, pterygoid muscle, base of tongue, or skin of neck

Neck

N0	No clinically positive nodes
N1	Single clinically positive homolateral node 3 cm or less in diameter
N2	Single clinically positive homolateral node > 3 cm, but not > 6 cm in diameter, or multiple clinically positive homolateral nodes, none > 6 cm in diameter
N2a	Single clinically positive node > 3 cm, but not > 6 cm in diameter
N2b	Multiple clinically positive homolateral nodes, none > 6 cm in diameter
N3	Massive homolateral node(s), bilateral nodes, or contralateral node(s)
N3a	Clinically positive homolateral node(s), one of which is > 6 cm in diameter
N3b	Bilateral clinically positive nodes
N3c	Contralateral clinically positive node(s) only

Metastases (M)

M0	No (known) distant metastases
M1	Distant metastates present — specify site(s)

Table 2
CLINICAL STAGES OF
ORAL CANCER

Stage I	T1 N0 M0
Stage II	T2 N0 M0
Stage III	T3 N0 M0
	T1,T2, or T3 N1 M0
Stage IV	T4 N0 or N1 M0
	Any T N2 or N3 M0
	Any T, any N M1

be necessary to modify further existing staging systems in order to improve their prognostic significance.

As detailed above there are three aspects to the most widely used staging system. Each will be dealt with briefly.

B. Evaluation of Primary Lesion (T)

The evaluation of the primary lesion is intended to determine not only the size of the carcinoma in centimeters but also whether contiguous structures, e.g., muscle, bone, etc. are involved. Bimanual palpation of all lesions will obviously yield far more useful, accurate information regarding size and extent than simple visual inspection. (If the lesion has been previously biopsied, accurate clinical assessment may be hampered by the tissue reaction to the biopsy). Other techniques which may be useful include having the patient protrude the tongue and examining for lack of mobility or lateral deviation which may give an indication of intrinsic muscle involvement. Bony involvement is harder to assess. Panoramic and periapical radiographs and radionuclide scanning have all been used in an attempt to

Table 3A
THE STNMP CLASSIFICATION FOR INTRAORAL CARCINOMATA

S (site)		T (tumor)		N (node)	
S1	Lip-skin	T1	Tumor < 20 mm in diameter	N0	No palpable nodes
S2	Lip-mucous membrane	T2	Tumor between 20 and 40 mm in diameter	N1	Equivocal node enlargement
S3	Tongue	T3	Tumor between 40 and 60 mm in diameter and/or extending beyond the primary region	N2	Clinically palpable homolateral regional node(s) not fixed
S4	Cheek				
S5	Palate	T4	Any tumor > 60 mm in diameter and/or extending to involve adjacent structures	N3	As N2 but fixed
S6	Floor of mouth				
S7	Alveolar process			N4	Clinically palpable contralateral or bilateral node(s) not fixed
S8	Antrum			N5	As N4 but fixed
S9	Central Ca of bone				

M (metastases)		P (pathology)	
M0	No distant metastases	P0	Hyperkeratotic lesion showing atypia
M1	Clinical evidence of distant metastases without definite histological and/or radiographic confirmation	P1	Carcinoma *in-situ*
		P2	Basal cell carcinoma
		P3a	Verrucous carcinoma
		P3b	Well-differentiated squamous cell carcinoma
M2	Proven evidence of metastases beyond the regional nodes	P3c	Moderately differentiated squamous cell carcinoma
		P3d	Poorly differentiated squamous cell carcinoma

Table 3B
ARITHMETIC VALUES FOR
STNMP CLASSIFICATION

T1	0	N0	0	M0	0		
T2	10	N1	10	M1	30		
T3	20	N2	20	M2	40		
T4	35	N3	30				
		N4	40				
		N5	40				
P0	0	S1	4	Stage I	0—30		
P1	5	S2	6	II	31—50		
P2	5	S3	8	III	51—70		
P3a	5	S4	10	IV	71—155		
P3b	10	S5	12				
P3c	15	S6	14				
P3d	20	S7	16				
		S8	18				
		S9	20				

determine bone involvement.[31-33,47] It seems that radionuclide scanning may be more sensitive than panoramic radiographs in determining mandibular bone involvement,[32,47] However, since most scans merely measure bone turnover the possibility of false positive results from conditions such as active periodontal disease should be considered.[32] The finding of mandibular bone involvement will alter therapeutic considerations, such as the specific surgical operation to be used.[32] Computed tomography (CT) scanning has recently been used, with some success, in assessing the extent of certain lesions.[34,48]

The size of the initial lesion (T) relates to the clinical staging by arbitrary grouping into

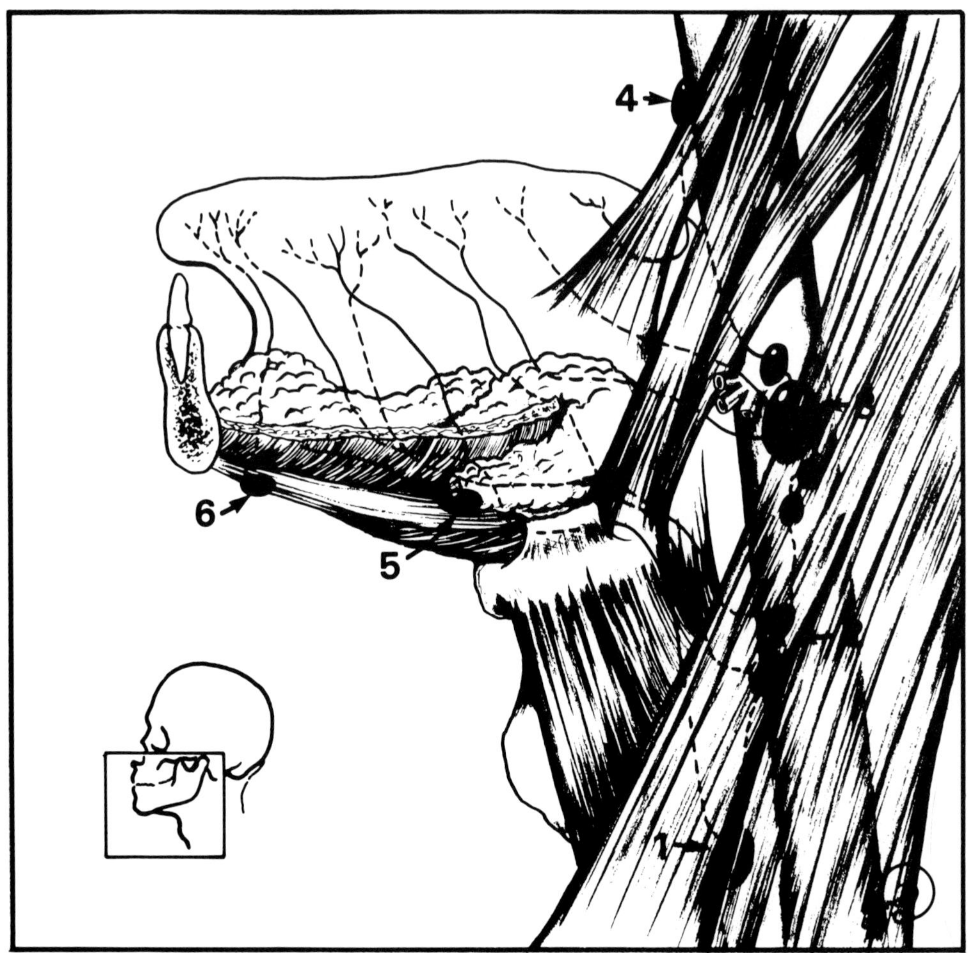

FIGURE 1.   A diagram showing the basic lymphatic drainage from the oral cavity: (1) jugulo-omohyoid lymph node, (2) deep cervical lymph node, (3) jugulo-digastric lymph node, (4) deep parotid lymph node, (5) submandibular lymph node, and (6) submental lymph node.

less than 2 cm, 2 to 4 cm, and greater than 4 cm. There may need to be modification of these size categories because of data such as that presented by Maddox.[27] He found, for lesions less than 1 cm, 1 to 3 cm, and over 3 cm actuarial 5-year survival rates of 100, 65, and 46%, respectively. Future studies correlating the size of the initial lesion with prognosis may help to clarify the size groupings in the clinical staging.

C. Regional Lymph Nodes (N)

The second essential part of the clinical staging is detailed assessment of the regional lymph nodes for the suspected presence of tumor. Obviously, this cannot be done without an accurate knowledge of regional lymphatic drainage patterns as they relate to the primary lesion. Reference should be made to standard anatomy texts or articles.[49] Figure 1 shows a simplified version of the major lymph nodes draining the oral cavity. The possibility of contralateral lymph node metastases especially from the tongue and floor of mouth must always be considered.

Each chain of lymph nodes should be examined individually. Certain techniques are useful. For example bimanual palpation of the submental lymph node will help to elicit more detail with regard to enlargement and texture. The lymph nodes along the anterior border of the sternocleidomastoid muscle can be best palpated with the finger tips by approaching the neck from behind with the muscle in a relaxed (not taut) position. It obviously takes experience to estimate not only lymph node size but also whether any enlargement is due to tumor or inflammation. Correlation should always be made with any subsequent pathological examination to confirm or refute the clinical impression.

The importance of the presence of lymph node metastasis can be judged by the marked difference in survival between those with and without regional disease. This is true regardless of anatomic site of the primary tumor. For example, carcinoma of the anterior two thirds of tongue without evidence of lymph node metastasis (stages I and II) has 5-year survival rates of between 50 to 65%, while when lymph node metastases are present (stage III and IV) this figure drops to 18 to 34%.[27,29,42] A similar trend, i.e., a marked worsening of prognosis once lymph node metastases are present, can be documented from the floor of the mouth[9,15,18,28,50] and from the lip.[12,14,16]

There are several other areas of concern regarding lymph node involvement in oral cancer. The first of these is the problem of false positive and false negative neck nodes[50-53] (see also Chapter 6). False positive neck nodes are those thought clinically to be malignant, but at pathological examination found not to contain tumor. The incidence of false positive nodes has ranged from 20 to 50%.[50] This may be due, in part, to the difficulty in differentiating an enlarged submandibular salivary gland from a lymph node containing tumor. Equally disturbing is the high frequency of false negative neck nodes, i.e., clinically negative nodes found to contain microscopic evidence of tumor. False negative rates (occult metastases) have been found to range from 20 to 37%.[50-53] Presumably it is this high rate of occult metastases together with the poor prognosis in patients who subsequently manifest neck metastases following apparent control of the primary lesion that has rekindled the debate regarding treating the clinically negative neck (Chapter 6). This topic has been recently reviewed for tongue and floor of mouth,[52] and there seems to be some evidence supporting elective neck dissections for lesions T2 or greater.

D. Distant Metastases (M)

Most treatment failures for oral cancer occur as a result of either local or regional recurrence rather than from distant metastases. There have been a number of studies on distant metastases from head and neck carcinomas,[54,55] with the incidence ranging from 5 to 57%.[55] This wide variation depends on whether the study was clinical or autopsy based. Platz et al.[56] found only a 2% incidence of clinically detectable distant metastases in over 1000 oral cancer cases. The most common sites of metastasis are lungs, bone, and liver[55] with other sites much less commonly involved. Probert et al.[55] stated that the larger, more advanced primary lesions were more likely to have distant metastases. However, Berger and Fletcher[54] found no correlation between size of the primary lesion and distant disease, but they did note that advanced nodal disease (N2, N3) was significantly more often associated with metastases than early nodal involvement (N0, N1). One study pointed out that control of primary disease was achieved in one half of the patients who later manifested distant metastases.[55]

If metastases are suspected, then whole lung tomograms, bone scans, and liver scans or hepatic ultrasound may be necessary to document distant disease.

E. Host Performance Scale

Host performance scale is a measure of the overall status of the patient. Although not part of the clinical staging procedure, it is important because it may have a bearing on treatment selection and overall prognosis. There are three scales mentioned in the AJC manual:[2] AJC Host (H), Karnofsky, and Eastern Cooperative Oncology Group Scale. In the AJC Host (H) scale, H0 is normal activity; H1, symptomatic and ambulatory; H2, ambulatory more than 50% of the time; H3, nursing care needed; and H4, bedridden.

IV. SECOND PRIMARIES

It is well known that a certain percentage of oral cancer patients will develop second primary tumors.[40,41] Whether this is due to a field cancerization effect, the cocarcinogenic effect of alcohol and tobacco, or a suppression of the immune system is not known.[40,41,57] A review of series of cases of oral cancer shows that up to 40% of patients in any series may develop second primaries.[9,11,15,18,28,29,41,42,58] These may present at the same time (synchronous) but in a different site; may develop subsequently in the mouth (Figure 2A, B) or upper aerodigestive tract;[41] or may be second primaries in other parts of the body. Regardless of the cause of these second neoplasms the clinician must be aware of the high percentage of oral cancer patients who develop them. They should be diligently sought not only at the initial evaluation but at all follow-up visits.

V. DENTAL STATUS EVALUATION

The proper evaluation of the dental status of oral cancer patients by a qualified expert in this area is a vital part of the overall work-up. The periodontal and pulpal status of all remaining teeth must be recorded. If radiation or chemotherapy is contemplated it may be necessary to restore or remove compromised teeth to avoid subsequent osteoradionecrosis or complications of infection.[35-39] Beumer et al.[39] recommended a fairly aggressive policy of dental extraction, especially in the mandible, for patients who were going to undergo radiation treatment. Advanced caries, periapical disease, or significant periodontal deficiencies, e.g., furcation involvement of mandibular molars, are considered indications for preradiation extraction. An estimation, based on previous experience, of the patient's willingness to maintain proper dental health will also play a role in deciding such things as extraction vs. restoration. Because of the potential for mandibular osteoradionecrosis following extractions in irradiated areas all possible efforts must be made to avoid this complication. It also behooves all people on the tumor board to have a knowledge of the oral complications of such treatments as radiotherapy or chemotherapy in order to assist in their management (Chapter 7).

If major surgery is contemplated as a primary treatment modality, properly mounted casts of both mandible and maxilla should be obtained prior to treatment as this will greatly aid the prosthodontist's post-treatment rehabilitation. It should be noted that on occasion dental appliances may predispose irradiated tissues to develop osteoradionecrosis.[39] Therefore, proper construction of appliances and their continued evaluation by a dentist is mandatory.

VI. GENERAL MEDICAL EVALUATION

The work-up of any oral cancer patient would not be complete without a full history and physical examination together with appropriate laboratory tests. The local disease must be viewed in the context of the whole patient. Many, if not most, oral cancer patients are over 50 years of age and a large number are, or will have been, prodigious users of tobacco and alcohol. Such a group of patients is obviously prone to other diseases, e.g., coronary artery disease and chronic obstructive lung disease. Obviously the general health of the patient must be considered when selecting treatment options. For example, an elderly patient with severe obstructive lung disease might be better treated by local radiation than by being subjected to a general anesthetic for surgical treatment.

There is no all-encompassing list of tests to be carried out, but included might be a complete blood count (CBC), prothrombin time (PT), partial thromboplastin time (PTT), SMAC, chest film, and urinalysis. A CBC provides a hemoglobin estimation, hematocrit, and platelet count as well as white cell count and differential. A CBC is routinely ordered

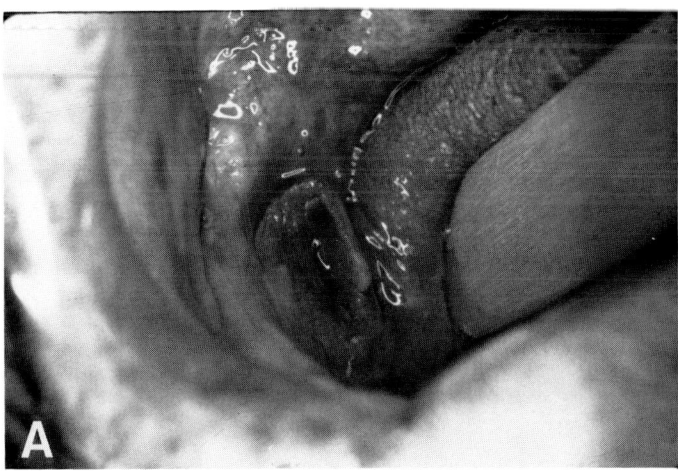

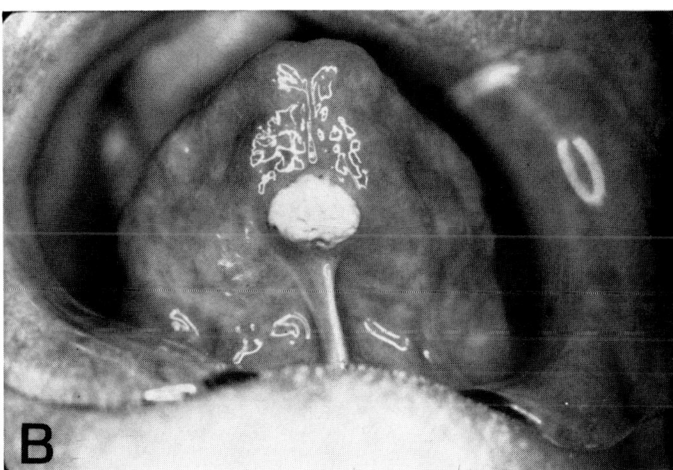

FIGURE 2.   (A) Illustrates a primary squamous cell carcinoma in the right retromolar floor of mouth region. (B) 18 months later the patient developed a second primary carcinoma on the ventral surface of tongue. (Courtesy of Dr. J. Bradfield.)

if surgery or chemotherapy is contemplated. PT and PTT are useful screening procedures for hemostasis. A SMAC or SMA-12 will give information regarding blood urea nitrogen and creatinine for renal function which is especially important if chemotherapy is contemplated. Raised alkaline phosphatase and serum calcium may prompt a search for distant metastases while elevated liver enzymes may indicate liver metastasis or intercurrent liver disease. An electrocardiogram may be indicated, especially if surgery is contemplated. A routine chest radiograph should be obtained as part of the evaluation of the respiratory system. If history, physical findings, or chest film suggest ongoing pulmonary disease, or if bleomycin chemotherapy is planned, then pulmonary function tests may be required. Other tests may be necessary depending on findings from the history and physical examination.

VII. PSYCHOLOGICAL STATUS

Finally, the assessment of the oral cancer patient would not be complete without a few remarks about the psychological status of the patient. The diagnosis of oral cancer has devastating implications for all but the most stoic of patients. All members of the "team" must be aware of this and continue to talk to the patient openly, honestly, and with understanding. Frequently family members will be involved and need sympathetic help in coming to terms with the disease.

Oral cancer, although quite uncommon in the overall scheme of cancer, has a profound effect on the patient. Unlike breast or colonic cancer, very often the effects of treatment cannot be hidden from the general public. Continuing discussion with the patient, and often with the immediate family, about the effects and outcome of a particular treatment modality will go a long way to help the patient understand, and ensure full patient cooperation with, planned treatment. There have been attempts recently to develop a series of tests for functional evaluation of oral cancer patients.[59] Publications such as this help to place emphasis on the post-treatment quality of life.

In general the overall prognosis for oral cancer, with the exception of carcinoma of the lip, is poor (as low as 20% survival at 5 years if regional nodes are involved). In these days of better patient education many want an honest and accurate assessment of their disease. Therefore, a realistic appraisal with emphasis on the positive side of things is probably the best approach. An honest approach of "I don't know what the future holds" might be more acceptable than inadvertently (or worse) deliberately misleading the patient.

Patients will often require a great deal of emotional support and want to ask a lot of questions. In many instances the surgeon or radiation oncologist may be too busy to provide this support. With in-patients, the nursing staff is an invaluable asset in helping patients come to terms with their disease. For out-patients the family physician can be a very valuable resource for the patient and his or her family. If the outlook appears bleak, hospice care may be appropriate, but should be involved as early as possible so that they are able to establish a rapport with the patient and the family.

VIII. CONCLUSION

Ideally, all patients should all be assessed by a tumor board and therapeutic decisions made with regard to all treatment modalities. However, it must be realized that not all these modalities will be available to all patients. Some will be referred to and treated by one specialist, e.g., surgeon, radiation oncologist. For some lesions this will not affect the outcome (see Chapter 6), while for others more complex decision making will be necessary.

REFERENCES

1. **Vaughan, C. W., Jr.,** Work-up treatment planning for head and neck cancer, *Otolaryngol. Clin.*, 18, 403, 1985.
2. **Beahrs, O. H. and Myers, M. H.,** *Manual for Staging of Cancer,* 2nd ed., American Joint Committee on Cancer, Eds., Lippincott, New York, 1983.
3. **Poleksic, S. and Kalwaic, H. J.,** Prognostic value of vascular invasion in squamous cell carcinoma of the head and neck, *Plast. Reconstr. Surg.*, 61, 234, 1978.
4. **Byers, R. M., O'Brien, J., and Waxler, J.,** The therapeutic and prognostic implications of nerve invasion in cancer of the lower lip, *Int. J. Radiat. Oncol. Biol. Phys.*, 4, 215, 1978.
5. **Frierson, H. F. and Cooper, P. H. ,** Prognostic factors in squamous cell carcinoma of the lower lip, *Hum. Pathol.*, 17, 346, 1986.
6. **Moore, C., Flynn, M. B., and Greenberg, R. A.,** Evaluation of size in prognosis of oral cancer, *Cancer,* 58, 158, 1986.
7. **Spiro, R. H., Huvos, A. G., Spiro, J. D., Wong, G. Y., Gnecco, C. A., and Strong, E. W.,** The predictive value of tumor thickness in patients with squamous carcinoma confined to the tongue and the floor of the mouth, in Abstracts, 32nd Annu. Meet., Society of Head and Neck Surgeons, Colorado, 1986.

8. **Mohit-Tabatabi, M. A., Sobel, H. J., Rush, B. F., Jr., and Mashberg, A.,** Relation of thickness of the primary to regional metastases in stage I and II floor of mouth cancers, in Abstracts, 32nd Annu. Meet., Society of Head and Neck Surgeons, Colorado, 1986.

9. **Kolson, H., Spiro, R. H., Rosewit, B., and Lawson, W.,** Epidermoid carcinoma of the floor of the mouth. Analysis of 108 cases, *Arch. Otolaryngol.,* 93, 280, 1971.

10. **Bertino, J. R., Boston, B., and Capizzi, R. L.,** The role of chemotherapy in the management of cancer of the head and neck: a review, *Cancer,* 36, 752, 1975.

11. **Gilbert, E. H., Goffinet, D. R., and Bagshaw, M. A.,** Carcinoma of the oral tongue and floor of mouth: fifteen years' experience with linear accelerator therapy, *Cancer,* 35, 1517, 1975.

12. **Wurman, L. H., Adams, G. L., and Meyerhoff, W. L.,** Carcinoma of the lip, *Am. J. Surg.,* 130, 470, 1975.

13. **Whitehurst, J. O. and Droulias, C. A.,** Surgical treatment of squamous cell carcinoma of the oral tongue. Factors influencing survival, *Arch. Otolaryngol.,* 103, 212, 1977.

14. **Hornback, N. B. and Shidnia, H.,** Carcinoma of the lower lip. Treatment results at Indiana University Hospitals, *Cancer,* 41, 352, 1978.

15. **Nakissa, N., Hornback, N. B., Shidnia, H., and Sayoc, E.,** Carcinoma of the floor of the mouth, *Cancer,* 42, 2914, 1978.

16. **Heller, K. S. and Shah, J. P.,** Carcinoma of the lip, *Am. J. Surg.,* 138, 600, 1979.

17. **Fu, K. K., Ray, J. W., Chan, E. K., and Phillips, T. L.,** External and interstitial radiation therapy of carcinoma of the oral tongue. A review of 32 years' experience, *Am. J. Roentgenol.,* 126, 107, 1976.

18. **Ildstad, S. T., Bigelow, M. E., and Remensnyder, J. P.,** Intra-oral cancer at the Massachusetts General Hospital. Squamous cell carcinoma of the floor of the mouth, *Ann. Surg.,* 197, 34, 1983.

19. **Stephens, F. O., Harker, G. J. S., and Hambly, C. K.,** Treatment of advanced cancer of the lower lip — the use of intraarterial or intravenous chemotherapy as basal treatment, *Cancer,* 48, 1309, 1981.

20. **Leipzig, B., Cummings, C. W., Johnson, J. T., Chung, C. T., and Sagerman, R. H.,** Carcinoma of the anterior tongue, *Ann. Otol. Rhinol. Laryngol.,* 91, 94, 1982.

21. **Pennacchio, J. L., Hong, W. K., Shapshay, S., Gillis, T., Vaughan, C., Bhutani, R., Ucmakli, A., Katz, A. E., Bromer, R., Willet, B., and Strong, S. M.,** Combination of cis-platinum and bleomycin prior to surgery and/or radiotherapy compared with radiotherapy alone for the treatment of advanced squamous cell carcinoma of the head and neck, *Cancer,* 50, 2795, 1982.

22. **Elias, E. G., Chretien, P. B., Monnard, E., Khan, T., Bouchelle, W. H., Wiernik, P. H., Lipson, S. D., Hande, K. R., and Zentai, T.,** Chemotherapy prior to local therapy in advanced squamous cell carcinoma of the head and neck. Preliminary assessment of an intensive drug regimen, *Cancer,* 43, 1025, 1979.

23. **Decker, D. A., Drelichman, A., Jacobs, J., Hoschner, J., Kinzie, J., Loh, J. J. K., Weaver, A., and Al-Sarraf, M.,** Adjuvant chemotherapy with cis-diamminodichloroplatinum II and 120-hour infusion 5-fluorouracil in stage III and IV squamous cell carcinoma of the head and neck, *Cancer,* 51, 1353, 1983.

24. **Ringborg, U., Ewert, G., Kinnman, J., Lundqvist, P. G., and Strander, H.,** Sequential methotrexate-5-fluorouracil treatment of squamous cell carcinoma of the head and neck, *Cancer,* 52, 971, 1983.

25. **Vikram, B. and Farr, H. W.,** Adjuvant radiation therapy in locally advanced head and neck cancer, *Ca.,* 33, 134, 1983.

26. **Bosi, G. J.,** Adjuvant chemotherapy in the management of stage III and IV tumors of the head and neck, *Ca.,* 33, 139, 1983.

27. **Maddox, W. A.,** Vicissitudes of head and neck cancer, *Am. J. Surg.,* 148, 428, 1984.

28. **Shaha, A. R., Spiro, R. H., Shah, J. P., and Strong, E. W.,** Squamous carcinoma of the floor of the mouth, *Am. J. Surg.,* 148, 455, 1984.

29. **Callery, C. D., Spiro, R. H., and Strong, E. W.,** Changing trends in the management of squamous carcinoma of the tongue, *Am. J. Surg.,* 148, 449, 1984.

30. **O'Brien, C. J., Lahr, C. J., Soong, S. -J., Gandour, M. J., Jones, J. M., Urist, M. M., and Maddox, W. A.,** Surgical treatment of early-stage carcinoma of the oral tongue — would adjuvant treatment be beneficial?, *Head Neck Surg.,* 8, 401, 1986.

31. **Front, D., Hardoff, R., and Robinson, E.,** Bone scintigraphy in primary tumors of the head and neck, *Cancer,* 42, 111, 1978.

32. **Baker, H. L., Woodbury, D. H., Krause, C. J., Saxon, K. G., and Stewart, R. C.,** Evaluation of bone scan by scintigraphy to detect subclinical invasion of the mandible by squamous cell carcinoma of the oral cavity, *Otolaryngol. Head Neck Surg.,* 90, 327, 1982.

33. **Welsman, R. A. and Kimmelman, C. P.,** Bone scanning in the assessment of mandibular invasion by oral cavity carcinomas, *Laryngoscope,* 92, 1, 1982.

34. **Muraki, A. S., Mancuso, A. A., Harnsberger, H. R., Johnson, L. P., and Meads, G. B.,** CT of the oropharynx, tongue base, and floor of mouth: normal anatomy and range of variations and applications in staging carcinoma, *Radiology,* 148, 725, 1983.

35. **Sapp, J. P.,** The role of the dentist in the management of patients irradiated for oral cancer, *J. Can. Dent. Assoc.*, 38, 104, 1972.
36. **Carl, W., Schaaf, N. G., and Chen, T. Y.,** Oral care of patients irradiated for cancer of the head and neck, *Cancer*, 30, 448, 1972.
37. **Rubin, R. L. and Doku, H. C.,** Therapeutic radiology — the modalities and their effects on oral tissues, *J. Am. Dent. Assoc.*, 92, 731, 1976.
38. **Beumer, J., III, Harrison, R., Sanders, B., and Kurrasch, M.,** Preradiation dental extractions and the incidence of bone necrosis, *Head Neck Surg.*, 5, 514, 1983.
39. **Beumer, J., Harrison, R., Sanders, B., and Kurrasch, M.,** Osteoradionecrosis: predisposing factors and outcomes of therapy, *Head Neck Surg.*, 6, 819, 1984.
40. **Wynder, E. L., Mushinski, M. H., and Spivak, J. C.,** Tobacco and alcohol consumption in relation to the development of multiple primary cancers, *Cancer*, 40, 1872, 1977.
41. **Tepperman, B. S. and Fitzpatrick, P. J.,** Second respiratory and upper digestive tract cancers after oral cancer, *Lancet*, ii, 547, 1981.
42. **Ildstat, S. T., Bigelow, M. E., and Remensynder, J. P.,** Squamous cell carcinoma of the tongue: a comparison of the anterior two thirds with its base, *Am. J. Surg.*, 146, 456, 1983.
43. Union Internationale Contre le Cancer *TNM Classification of Malignant Tumors,* 3rd ed., Union Internationale, Contre le Cancer, Geneva, 1978.
44. **Platz, M., Fries, R., Hudec, M., Tjoa, A. M., and Wagner, R. R.,** Carcinomas of the oral cavity: analysis of various pretherapeutic classifications, *Head Neck Surg.*, 5, 93, 1982.
45. **Rapidis, A. D., Langdon, J. D., Patel, M. F., and Harvey, P. W.,** STNMP: a new system for the clinico-pathological classification and identification of intra-oral carcinomata, *Cancer*, 39, 204, 1977.
46. **Rich, A. M. and Radden, B. G.,** Prognostic indicators for oral squamous cell carcinoma: a comparison between the TNM and STNMP systems, *Br. J. Oral Maxillofac. Surg.*, 22, 30, 1984.
47. **Pretorius, D. and Taylor, A., Jr.,** The role of nuclear scanning in head and neck surgery, *Head Neck Surg.*, 4, 427, 1982.
48. **Shaefer, S. D., Merkel, M., Diehl, J., Maravilla, K., and Anderson, R.,** Computed tomoghraphic assessment of squamous cell carcinoma of oral and pharyngeal cavities, *Arch. Otolaryngol.*, 108, 688, 1982.
49. **Droulias, C. and Whitehurst, J. O.,** The lymphatics of the tongue in relation to cancer, *Am. Surg.*, 42, 670, 1976.
50. **Crissman, J. D., Gluckman, J., Whitely, J., and Quenelle, D.,** Squamous-cell carcinoma of the floor of the mouth, *Head Neck Surg.*, 3, 2, 1980.
51. **Ali, S., Tiwari, R. M., and Snow, G. B.,** False-positive and false-negative neck nodes, *Head Neck Surg.*, 8, 78, 1985.
52. **Teichgraeber, J. F. and Clairmont, A. A.,** The incidence of occult metastases for cancer of the oral tongue and floor of the mouth: treatment rationale, *Head Neck Surg.*, 7, 15, 1984.
53. **Grandi, C., Alloisio, M., Moglia, D., Podrecca, S., Sala, L., Salvatori, P., and Molinari, R.,** Prognostic significance of lymphatic spread in head and neck carcinomas: therapeutic implications, *Head Neck Surg.*, 8, 67, 1985.
54. **Berger, D. S. and Fletcher, G. H.,** Distant metastases following local control of squamous-cell carcinoma of the nasopharynx, tonsillar fossa, and base of tongue, *Radiology,* 100, 141, 1971.
55. **Probert, J. C., Thompson, R. W., and Bagshaw, M. A.,** Patterns of spread of distant metastases in head and neck cancer, *Cancer*, 33, 127, 1974.
56. **Platz, H., Fries, R., Hudec, M., Tjoa, A. M., and Wagner, R. R.,** The prognostic relevance of various factors at the time of the first admission of the patient, *J. Maxillofac. Surg.*, 11, 3, 1983.
57. **Wanebo, H. J., Jun, M. Y., Strong, E. W., and Oettgen, H.,** T-cell deficiency in patients with squamous cell cancer of the head and neck, *Am. J. Surg.*, 130, 445, 1975.
58. **Moore, C.,** Cigarette smoking and cancer of the mouth, pharynx, and larynx. A continuing study, *JAMA*, 218, 553, 1971.
59. **Teichgraeber, J., Bowman, J., and Goepfert, H.,** New test series for the functional evaluation of oral cavity cancer, *Head Neck Surg.*, 8, 9, 1985.

Chapter 6

TREATMENT OF ORAL CANCER

John M. Wright, John C. O'Brien, Zelig H. Lieberman, John S. Bradfield, and Robert G. Mennel

TABLE OF CONTENTS

I. INTRODUCTION

Surgery and radiation are the primary modalities of therapy for patients with early stage intraoral carcinomas. In some instances, surgery and radiation are equally efficacious, and the decision as to which modality is selected may be based on other factors.

Patients with advanced disease require a multidisciplinary approach to achieve local and regional control. Surgical ablation with radiation and chemotherapy can improve disease control. The role of chemotherapy is still investigational, but its use holds promise for the future. Modalities such as photodynamic therapy[1] and laser surgery[2] are presently being evaluated.

II. SURGICAL ABLATION FOR HEAD AND NECK CANCER

Surgical ablation is the treatment of choice for many patients with oral carcinoma. Excellent disease control rates with good oral function and cosmetic appearance are achieved when treating patients with early localized lesions. Surgery is used with other modalities for patients with advanced disease.

No patient should ever receive treatment without microscopic tissue evaluation and pathologic confirmation of the diagnosis of malignancy. This is best accomplished with a punch or incisional biopsy. It is essential to obtain an adequate amount of representative tissue in order for the pathologist to render a definitive diagnosis. However, larger biopsies, and even suturing, cause tissue reactions that make subsequent clinical evaluation of the lesion more difficult. An adequate biopsy can often be obtained without suturing, and bleeding controlled with pressure or chemical or electrocoagulation. Excisional biopsy should be performed only by a clinician who is prepared to remove the entire lesion adequately and have its margins examined microscopically to ensure complete removal of the lesion[3,4] (see also Chapter 4). If a lesion is suspected to be malignant clinically, the patient is best referred for biopsy to the clinician who will provide the definitive therapy.

Once a positive diagnosis of malignancy is established microscopically, each patient must be clinically staged (see Chapter 5). Clinical staging plays a major role in determining treatment and prognosis. The initial evaluation also includes assessment of cardiovascular, pulmonary, and renal functions, nutritional and functional status, as well as psychosocial aspects of the patient.

It is at this phase of the evaluation just prior to the strategic planning that these factors are taken into consideration and thoroughly evaluated for their influence on the treatment plan. The most important factors are the patient performance status and the support systems available to ensure success of treatment and rehabilitation of the patient.

A. Strategic Planning for Treatment Selection Phase (Integrated Management)

It is essential that a multidisciplinary oral cancer treatment team be organized.[5] It is important that all members of this team examine the patient and review the diagnostic tests, including the pathologic material available, at the time of the initial evaluation. This allows the expertise of each team member to influence the selection of the most appropriate treatment plan for each individual patient.

A support team must also be available to assist the patient and his or her family during the treatment phase, especially during rehabilitation to achieve a return to maximum performance and enable the patient to return to his previous lifestyle and occupation. We use the term integrated management to identify this multidisciplinary approach to the treatment of these patients. Integrated management can result in proper ablation of the patient's carcinoma with appropriate concern and attention given to restoration of function, cosmetic appearance, and rehabilitation.

During the strategy-planning stage the multidisciplinary team reviews treatment options with regard to each individual case. If two modalities are of equal efficacy in the treatment of a particular case, patient factors and preferences may play a role in determining which form of therapy will be used. If one form of treatment is superior, then this will be strongly recommended to the patient and his or her family, realizing that the ultimate decision will be made by the patient.

There are times when the treatment team must recommend that no treatment be given because of mitigating circumstances. No treatment may be better than the misapplication of powerful therapeutic modalities by a well-meaning, overzealous practitioner.

B. Selection of Treatment

Oral cavity carcinomas can be divided into two major categories: early and late stage disease. Selection of treatment for these categories differs and will be addressed individually.

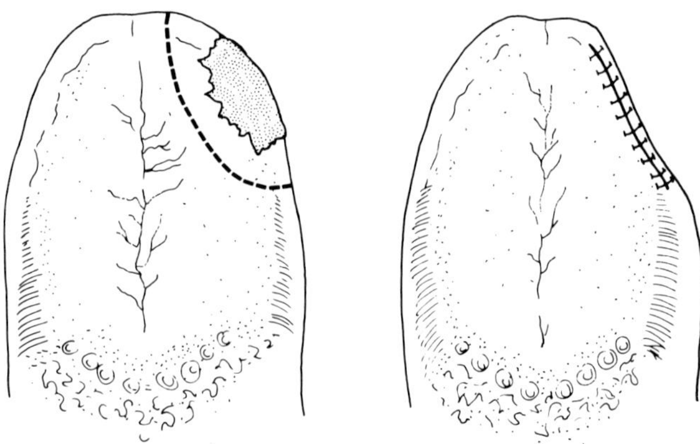

FIGURE 1.   Local resection for small anterior lateral tongue carcinoma with primary closure.

C. Early Stage Disease (Stage I and II)

Stage I (T1, N0, M0) and stage II (T2, N0, M0) carcinomas are small (0 to 2 cm) to moderate (2 to 4 cm) in size with clinically negative nodes. Selection of the treatment modality depends on the type and size of tumor, the patient's personal habits, the potential for developing another primary malignancy, and the availability of facilities and clinicians with experience in the various treatment modalities.

Patients with oral cavity cancer have approximately a 15 to 30% chance of developing a second primary malignancy in the upper aerodigestive tract[6,9] (40% chance for a second primary if the patient continues to smoke and 6% if he or she ceases smoking).[7]

As surgery and radiation generally have equal effectiveness in the treatment of early stage oral cancer,[8] other factors may influence the choice of treatment.

1. Factors Affecting Treatment Selection
a. Type and Size of Tumor

T1 lesions can be resected surgically, and the surgical defect can be closed primarily in most cases (Figure 1) or with a local tissue flap or split thickness skin graft. The amount of tissue which is removed is generally not sufficient to cause major dysfunction of the oral cavity. Rehabilitation is immediate and the patient can resume his life quickly.

Surgical resection of T2 lesions, on the other hand, can potentially cause significant dysfunction of the oral cavity, interfering with speech, handling of saliva, and eating due to loss of substance of the tongue or floor of mouth. There is increased need for grafts and flap reconstruction.

Surgical resection is the treatment of choice for verrucous carcinomas which tend to grow slowly, exophytically, and rarely metastasize.

b. Patient Habits and the Possibility of a Second Primary

Patients who intend to continue using tobacco and alcohol should be treated surgically, if possible, because they have a 40% risk of developing a second primary malignancy.[7] Radiation therapy can generally be given only once in therapeutic dosage. So, if radiation were used for the original small primary, then it would not be available should the patient develop another cancer. Tobacco and alcohol use also increases the severity of the local intraoral reaction to radiation therapy.

c. Availability of Physicians and Facilities

If patients have access to both radiation facilities and experienced surgeons, other factors

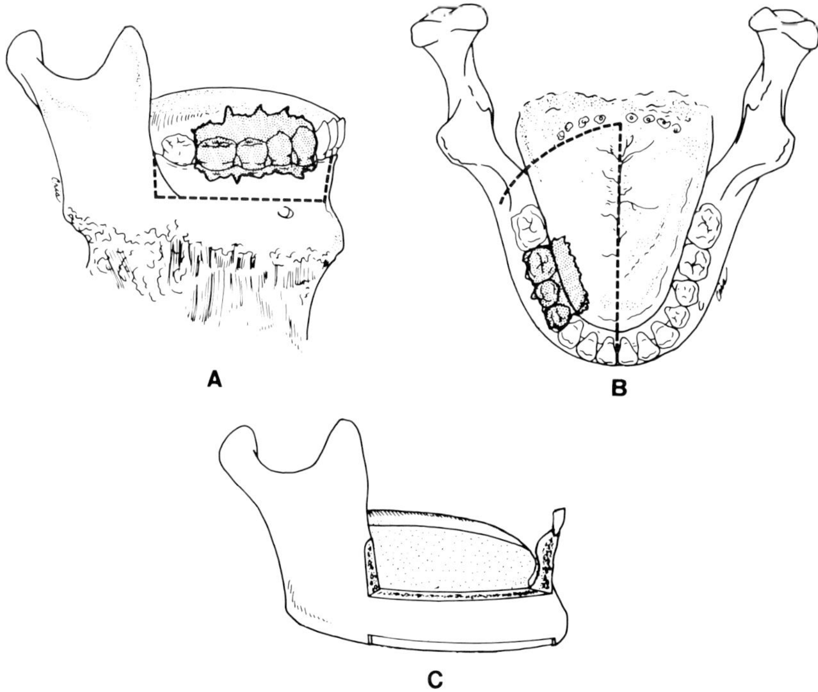

FIGURE 2. (A and B) Planned resection (dotted lines) for carcinoma (shaded) of the lateral tongue, floor of mouth, and mandible. (C) Surgical defect with preservation of the lateral and inferior border of the mandible.

may influence the choice of treatment. However, surgery is often the only choice because remote communities may not have adequate radiation facilities.

d. Patient Preference

If both surgery and radiation offer an equal opportunity to cure the patient, then factors such as occupation and patient preference may affect the choice of treatment modality. A lawyer with a 4-cm carcinoma of the tongue might prefer treatment by radiation to preserve his oral function and speech. A laborer, however, might choose surgery, which could result in altered speech, so that he could return to work more quickly.

e. Surgery vs. Radiation

Surgery is often chosen for early stage disease (to reserve radiation for a possible second primary), for inveterate tobacco and alcohol users, and in patients who desire a shorter treatment and rehabilitation time. Surgery is also indicated in patients with bone involvement. The extent of bone invasion will determine whether marginal resection (Figure 2) or segmental resection of the jaw is performed. A major advantage of surgery is that it does not alter taste or salivary function.

Radiation therapy is chosen for moderate-sized lesions (2 to 4 cm); those lesions with a high probability for nodal metastasis (T2 tongue and floor of mouth)[9] because the primary lesion and draining nodes can be treated; patients who have an occupational or psychological need to maintain the integrity of the function of the oral cavity; and surgical patients with inadequately resected (involved margins) tumors and/or nodal disease, vascular invasion, or perineural involvement.[10-13] Poorly differentiated squamous carcinomas, posterior location, and an exophytic nature are instances where radiation has a high rate of cure. Radiation is also indicated for patients in whom general anesthesia is contraindicated. Xerostomia, increased caries incidence, dysgeusia, and osteoradionecrosis are potential problems following radiation therapy[14,15] (see also Chapter 7).

D. Late Stage Disease (Stage III and IV)

Planned combined therapy of surgery and radiation has resulted in the best local and regional control rates and survival for patients with large cancers and/or metastatic disease.[16]

The timing of radiation can precede or follow surgery with no series showing a decided advantage for either sequence.[8,10,17] Most radiation is now being given in the postoperative period because (1) of the ease of surgery in nonirradiated tissues, (2) full doses of radiation can be given postoperatively whereas doses of 4500 to 5000 rad in the preoperative period can lead to a high incidence of postoperative complications, (3) the extent of disease is better defined by surgery, and (4) the disease is reduced to the microscopic level where radiation is more effective. Proponents of preoperative radiation state that cells are better oxygenated and more radiosensitive when the tumor vascularity is undisturbed by surgery. Certainly, impressive tumor shrinkage can be seen with preoperative radiation.

Surgery is most likely to fail at the periphery of large tumors[16] where the more rapidly growing cancer cells are better oxygenated and, if left behind, can cause local or regional recurrence. Radiation is most likely to fail in the hypoxic center of large cancers[16] where the malignant cells are furthest from the blood supply of the tumor and, hence, less radiosensitive. Thus surgical ablation is used to remove all clinically detectable tumor, and radiation is then used to kill any residual tumor cells.

Patients with large tumors and no clinical nodal disease, but who have a high risk of developing neck node metastasis can be treated with elective postoperative radiation to decrease this risk[10,18] (e.g., T3, N0 tongue has a 50 to 60% chance of having positive nodes).

Patients with perinodal involvement, soft tissue disease, jugular vein or carotid artery involvement, and multiple nodes containing metastatic tumor have a high recurrence rate which can be decreased by postoperative radiation.[8,10,18]

At the present time, in an effort to improve local/regional/distant control, protocols are being studied which use adjuvant chemotherapy, pre- and/or postoperatively.[19-24] As with preoperative irradiation, preoperative chemotherapy may dramatically decrease the size of the tumor. The resection is planned at the initial tumor evaluation and is not altered by the response of the tumor to chemotherapy. Tattooing[25] with India ink can ensure that the entire original tumor bed is resected.

Cervical lymph node dissection is indicated for clinically positive lymph nodes (Figure 3). Confirmation of metastatic disease can be obtained by fine needle aspiration which is extremely accurate in the hands of experienced pathologists (90 + %).[26-28]

Elective or prophylactic neck node dissection is recommended: (1) for cases in which the neck will be entered to facilitate the removal of intraoral tumors; (2) if the patient is at high risk of developing nodal disease (e.g., T2 or T3, N0 of tongue or floor of mouth); and (3) in some cases if the patient will not or cannot return for follow-up.[29] Elective node dissection allows accurate pathologic staging of the disease and can identify patients with a high risk of recurrence. These high risk patients can receive adjunctive postoperative radiation.

In high risk patients with clinically negative nodes or only one positive node (70% accuracy rate of clinical diagnosis),[30] some form of modification of the neck dissection can be performed with acceptable neck recurrence rates.[31] Most modifications[32-34] include preservation of the spinal accessory nerve (XI) to the trapezius. Resection of this nerve causes shoulder drop which is a major aspect of postradical neck dissection morbidity.[35-36] Modified or functional neck dissection for advanced nodal disease (N2 to N3) has a high recurrence rate,[37-38] and this is not recommended.

At times, because of the size of the tumor and involvement of contiguous structures, the proposed resection may achieve heroic proportions. Proper patient selection is imperative.

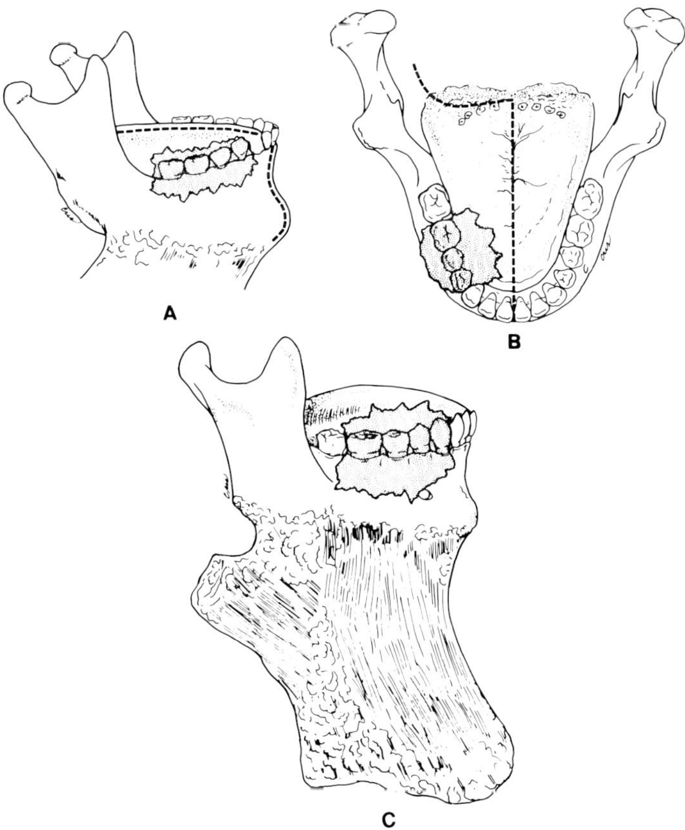

FIGURE 3. (A and B) Planned composite resection (dotted lines) with neck dissection for T3, N1, M0, carcinoma (shaded) of the tongue, floor of mouth, and mandible. (C) Surgical specimen after resection.

If the patient is judged unfit either physically or psychologically for a resection of this magnitude, then radiation and/or chemotherapy may be offered in an attempt at local control.

Patients with advanced disease require careful planning, proper sequencing of treatment modalities, and exacting attention to detail in the ablative portion of the surgical procedure.

E. Follow-Up Phase

After treatment for oral carcinoma, the patient must be followed closely. One member of the treatment team should be designated as the clinician in charge of follow-up. Many members of the team may desire to see the patient following treatment, but one clinician must assume the responsibility. Occasionally, each member of the team believes that another member is following the patient when in actuality no one is following the patient.

Our routine surveillance in the posttreatment phase is an office visit every 2 to 3 months for the first 2 years. During this time, 80 to 90% of all recurrences will occur.[39] Particular attention is paid to local and regional areas with inspection and palpation. Questions about nutrition, weight loss, bone pain, etc. are asked. Chest X-rays at 6 to 12 month intervals are obtained.

After the first 2 years, follow-up is every 6 months for the next 3 years. After 5 years, patients are seen yearly. Late recurrences are uncommon after 5 years, but second primaries are not. It is imperative to examine all mucosal surfaces during each visit in order to detect second primary malignancies.

F. Nutrition

Not uncommonly, patients with head and neck cancer present in a poor nutritional state. Weight, hemoglobin, serum albumin, hepatic function, and delayed hypersensitivity reaction are depressed.

Intravenous total parenteral nutrition (TPN), nasogastric feeding tube, tube jejunostomy, gastrostomy, or peripheral TPN can be used to improve the patient's tolerance to any form of therapy.[40-43] We prefer to use the alimentary tract rather than an i.v. route, if at all possible, as this method is easiest, least expensive, and can generally be performed by the patient and his or her family. TPN necessitates a central venous catheter, expensive parenteral solution, and skilled help in maintaining proper sterile technique. Nevertheless, many patients can be taught home hyperalimentation with visiting nurse support.

G. Laser Surgery

Lasers, both carbon dioxide and argon, are currently being used in the treatment of benign lesions of the oral cavity and protocols involving the treatment of carcinoma *in situ*, and some minimally invasive carcinomas are under investigation.

Several advantages for laser therapy are[1,44] (1) less destruction of normal tissue, (2) less pain, (3) less blood loss, and (4) lymphatics are sealed. The carbon dioxide laser can be used to cut or vaporize tissues. Good visibility is an essential requirement. The field must be dry and vessels larger than 0.5 mm cannot be coagulated by the beam. A disadvantage is that tissue vaporized with superficial treatment is not available for pathologic evaluation.

III. RADIATION THERAPY FOR ORAL CANCER

Malignant tumors of the oral cavity are particularly suitable for treatment by ionizing radiation. These malignancies are easily examined and allow flexibility in choosing radiation therapy from an external source, i.e., a linear accelerator or radiation from an internally implanted isotope such as ^{192}Ir. These two modes of delivering ionizing radiation may be used either alone or in combination.

A. Physical Principles[45]

Ionizing radiation dissipates its energy in tissues by interacting with the loosely bound, outermost orbital electrons of the atoms of the tissue radiated. X-rays from a high energy (4 to 25 million eV) linear accelerator or γ-rays (1.17 and 1.33 million eV) from a ^{60}Co teletherapy unit are the most common types of external radiation used in the treatment of cancer of the oral cavity. X-rays and γ-rays comprise that end of the electromagnetic spectrum with the highest energy. Ionizing radiation useful for radiotherapy may be of relatively low energy (less than 1000 KeV) and is called orthovoltage radiation or may be of higher energy (usually 4 to 25 million eV) and is called supervoltage radiation. Orthovoltage X-rays have limited tissue penetration and may be useful in treating carcinomas of the skin and lip; supervoltage X-rays are more penetrating and are used in the treatment of carcinoma of the oral cavity. Supervoltage has the advantage of a "skin sparing" effect; that is, the point of maximum energy deposition (Dmax) is below the skin and delivers a greater dosage at 5 cm depth (a typical midplane point of calculation for intraoral carcinoma).

In addition to electromagnetic ionizing radiation, electrons, protons, α-particles, neutrons, negative pi-mesons, and heavy charged ions may be used as particulate radiation. The most useful of these is the electron beam generated from a linear accelerator at energies commonly ranging from 6 to 21 million eV. Electron beams are useful in treating neck nodes while sparing underlying critical structures.

B. Unit of Dose

The biological changes that occur in tissues as a result of ionizing radiation are dependent on the amount of energy absorbed in those tissues, and a measure of this energy deposition is defined as the rad (an acronym for "radiation absorbed dose"), where 1 rad = 100 ergs/g = 10^2 J/kg. In the international system of units, the gray (Gy) is defined as 1 Gy = 1 J/kg and 1 Gy = 100 rad.

C. Radiobiological Principles[46]

Macromolecules, i.e., DNA, RNA, and complex proteins within the cell, can be directly ionized and result in cell death, but most radiation-induced cellular injury occurs by indirect action. Radiation ionizes water molecules which leads to a series of reactions that gives rise to free radicals. The free radicals may combine to form free water, hydrogen peroxide, (itself toxic to cells), or additional free radicals. The formation of free radicals is the major factor in radiation-induced cell injury. Radiation in the electromagnetic spectrum primarily exerts its lethal effects indirectly by the formation of free radicals while particulate radiation affects cells more directly.

The role of oxygen in the response of malignant tumors to radiation is critical, since the ionization of water and subsequent formation of free radicals is strongly dependent upon the presence of oxygen in the tissues which are being irradiated.

D. Dose Response Curves

Intuitively one would suspect that the higher the radiation dose the greater the number of cells killed within the volume radiated. This cell response to radiation dose is not linear, however, and follows a log-linear response first described in vitro by radiating cells in tissue culture.[47] Cells exposed to ionizing radiation in the electromagnetic spectrum under anoxic conditions are much more radioresistant than oxygenated cells. Doses of 150 to 300 rad are required to expect killing of cultured mammalian cells on the straight-line portion of the dose response curve. The presence of oxygen has less effect on cell killing with α-particles since particulate radiation exerts its effects directly.

E. The Four Rs of Radiobiology

1. Redistribution

The sensitivity of a cell to radiation is dependent on its position in the cell cycle. The cell cycle consists of mitosis (M) and DNA synthesis (S) separated by two gaps (G1 and G2). Tumor cells are significantly more radiosensitive during mitosis, the junction of G1 and S, and in late G2. At any given time, the cells of a tumor are in all positions of the cell cycle. At the time of radiation, cells in the radiosensitive phases of the cell cycle will be killed while many cells in the radioresistant phases will be spared. These surviving cells would be more responsive to future courses of radiation therapy as they enter more radio-sensitive stages of the cell cycle. This redistribution of cells within the cell cycle contributes to the effectiveness of daily or fractionated radiotherapy.

2. Repair of Sublethal Damage

An optimal time interval between doses of radiation cannot be estimated for a given asynchronous cell population in a human tumor. There are some differences in surviving fraction of cells with increasing intervals between doses of radiation for asynchronous cells irradiated in vitro. An increase in surviving fraction is noted up to 4 hr between two doses of radiation. This phenomenon, repair of sublethal damage, may progress more rapidly and to a greater degree in normal tissues than in (hypoxic) malignant tumors. This differential response is the basis for altered fractionation schemes, i.e., hyperfractionation (dividing a daily dose into two or three smaller doses given at intervals during the day) or accelerated fractionation (giving two conventional daily doses in the same day at less than 12 hr intervals).[48]

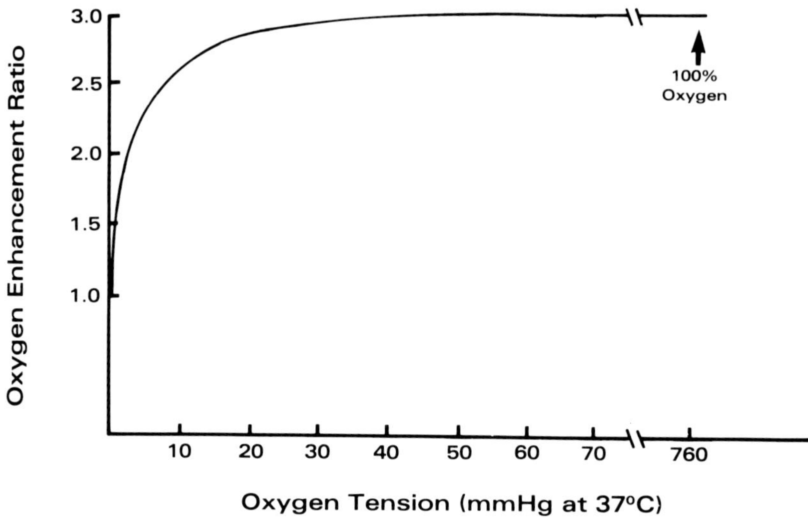

FIGURE 4.   Enhancement of radiation sensitivity by increasing oxygen tension.

3. Repopulation

The third factor in the contest for survival between normal and malignant cells exposed to ionizing radiation is repopulation. A "feedback" control that stimulates the regrowth of normal cells lost by radiation injury does not exist for malignant cell populations. This situation then favors the repopulation or regrowth of normal cell populations over malignant cells with fractionated radiotherapy.[49]

4. Reoxygenation

Cells irradiated at extremely low oxygen concentrations are relatively radioresistant. Figure 4 demonstrates the relative radiosensitivity of cells irradiated at varying oxygen tensions and demonstrates that there is a 2.5- to 3.0-fold increase in radiosensitivity of well-oxygenated cells over cells irradiated under anoxic conditions. This multiple (2.5 to 3.0) is called the oxygen-enhancement ratio (OER).

Solutions to the problem of radioresistant hypoxic tumor cells have been a major goal of research in radiation biology. Partial solutions to tumor hypoxia have evolved in the treatment of cancer of the oral cavity, but the mainstay of improved oxygenation (and thus improved radiosensitivity) is fractionated radiotherapy. As the better oxygenated, radiosensitive cells within the tumor (presumably cells close to tumor vasculature) are killed and removed from the tumor site, more hypoxic radioresistant cells acquire a position of better oxygenation with decreasing tumor volume.

Other approaches to the problem of hypoxic, radioresistant tumor cell populations that are applicable in the treatment of cancer of the oral cavity are densely ionizing, particulate radiation beams, especially fast neutrons,[50] and heavy charged particles whose dose response shows no difference between well-oxygenated and hypoxic cells; surgery as an adjunct to radiation to remove large, hypoxic cell populations after radiotherapy, i.e., in poorly responsive large (greater than 3 cm) neck nodes;[51] hypoxic cell sensitizers analogous to misonidazole which mimic the action of oxygen by "fixing" the damage to macromolecules induced by radiation;[52] and the combination of hyperthermia and interstitial radiotherapy.[53] Hyperthermia is complementary to ionizing radiation in that hypoxic cells and cells in radioresistant phases of the cell cycle are preferentialy killed by hyperthermia (greater than 42.5°C).[54] All of these approaches are investigative, but offer promise for the future.

Table 1
FREQUENCY OF CERVICAL METASTASIS IN T1 AND T2

	T1	T2
Clinically palpable	5/67	7/43[a]
	(7.5%)	(16.3%)
Clinically negative but neck dissection positive	3/67	5/43
	(4.5%)	(11.6%)
Total with neck nodes at presentation	8/67	9/43
	(12%)	(20.9%)
Subsequent to treatment (clinically negative neck)	6/62	6/36
	(9.6%)	(16.7%)
Total T1, N0; T2, N0 (lines 2 and 4)	9/62	11/36
	(14.5%)	(30.6%)
Total T1, Nx; T2, Nx (lines 1,2, and 4)	14/67	15/43
	(20.9%)	(34.9%)

[a] Includes three patients with palpable neck nodes, but no node metastases at time of neck dissection (these three patients are not included in final totals).

Table 2
FREQUENCY OF CERVICAL METASTASIS IN T1 BY SIZE OF PRIMARY

	T1a ($\leq$1.0 cm)	T1b ($>$1.0 cm)
Clinically palpable	2/33 (6.1%)	3/34 (8.8%)
Clinically negative but neck dissection positive	0/33 (0%)	3/34 (8.8%)
Total with neck nodes at presentation	2/33 (6.1%)	6/34 (17.6%)
Subsequent to treatment (clinically negative neck)	3/31 (9.7%)	3/31 (9.7%)
Total T1 N0 (lines 2 and 4)	3/31 (9.7%)	6/31 (19.4%)
Total T1, Nx (lines 1,2, and 4)	5/33 (15.2%)	9/34 (26.5%)

F. Clinical Applications

Treatment volume is determined by the precise tumor volume and its localization. Treatment planning for radiation therapy is, therefore, dependent on meticulous physical evaluation of the patient (Chapter 5). As treatment progresses, the mouth allows direct observation of the response of both normal and malignant tissues. The small volume of the mouth and severity of normal tissue response to radiation demand that the treatment volume be precisely defined and daily treatments reproduced accurately.

Despite careful physical examination and increasingly sophisticated imaging studies, it remains difficult to estimate the risk of occult spread of carcinoma of the oral cavity to the neck. As a model of that relative risk, a study of the patients with squamous cell carcinoma of the anterior two thirds of the tongue treated at Baylor University Medical Center[55] indicates that the risk of occult, nonpalpable cervical metastases is approximately 14.5% in patients with T1 primaries and 30.6% in patients with T2 primaries (Table 1). If the patients with T1 primaries are further subdivided by size, then those patients with primary lesions less than or equal to 1.0 cm have a 9.7% risk of occult cervical metastases, and those patients whose primary lesions are greater than 1.0 cm have a 19.4% risk of occult cervical metastases (Table 2). Vermund et al.[56] reported that the ultimate control rate in the neck for patients who were initially N0, but developed cervical metastasis subsequent to primary therapy was 33% in T1 patients and 16% in T2 patients. The decision, then, to irradiate the neck (or treat it surgically) depends in part on the size of the primary tumor and the ability to salvage the patient who does recur in the neck. The relative risk of failure in the neck, if untreated, must be weighed against the risks of complications secondary to large field neck radiation (Chapter 7).

1. Dose Prescriptions

The dose prescribed for control of the majority of early (T1 and T2) squamous cell carcinomas of the oral cavity ranges from 6500 to 7000 rad given in 33 to 35 fractions at a rate of 180 to 200 rad/day over $6^{1}/_{2}$ to 7 weeks. More advanced lesions are usually treated in combination with chemotherapy and surgery. If treated with radiation alone, advanced lesions will require doses approximating 7500 rad in 35 to 40 fractions over $7^{1}/_{2}$ to 9 weeks. This dose range is very narrow and errors of 10% will result in either local failure if too low or complications if too high. Mathematical models have been developed which can predict the probability of local control based on T stage, N stage, site of tumor, and the patient's grouped Karnofsky performance status.[57]

In order to achieve these high doses to the primary tumor yet cover areas potentially at risk but clinically uninvolved (i.e., the clinically negative neck in a T2, N0 carcinoma of the anterior two thirds of the tongue), methods have been developed to increase the dose of radiation to the obvious tumor. The simplest of these is a "reducing-field" technique whereby the treatment field size is reduced in one or more stages as the treatment progresses. A more common boost technique in cancer of the oral cavity is interstitial therapy with radioactive isotopes. This is discussed in a later section.

It is desirable to describe the radiation dosage at multiple points within a patient and, in fact, to give a pictorial representation of an infinite number of points for the distribution of radiation. Isodose curves (Figure 5) give us that picture and are so called because the dose at each point on a given line is the same. The contour of the patient will affect the distribution of the radiation since thinner body parts (the anterior portion of the oral cavity) will receive more radiation at the midline than thicker body parts (the posterior portion of the oral cavity). The patient's contour, normal anatomy, and tumor volume, whether drawn free-hand or derived from computed axial tomography, are included in the calculation of the isodose curves. Computers assist the radiation oncologist in rapidly deriving several sets of isodose curves from which he selects the one treatment plan that maximizes tumor dose and minimizes the dose to normal tissues. The dose may be prescribed to the mid-plane or to a volume encompassed by a percent isodose.

2. Daily Treatment Delivery: Accuracy vs. Reproducibility

The data acquired at simulation and treatment planning must be transferred to the treatment unit, and daily treatments performed in an accurate and reproducible fashion. The importance of this is illustrated in Figure 6. Despite accurate simulation and treatment planning, the patient in Figure 6A will fail treatment because of the lack of reproducibility of daily treatments. A relatively small portion of the intended treatment volume is included in each daily treatment. The patient in Figure 6B will also fail treatment because, despite reproducible daily treatments, errors were made in the initial simulation and treatment planning phase, and a portion of the tumor volume is never treated. The patient in Figure 6C has the best chance for control of tumor since, although there are minor variations of the treatment boundary with daily treatment, all of the tumor volume is included in each daily treatment.

Accuracy in the simulator is dependent on thorough clinical evaluation and correlation of imaging studies by the radiotherapist. Treatment accuracy and reproducibility can be enhanced by various patient immobilization devices, i.e., a bite-block made from a paraffin impression of the patient's teeth which is mounted to the treatment couch. Other devices, i.e., plaster casts, lasers, and Polaroid® photos of the patient in the treatment position, improve treatment accuracy and reproducibility.

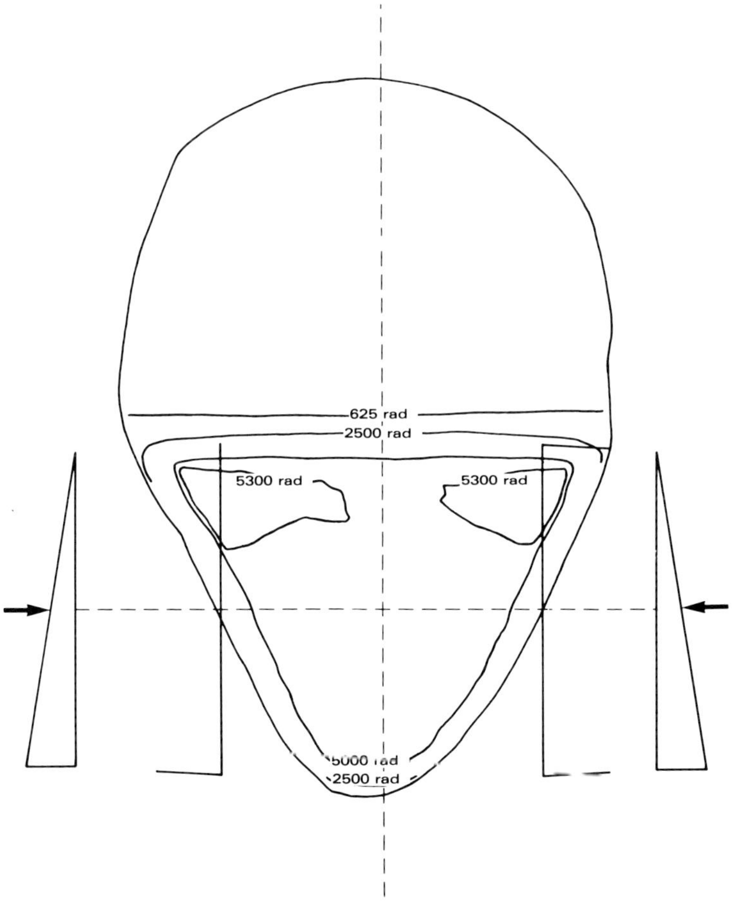

FIGURE 5. Isodose curve showing distribution of radiation in the oral cavity using opposed, wedge 4 mV X-ray fields.

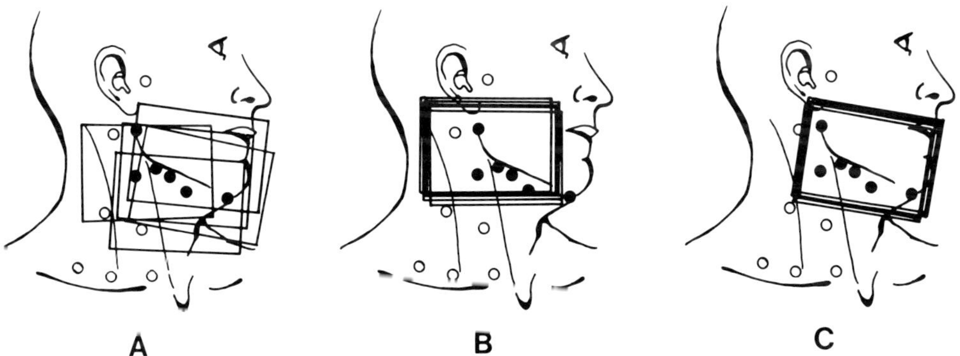

FIGURE 6. Accuracy of tumor assessment and reproducibility of daily radiation doses. (A) Lack of reproducibility. (B) Reproducible, inaccurate assessment of tumor volume. (C) Reproducible, accurate assessment of tumor volume.

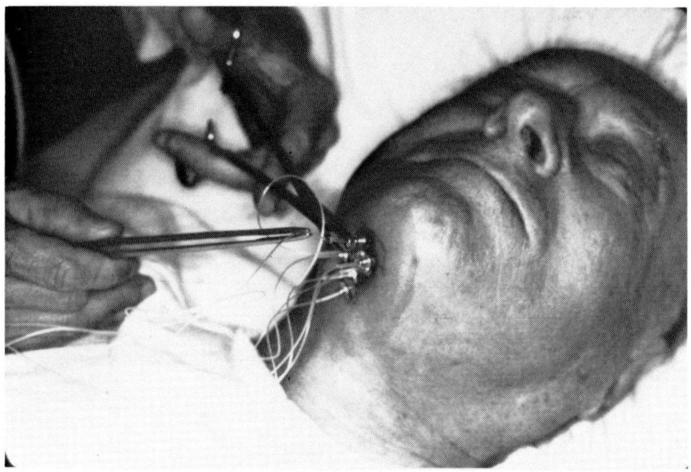

FIGURE 7. Active implants being placed via catheters.

3. Interstitial Radiotherapy

Interstitial radiotherapy, the implantation of radioactive isotopes into tissue, has application both as the primary therapy for selected, early carcinomas and as a boost for larger lesions treated with external radiotherapy. Radium needles have been used traditionally as a temporary implant which, when inserted according to certain patterns and strengths, gives a predictable distribution of radiation to the volume implanted. The Quimby method[58] provides a regular distribution of radium with a nonhomogeneous, but predictable, pattern of dose distribution. The Patterson-Parker method[59] provides a homogeneous distribution of dose when the radium is inserted according to prescribed rules. Since the intensity of radiation decreases inversely as the square of the distance from the source of radiation, structures such as the mandible and parotid salivary glands receive relatively little radiation.

Radium as an isotope for interstitial therapy in oral cavity cancer is being supplanted by ^{192}Ir.[60] This isotope is available as seeds embedded in plastic ribbons which may be inserted into tissues by an afterloading technique. With the afterloading technique, stainless steel 17-gauge needles are inserted under general anesthesia without radiation exposure to the physician and operating room personnel. Flexible catheters are then inserted via the path of the needles as the needles are removed. Upon recovery from anesthesia, orthogonal films are made of the patient's implant with inactive seeds placed in the catheters. Rapid calculation of the isodose curves may then be produced with a computer based on the arrangement of the inactive seeds. The active ^{192}Ir is then placed via the catheters, thus minimizing radiation exposure to personnel and allowing more flexibility in the positioning of the isotope (Figure 7). When combined with external radiation of 5000 rad in 25 fractions, an interstitial implant of 2500 rad may be given as a boost to the primary site of 40 to 50 rad/hr in 50 to 62.5 hr.

^{125}I, an isotope emitting a very low energy γ-ray and having a low dose rate, may be used as palliative therapy in patients who have local recurrence despite high dose radiation and surgery. This type of permanent implant is associated with minimal patient discomfort and infrequent complications.[61]

Although interstitial radiotherapy is applicable to the treatment of both carcinomas of the anterior two thirds of the tongue and the floor of the mouth, such therapy entails greater risk for the patient with carcinoma of the floor of the mouth since the implanted volume is closer to the mandible with the attendant risks of gingival ulceration and exposure of the mandible. Despite these risks the implant must include deep tumor extension into the soft tissues from the floor of the mouth either with a "pallisading" technique using radium needles[62] or an afterloading technique with ^{192}Ir.

Table 3

**CARCINOMA ANTERIOR TWO THIRDS OF
TONGUE LOCAL CONTROL WITH
RADIATION AS INITIAL THERAPY**

Author/stage	T1	T2	T3	
Delclos[66a]	18/18	56/57	22/27	(All T1—3)
(2 yr FU)	(100%)	(98%)	(81%)	
Fu[67]	10/12	28/38	3/8	(All T1—3)
(3 yr FU)	(83%)	(74%)	(38%)	
Gilbert[68a]	10/11	5/8	13/36	(All T1—3)
(5 yr FU)	(91%)	(63%)	(36%)	
Marks[70a]	14/16	10/19	1/3	(T1—3, N0)
(2 yr FU)	(88%)	(53%)	(33%)	
Mendenhall[69a]	8/8	22/27	12/22	(T1—3, N0)
(2 yr FU)	(100%)	(81%)	(55%)	
BUMC[55a]	16/16	12/17	—	(T1, 2, N0)
(2 yr FU)	(100%)	(71%)		

[a] Includes ultimate control with surgical salvage (contributes approximately 10% to local control when all series and stages are summed).

4. Intraoral Cones

In edentulous patients with small anterior lesions of the tongue and floor of the mouth, treatment may be given with an intraoral cone.[63-65] The cone is positioned by a stent placed in the mouth which fixes the relationship of the cone to the lesion. This approach has been used both with orthovoltage X-ray and electron beam and may be used alone for a small lesion or as a boost in combination with external radiotherapy.

G. Goals of Therapy

Local tumor control and cure of the patient are the first considerations in selecting the method of treatment for oral cancer patients. Nevertheless, one must also consider the side effects and morbidity associated with each modality of therapy.

If radiation is selected, is the loss of taste and salivary gland function and the risk of osteoradionecrosis worth the preservation of speech and deglutition offered by radiation therapy? Additionally, one must consider the cosmetic result of treatment. The absence of surgical deformity makes radiotherapy appealing to some patients; however, subcutaneous edema and fibrosis are definite functional and cosmetic side effects. The acute and chronic sequelae of radiation therapy will be discussed in Chapter 7.

Many patients with oral cancer are not curable. The goal of therapy may be palliation in patients with advanced local disease, distant metastasis, or poor general health. Palliation still requires 5500 to 6000 rad or more for local tumor control. Local control in this circumstance means control of the tumor at the primary site for the duration of the patient's life. Distant metastasis may also be palliated effectively with radiation therapy.

H. Results of Treatment

1. Carcinoma of the Anterior Two Thirds of the Tongue and Floor of Mouth

The results of treatment of carcinoma of the anterior two thirds of the tongue and floor of mouth have shown that satisfactory results may be obtained in early lesions (stage I and II) with radiation alone (Tables 3 and 4). Local control rates of 83 to 100% for T1 lesions and 59 to 98% for T2 lesions of the anterior two thirds of the tongue have been reported.[55,66-70] If an excisional biopsy has been done for small lesions of the tongue or floor of

Table 4
CARCINOMA OF THE FLOOR OF MOUTH
LOCAL CONTROL WITH RADIATION AS
INITIAL THERAPY

Author/stage	T1	T2	T3	
Aygun[62a]	15/18	17/20	4/9	(T1—3, N0)
(2 yr FU)	(83%)	(85%)	(44%)	
Delclos[66a]	9/10	22/24	8/9	(All T1—3)
2 yr FU	(90%)	(92%)	(89%)	
Fu[72a]	33/37	24/31	4/8	(T1—3, N0)
(2 yr FU)	(89%)	(77%)	(50%)	
Gilbert[68a]	22/26	7/14	3/15	(All T1—3)
(5 yr FU)	(84%)	(50%)	(20%)	
Marks[73a]	11/14	12/15	1/4	(All T1—3)
(2 yr FU)	(79%)	(80%)	(25%)	
Mendenhall[69]	14/16	16/17	17/25	(All T1—3)
(2 yr FU)	(87%)	(94%)	(68%)	

[a]   Includes ultimate control with surgical salvage (contributes approximately 10% to local control when all series and stages are summed).

mouth, one may expect a high probability of local control (100%) with interstitial therapy alone at doses in the range of 5500 to 6000 rad. At this dose soft tissue and bone necrosis is rare and function is preserved.[71] The combination of external radiotherapy with interstitial therapy may compensate for dose inhomogeneity of an implant alone, especially for large lesions,[66] but an implant alone allows for greater dose over a shorter period of time with theoretical improvement in local control.[69] Local control rates of 83 to 92% for T2 carcinomas for the floor of the mouth have been reported.[62,66,68,69,72,73] The above data are based on 2-year minimum follow-up and include up to 19% of patients surgically salvaged after local recurrence following radiation alone. A broader view of the results of radiotherapy for squamous cell carcinoma of the oral tongue and floor of mouth may be obtained from the Patterns of Care Study initiated in 1971 to improve quality and accessibility of radiation therapy care in the U.S. This study provided a profile of the results of radiotherapy for 434 patients treated in 97 institutions in 1973. By stage, 75% of stage I, 59% of stage II, 43% of stage III, and 21% of stage IV patients are free of recurrence at 4 years.[74]

2. Retromolar Trigone and Anterior Tonsillar Pillar

Squamous cell carcinomas of the retromolar trigone and anterior tonsillar pillar may be treated with radiation alone in early stages (I and II). Care must be taken, however, to exclude involvement of the mandible by Panorex radiographs or computed tomography (CT) scanning. Lower cervical and contralateral neck involvement is quite rare in early lesions of the retromolar trigone and anterior tonsillar pillar. Stage I and II cancers, therefore, may be treated with external beam radiation. The goal of therapy is to deliver 6500 to 7000 rad in 33 to 35 fractions over $6^{1}/_{2}$ to 7 weeks. Field arrangement can allow the primary lymphatic drainage on the ipsilateral side to be included in the treatment volume. Patients with T1 and T2 primaries, but limited (N1) cervical metastases, may be treated with radiation alone or a combination of chemotherapy and radiation. In this circumstance the lower neck and contralateral neck must be prophylactically treated to 5000 to 5500 rad. More advanced disease (T3, 4 and/or N2, 3) requires a multimodality approach with chemotherapy, surgery, and radiotherapy. One may expect to control approximately 80% of T1 and 70% of T2 lesions of the retromolar trigone with radiation alone (Table 5).[75-78]

Table 5
CARCINOMA OF THE LATERAL ORAL CAVITY LOCAL
CONTROL BY RADIATION WITHOUT SURGICAL SALVAGE

	Retromolar trigone		Lower gum		Buccal mucosa	
Author/site	**T1**	**T2**	**T1**	**T2**	**T1**	**T2**
Fletcher[75,76]	22/26 (85%)	83/103 (81%)	8/9 (89%)	18/21 (86%)	10/10 (100%)	30/33 (91%)
Million[77]	4/4 (100%)	2/8 (25%)	1/1 (100%)	1/5 (20%)	—	—
Wang[78a]	20/26 (77%)	54/91 (59%)	7/11 (64%)	4/16 (25%)	1/4 (25%)	13/31 (42%)

[a] NED.

3. Gingiva and Hard Palate

Treatment of gingival lesions with radiation is limited to small, mobile lesions with no radiographic evidence of bone involvement. Bone involvement precludes radiation therapy as the primary treatment modality. Treatment of early lesions delivers 4500 to 5000 rad to the entire bone, boosting the primary site to 6500 to 7000 rad via a reducing field technique. Alternatively, an intraoral cone may be used in an edentulous patient either as the only therapy or, preferably, as a boost. Limited data in the literature suggests that approximately 75% of T1 and 55% of T2 lesions of the lower gum may be controlled with radiation alone (Table 5).[75,76,78]

The rare patient with squamous cell carcinoma of the hard palate is best treated surgically, although occasional patients with small lesions have been treated with external beam therapy and boosting with an intraoral cone.

4. Buccal Mucosa

Early T1 lesions of the buccal mucosa are most expediently treated with wide local excision with little functional or cosmetic impairment to the patient. A combination of chemotherapy, surgery, and radiation is indicated for patients with advanced (T3, 4 or any N) lesion. Selected patients with T2 squamous cell carcinomas of the buccal mucosa may be treated with a combination of electron beam and photons to deliver 5000 to 5500 rad in 25 to 30 fractions in 5 to 6 weeks (Figure 8). A boost is given with interstitial ^{192}Ir, the isotope being inserted via catheters placed externally through the skin. This approach through the skin allows better coverage of the superior and inferior margins of the tumor than an intraoral technique. Care must be taken that the primary site does not involve the gingiva or retromolar trigone in which case interstitial therapy would not be satisfactory. Buccal mucosal carcinomas frequently spread to the cervical lymph nodes[79] which must be treated, even if negative by palpation. Approximately 80% of T1 and 65 to 70% of T2 carcinomas of the buccal mucosa are controlled by radiation alone (Table 5).[75,78]

5. Soft Palate

Squamous cell carcinomas of the soft palate and uvula are very amenable to radiation therapy. These cancers are frequently associated with premalignant lesions. Patients selected for treatment with radiation must be observed closely in the first 2 weeks of therapy to detect early mucosal reaction or "tumoritis". This sign of occult mucosal involvement will help the radiotherapist judge the adequacy of his treatment volume. Opposed, lateral X-ray fields treating to the midline to give 6600 to 7000 rad in 33 to 35 fractions over $6^{1}/_{2}$ to 7

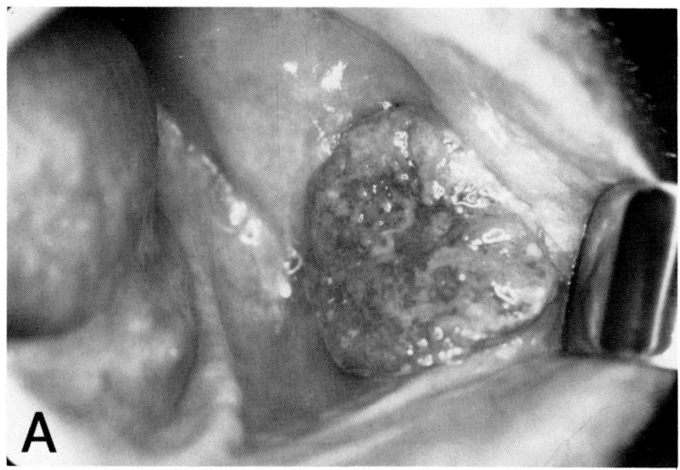

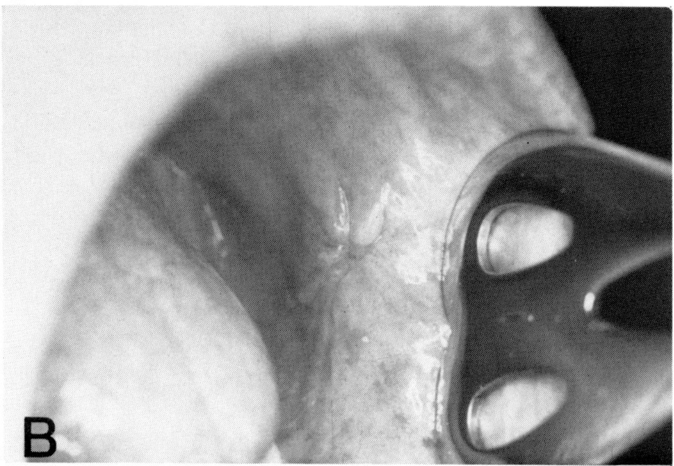

FIGURE 8.   (A)T2 carcinoma of the buccal mucosa. (B) Resolution of the lesion following treatment with radiotherapy.

weeks are indicated for early T1 and T2 lesions. The lower neck need not be treated in N0 patients. However, the upper cervical nodes should be treated to 5000 rad reducing the fields at that dose to deliver a boost to 7000 rad to the primary site. Greater than 90% of T1 patients and 70% of T2 patients have no detectable disease at 3 years.[78]

6. Lip

Squamous cell carcinoma of the lip involves the lower lip in approximately 90% of the cases. The majority of these lesions are small (less than one third of the lip), well-differentiated squamous cell carcinomas in men subjected to chronic sun exposure. Cancers of this size and differentiation may be treated most expediently with surgical V-excision or some modification of that approach. Although radiotherapy may be used in small lesions of the lower lip, the cosmetic result, because of radiation fibrosis, is usually inferior to excision.

Larger lesions (greater than one third of the lip) are best treated with fractionated radiotherapy. Doses of 5000 to 6000 rad in 4 to 6 weeks (20 to 30 fractions) will result in a high probability of local control and a satisfactory functional and cosmetic result. An intraoral shield of wax-coated lead is inserted between the lip and gingiva to protect the underlying gum. Interstitial radiotherapy may be used alone for small lesions or as a boost for larger lesions when combined with external radiotherapy.

Massive lesions of the lower lip involving the mandible, mental nerve, and the commissures of the lip or tumors with extensive soft tissue defects are best managed surgically with reconstruction and then followed by postoperative radiation.

Patients who present with nodal metastases are best treated with surgery to remove both the primary lesion and the nodal disease followed by postoperative radiation.

Squamous cell carcinoma of the upper lip, even when clinically small, may be treated with fractionated radiotherapy to achieve a satisfactory functional and cosmetic result. Care must be taken to include the primary site with generous margins, particularly if the primary is adjacent to the nasal ala or near the commissure of the lip.

Whether treated with radiation or surgery, the prognosis is excellent for squamous cell carcinoma of the lip. One can expect a 5-year determinate survival of 95% for patients with T1 and T2 lesions.[80] Even patients with more advanced lesions or those who recur can be salvaged with combined modality therapy and careful treatment planning.

IV. CHEMOTHERAPY

The use of chemotherapy for head and neck cancer is relatively new and, at present, is generally considered investigational.[81-84] No drug or combination of drugs has been shown effective as a single therapeutic modality for head and neck cancer. Chemotherapy is primarily used for patients with systemic metastasis or as an adjunct to surgery and radiation in stage III and IV disease.

A. Biological Rationale for Using Chemotherapy

Ideally, controlling oral cancer is based on exploiting differences between normal and neoplastic cells. Tumor cell replication outpaces that of normal cells and is accompanied by an increase in nucleic acid synthesis and replication. A variety of drugs effectively alter the structure and/or function of DNA and result in cytotoxic damage and cell death. Unfortunately, chemotherapeutic agents cannot distinguish between dividing tumor cells and normal cells (see complications, Chapter 7).

At any given time, the cells of a malignancy are in all stages of cellular replication. The different categories of chemotherapeutic agents exert their cytotoxic effects at different stages of the cell cycle or at different stages of DNA or RNA production. Many tumors, therefore, respond more completely to a combination of drugs. Drug regimens are also commonly given sequentially to allow time between treatments for the reversal of the cytotoxic effects on normal cells.

B. Theoretical Considerations

Failure of surgery and/or radiation therapy to control oral cancer is generally due to local recurrence or regional metastases. Patients with stage III and IV head and neck cancer have a 70% incidence of local recurrence and a 30% incidence of systemic metastases,[85,86] and the rationale for using chemotherapy is to reduce the incidence of these causes of failure. Since the survival of patients with recurrent disease or systemic metastases averages only 3 to 4 months, there is clearly a potential role for systemic treatment in these patients. There are some patients with early stage disease (stages I and II) who are at high risk for recurrence who might also benefit from chemotherapy. Prognostic factors which have been shown in other studies to identify this high-risk group include the primary site, tumor grade, nutritional status, and performance status,[87-93] regardless of their clinical stage.

Excluding the treatment of systemic metastases, the major use of chemotherapy has been prior to surgery or radiation therapy in stage III and IV disease. The rationale for this is to

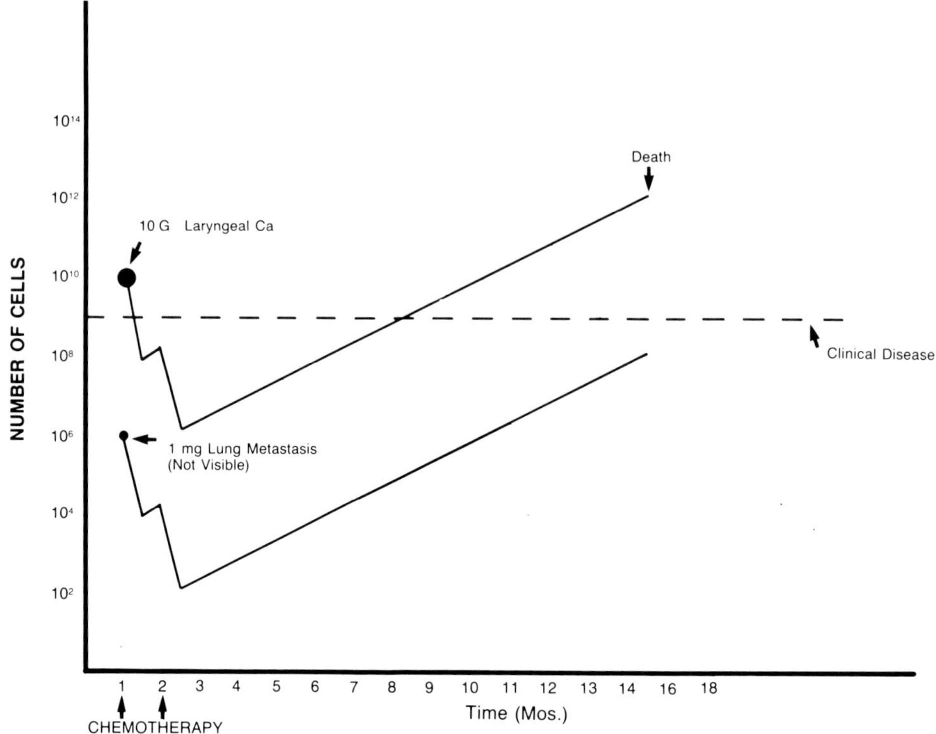

FIGURE 9.   Theoretical effect of two courses of chemotherapy on a nonresistant tumor when each course kills 99% of the tumor cells.

reduce the high recurrence rate in late stage head and neck cancer. Since most of these patients are clinically disease free after surgery or radiation therapy, recurrence must result from residual microscopic disease. It has been demonstrated that a significant tumor burden can be undetectable clinically. The log kill hypothesis states that a fixed percentage, not a fixed number of tumor cells, is killed each time a particular patient is treated with the same dose of a cytotoxic drug. Therefore, chemotherapy could eradicate microscopic disease at distant sites and reduce the primary tumor to microscopic, residual disease. Theoretically, surgery or radiation therapy could then be employed to eliminate the residual, primary disease and reduce the chance of local failure. Figure 9 demonstrates a theoretical course that a nonresistant tumor with microscopic lung metastases might follow if treated with two courses of chemotherapy when each course of chemotherapy kills 99% of the tumor. Although the two courses of chemotherapy are not curative, the therapy provides a 7-month disease-free interval. Theoretically, the patient might be cured if additional chemotherapy was given and the primary tumor was resected. Figure 10 demonstrates complete resolution of a primary tumor after chemotherapy.

The majority of studies have been designed with chemotherapy given prior to surgery or radiation therapy, because the delivery of chemotherapy to the tumor requires an intact vasculature, which surgery and radiation therapy disrupt. On the other hand, radiation therapy prior to chemotherapy may actually enhance the cytotoxic effect of the drug. Neoplastic cells in hypoxic areas of large tumors have a reduced replication rate and are, therefore, more drug resistant. As discussed in radiation biology, radiation may shrink large tumors and increase oxygenation and replication, thereby rendering the tumor more drug sensitive. The ideal sequencing of chemotherapy with other treatment modalities has not been established in humans. One study failed to show an advantage of surgery and pre- vs. postoperative chemotherapy.[94] Although there is no good evidence to prove the effectiveness of pre- or

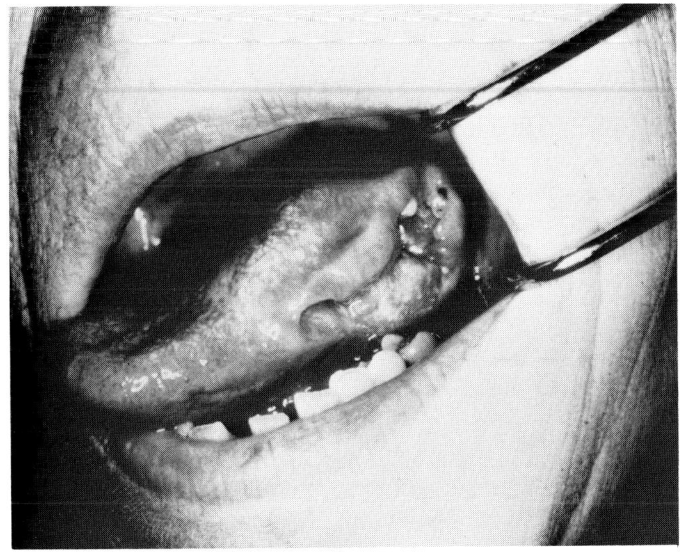

A

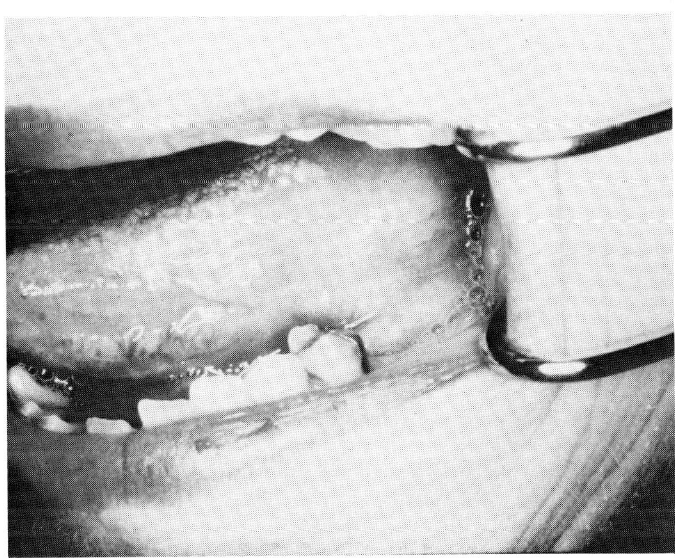

B

FIGURE 10.   (A) Carcinoma of the lateral border of the tongue. (B) Resolution of the lesion following chemotherapy.

postoperative chemotherapy in human head and neck cancer, other human cancers have benefited from this technique.[95-98] Figure 11 shows how the combination of surgery and chemotherapy as an experimental model gives a substantial cure rate where neither was effective by itself.

There have also been a few investigators that have proposed the use of chemotherapy to reduce bulky primary tumors to a size that could be managed with radiation alone, thereby eliminating major surgical procedures.[99] Such an approach could greatly improve the care

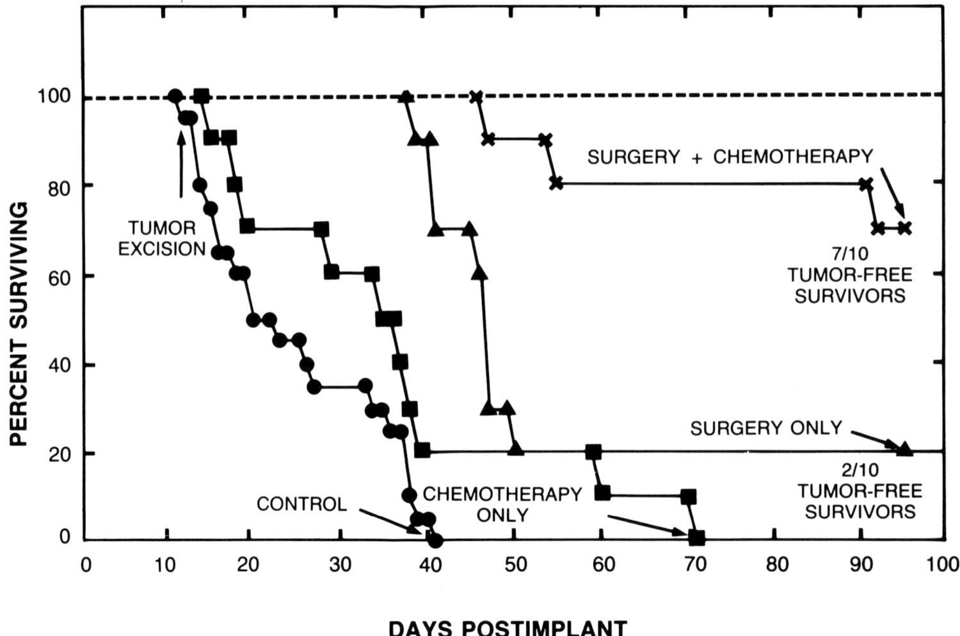

FIGURE 11.   Survival of mice implanted with melanoma comparing surgery alone, chemotherapy alone (semustine), or combination of surgery and chemotherapy. (From *Cancer Treat. Rep.*, 70, 81, 1986. With permission.)

of patients with late stage disease, because most surgeons proceed with the same radical surgery that was planned for the original tumor regardless of its response to chemotherapy. At present, it is not known whether less extensive surgery following chemotherapy adversely affects prognosis. The deletion of radical surgery for the primary tumor is not a new concept in oncology and has been used extensively in the treatment of early stage breast cancer.[100]

A well-accepted use of chemotherapy has been for patients with local recurrence and/or distant metastases. Chemotherapy is more readily accepted by some physicians in this group of patients because surgery and radiation have less to offer in these circumstances. Unfortunately, chemotherapy is also more likely to fail in this group of patients. The patient with metastases most likely has multiple macroscopic nodules, and the patient with recurrent disease has often received both surgery and radiation which inhibit delivery of drugs to the tumor. In some instances, these patients have also had preoperative chemotherapy which may increase the chance for resistance to other drugs. The expected poor outcome in this group is verified by a median survival of 3 to 5 months for patients with local recurrences and 4 months for patients with distant metastases.[86]

C. Interpreting Studies on Chemotherapy for Oral Cancer

A major goal of this section is to determine the appropriate role of chemotherapy by comparing and interpreting previously published studies which are nonparametric and from which it is very difficult to draw conclusions. Several problems contribute to this difficulty.

The majority of studies report results by grouping all head and neck cancer as one disease because most institutions do not have enough patients to randomize according to anatomic site. Yet it has been documented that cancers in different areas have different prognoses. Grose and Dixon[86] showed that the disease-free survival (DFS) from diagnosis to the first metastasis varied from 5.3 to 23 months depending on the site of the primary tumor.

Another major problem in chemotherapy studies is that results are usually compared to historical controls or no controls at all. The reporting of data compared to historical controls may give the impression that chemotherapy is more effective than it actually is. For instance, one of the major causes of death in oral cancer has been starvation,[101] so currently i.v. hyperalimentation and jejunostomy feedings are employed for some patients. It is possible that the increased survival of patients treated with chemotherapy for head and neck cancer, compared to historical controls, may reflect the effect of better nutrition and not that of chemotherapy.

Most studies are not randomized or stratified for prognostic variables. At least five variables which affect the outcome of treatment have been identified. These include the site of the primary tumor,[87-91] the nutritional status of the patient,[87-93] the performance status,[87-93] tumor grade,[92] and whether the patient has been treated previously.[90] A study which would stratify for the primary sites plus prognostic variables would be monumental and require approximately 600 patients to reach any statistical significance in a simple randomized two-arm study. With one exception[102] this has not been done.

It is difficult to make generalizations about the effectiveness of chemotherapy in oral cancer because many different drugs are used. Some of these drugs appear effective, while others do not. Even when the same drugs are used, they are not given by uniform methods or doses. For example, the combination of *cis*-platinum and 5-fluorouracil (5-FU) is probably the most active for head and neck cancer. However, infusing 5-FU for 96 hr for two courses vs. 120 hr for three courses alters the complete response rate from 19 to 54%.[103] Many more examples of the same combination of drugs varying with respect to doses of the drugs, routes of administration, sequences of the drugs, and duration of administration can be given. This makes it very difficult to draw conclusions about the effect of a particular combination of drugs.

In addition, oral cancer often affects patients from a lower socioeconomic group. Follow-up for this group of patients may be more difficult,[102,104] thus further affecting the possibility of drawing accurate conclusions with regard to success of treatment modalities.

Many of the problems contributing to the difficulty of interpreting studies on the efficacy of chemotherapy for treating head and neck cancer patients can be overcome by multi-institutional, randomized clinical trials. To date, few have been done.[102,105]

D. Chemotherapeutic Agents

There are six chemotherapeutic agents which have efficacy in the treatment of head and neck carcinomas. These include *cis*-platinum, methotrexate, bleomycin, 5-FU, vinblastine, and vincristine. The mechanism of action of these drugs is summarized in Figure 12.

1. cis-Diaminedichloroplatinum (CDDP)

cis-Platinum is one of the most effective drugs in treating oral cancer. It is an alkylating agent with its major action on DNA and RNA. When CDDP reacts with water, the two chlorine groups are lost and form a doubly positively charged diaquo compound.[106] This diaquo compound has a strong affinity for the negatively charged bases found in DNA and RNA. This bifunctional covalent bond can lead to inter- and intrastrand cross-links which can interfere with DNA replication and thus lead to cell death.[107,108]

2. Methotrexate (MTX)

MTX has had a long usefulness in the treatment of oral cancer and is the standard against which other single agents are judged. MTX is an antimetabolite, specifically an antifolate, which exhibits its cytotoxic effect by interfering with the metabolism of the reduced folates. The folates are very important because their reduction and subsequent oxidation contributes the one carbon building blocks necessary for the production of purines and thymidylate which are necessary for DNA and RNA production. As an inhibitor of nucleic acid and

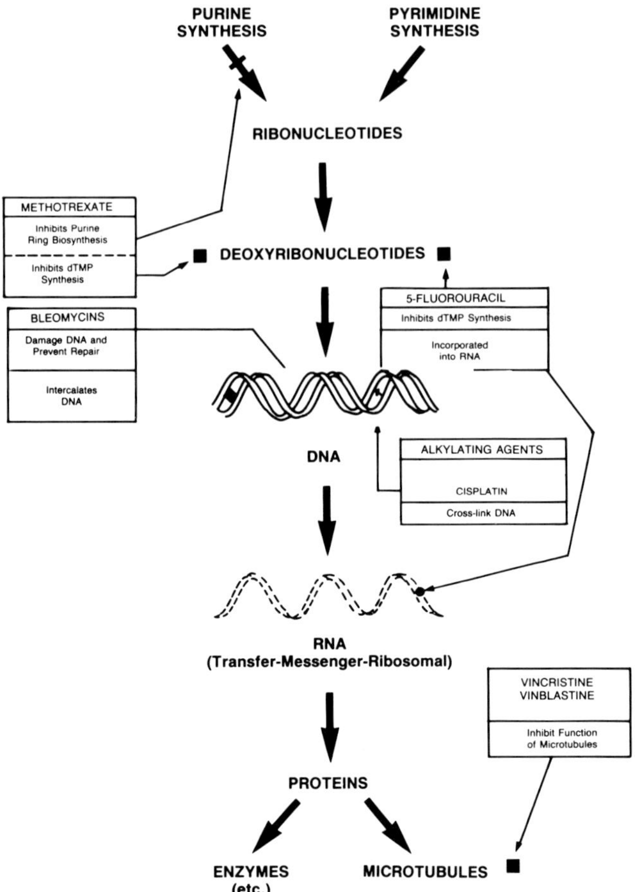

FIGURE 12.   Schematic representation of the mechanism of action of the drugs used to treat carcinomas of the head and neck.

thymidylate synthesis, MTX is a potent inhibitor of DNA and RNA synthesis and results in cell death.[109]

The effect of the antifolates can be overcome by supplying the cell with a reduced folate, i.e., leukovorin (D-L-N^5-formyl-tetrahydrofolic acid). If the leukovorin is given 24 hr after the MTX, its ability to "rescue" a cell from the cytotoxic effect of the MTX is much greater for normal cells than tumor cells. This increases the therapeutic to toxic ratio for MTX and has allowed higher dosages with acceptable toxicity.[110]

3. Bleomycin (BLM)

BLM is a chemotherapeutic agent which belongs to the antitumor antibiotic class of agents. It exerts it cytotoxic effects through at least two mechanisms. First, BLM can insert itself, by a process called intercalation, between two base pairs on the DNA.[111] The intercalation usually occurs between the guanine/thymine sequence, which causes an unwinding and lengthening of the DNA and interferes with the orderly unwinding of the DNA.[112] The second cytotoxic mechanism ascribed to BLM is its ability to cause breaks in the DNA chain at the 3' side of the guanine/thymine linkage.[113] When BLM forms a complex with the ferrous ion, it has the capability of forming a free radical which can break DNA at the site of intercalation.

4. 5-Fluorouracil (5-FU)

5-FU has two sites of action which could prove lethal to the cell, but it is not known which mechanism is the more important. The first is the inhibition of thymidylate synthetase by 5-dUMP.[114] This forms a tight bond with thymidylate synthetase and prevents the conversion of $N^{5,10}$-methylene tetrahydrofolic acid to dihydrofolic acid, thus inhibiting purine synthesis.

The second site of action is the incorporation of 5-FU into RNA, but the role this plays in the cytotoxicity of 5-FU is not clearly understood. In some models, the incorporation of 5-FU into RNA may be the major cytotoxic reaction. Santelli and Valeriote[115] showed that if 5-FU and thymidine were given concomitantly, the effect of 5-FU on thymidylate synthetase was blocked, that the incorporation of 5-FU into RNA was increased, and that cytotoxicity was enhanced.

5. Vinblastine and Vincristine

Vinblastine and vincristine are vinca alkaloids which avidly bind to tubulin. Tubulin is a protein that forms the building blocks for microtubules within the cell. Microtubules form the spindle which allows the orderly transport of chromosomes to daughter cells, as well as transporting proteins from the ribosomes to the cell membranes. They also transport neurotransmitters along the neuronal axons.[116] The vinca alkaloids can effectively bind tubulin at very low concentrations,[117] thus preventing the formation of microtubules.[118] Vincristine and vinblastine can, therefore, prevent the formation of a spindle or actually cause dissolution of the spindle.[119] An ineffective spindle can cause cell death by preventing the orderly transmission of vital genetic information to each daughter cell.

E. Treatment of Primary Disease with Chemotherapy

As a measure of the response of a tumor to chemotherapeutic agents, a complete response (CR) is the complete disappearance of all clinically detectable disease. A partial response (PR) is defined as a 50% or greater reduction in the product of cross-sectional diameters of all measurable disease.

1. Single Agents

a. MTX

MTX has been the standard against which many drugs have been compared. It has had a response rate (CR and PR) that has varied from 8 to 50%.[82] Most authors would agree that weekly doses (40 to 60 mg, i.v.) are superior to lower daily or higher monthly doses. In an attempt to increase the effectiveness of MTX by overcoming resistance, a number of investigators have looked at the use of high dose MTX with leukovorin rescue,[120-122] as originally postulated by Goldin et al.[123] In oral cancer the use of high dose MTX has not been shown to have an advantage over standard dosage.[120,122,124]

b. BLM

The appeal of BLM is that it has very little bone marrow suppression and is active against squamous cell carcinoma of the cervix. Its major disadvantage is that cumulative doses may lead to pulmonary fibrosis. This is especially undesirable for patients with oral cancer since most are cigarette smokers who have some degree of chronic obstructive lung disease before therapy. The response rate to BLM has been about 20% and lasts 2 to 3 months.[87] Although there are some studies to suggest increased response rates[125] and decreased pulmonary toxicity[120] with prolonged infusions of bleomycin, the best method of administering BLM (i.v. bolus, i.m. or i.v. infusion) has not been determined.[126]

c. cis Platinum

This drug has produced responses in squamous cell carcinoma of esophagus and uterine cervix; lesions which previously rarely responded to chemotherapy. It has also proved to be a very effective drug in oral cancer with a single agent response rate of 30%.[127] The responses have lasted 4 to 8 months. As with BLM, the optimal dose of *cis*-platinum and method of administration have not been determined.[82]

2. Combination Chemotherapy

There have not been many convincing studies of oral cancer to show the superiority of combination chemotherapy over single agent treatment. However, because of the much higher and complete response rate with combination chemotherapy for other malignancies, most investigators feel that combination chemotherapy will be more effective than using single agents. The major application of combination chemotherapy in head and neck cancer has been in induction chemotherapy.

3. Induction (Neoadjuvant) Chemotherapy

Induction chemotherapy is the use of chemotherapy to decrease gross disease to clinically undetectable or microscopic disease. This has been the most common method of employing chemotherapy in head and neck cancer. Table 6 summarizes the studies which have been done with previously untreated patients prior to surgery and/ or radiation.[103,105,128-143] The difficulties encountered interpreting clinical studies, as discussed previously, are especially true in these studies, but a few generalizations can nevertheless be made. The number of patients in each study is small, and the median follow-up when recorded is generally short. Patients have a high response rate (37 to 93%), but a relatively low complete response rate (0 to 54%). Very few studies are controlled with a randomly selected group of patients receiving no chemotherapy, and, therefore, it is impossible to tell whether the use of induction chemotherapy improves survival in late stage oral cancer over surgery and/or radiation therapy alone.[102]

These studies do provide preliminary information which may help in the management of patients with late stage disease. Some studies have shown that the duration of local and regional control is much better in those patients who achieve a complete response with chemotherapy as compared to surgery and radiation therapy.[132,135,144] For example, Fallon et al.[144] looked at all patients who achieved a CR after surgery and radiation and showed that the local and regional control correlated significantly (p <0.0001) with the response to chemotherapy. The local and regional recurrences were 16% in complete responders to chemotherapy, 53% in partial responders, and 100% in nonresponders. Improvement in local and regional control would be a major advance for chemotherapy since local recurrences are a major cause of failure in patients with head and neck cancer. Additionally, pathologic complete responses to chemotherapy may indicate an increased chance of survival in late stage disease. Three separate studies have shown very low recurrence rates (10 to 18%) in patients who have had pathologically complete responses with chemotherapy.[99,132,140]   It is not known at present, however, whether this reduced recurrence rate is the direct effect of chemotherapy or whether these patients would have been cured by surgery and/or radiation alone. Table 6 shows that there is a very high response rate which will probably have some impact on patient survival. However, this has not been proved by these or any other studies.

4. Adjuvant Chemotherapy

Adjuvant chemotherapy is the use of chemotherapy following surgery or radiation therapy in patients at very high risk for recurrence. Late stage oral cancer has a high recurrence rate,[85,86] and adjuvant chemotherapy could theoretically reduce recurrence and increase survival. Animal and human studies have shown an advantage for adjuvant chemotherapy in other tumors.[95-98] There are dissenting reports regarding the usefulness of adjuvant chemotherapy for head and neck cancer,[143,144] and at present, its effectiveness is not known.[144]

Table 6
TRIALS OF INDUCTION CHEMOTHERAPY IN PREVIOUSLY UNTREATED PATIENTS WITH HEAD AND NECK CANCER

No. of patients	Chemotherapy	Response rate		Median follow-up time (months)	No. without recurrence	Median survival (months)	Disease free survival (months)	Ref.
		Overall %	Complete %					
39	DDP, BLM	76	20	9.5	20	—	—	128
21	DDP, BLM	71	19	—	2 (24, 25 months)	—	—	129
9	DDP, BLM, HDMTX	50	0	—	2 (17, 18 months)	—	—	129
21	DDP, BLM, VLB, MTX	48	0	—	—	—	—	129
22	DDP	40	4	—	—	—	—	129
23	DDP, BLM	37	0	14.5 mean	12	—	—	130
113	DDP, BLM	49	7	—	—	—	—	131
68	DDP, BLM	59	13	13.2 mean	38	—	—	132
15	DDP, BLM, MTX	69	30	—	—	11	—	133
19	DDP, BLM, MTX	74	21	—	6	14.4	—	134
114	DDP, BLM, MTX	78	26	9.2	48	—	—	135
33	DDP, BLM, MTX	60	9	16	8	—	—	136
22	DDP, BLM, HDMTX	72.7	18	6—18	10	—	—	137
77	DDP, VCR, BLM	81	29	18	30 (40%)	15	—	103
26	DDP, 5-FU, 96 hr × 2	88	19	18	11 (40%)	13	—	103
61	DDP, 5-FU, 120 hr × 3	93	54	18	46 (62%)	18 +	—	103
47	DDP, VCR, BLM	85	23	14—20	27	—	—	138
32	VCR, BLM, MTX	80	34	—	—	22 + CR	15 +	139
58	DDP, VCR, MTX, BLM	66	28	—	—	—	—	140
31	DDP, 5-FU	84	23	—	—	—	10 +	141
34	DDP, VCR, BLM	67	32	—	—	—	24	
50							(For CRs)	142
Randomized to DDP and 5-FU or nothing	DDP and 5-FU	87	17	11	(53%)	—	—	105
	Nothing	—	—	11	(56%)	—	—	105
70	DDP + 5-FU	87	37	12—36	—	22.5	—	143

Note: BLM = bleomycin, DDP = *cis*-diaminedichloroplatinum, MTX = methotrexate, HDMTX = high dose methotrexate, VLB = vinblastine, VCR = vincristine, and 5-FU = 5-fluorouracil.

5. Intraarterial Chemotherapy

Oral carcinomas tend to remain localized and regionalized until very late in their course. Therefore, the direct instillation of a drug into the artery that supplies the tumor and its regional drainage would theoretically improve the response and cure rate of the tumor and decrease systemic toxicity by delivering much higher levels of the drug to the tumor bed. Studies have addressed the use of intraarterial chemotherapy in head and neck cancer,[145-147] but to date, there has been no controlled trial showing that intraarterial chemotherapy is better than systemic chemotherapy.

F. Treatment of Recurrent Disease with Chemotherapy

As mentioned previously this group of patients is often the domain of chemotherapy because other modes of therapy have failed. Unfortunately, patients with recurrent and metastatic disease are the group that does most poorly. Response rates vary from 7 to 67% with complete responses varying from 9 to 25%.[148-152] The median duration of responses has been short, averaging 2 to 7 months. The possible reasons for a poor response with chemotherapy include the large amount of tumor, the disruption of drug delivery to the tumor by previous surgery and radiation, and a higher incidence of drug resistance, probably secondary to previous drug exposure. Although chemotherapy is commonly used in patients with recurrent disease, because of systemic toxicity and poor results, its routine, noninvestigational use is questionable.

G. Newer Concepts

1. Chemotherapy as a Radiation Sensitizer

Major advances in radiation therapy in the next decade may occur as a result of the use of radiation sensitizers. Earlier radiation sensitizers, i.e., misonidazole, have been used in head and neck cancer with variable results. Two chemotherapeutic agents, *cis*-platinum and 5-FU, are also effective radiosensitizers.[153-155] The concomitant use of *cis*-platinum and 5-FU with radiation has a number of theoretical advantages. The first is that the radiosensitizing capabilities of the chemotherapy should increase the effectiveness of radiation. The second is that as the radiation reduces the size of the tumor, it increases the growth fraction, thereby increasing the effectiveness of the chemotherapy. The third is that the chemotherapy should eliminate microscopic distant metastases while sensitizing for the radiation therapy. This radiosensitizing effect of chemotherapy has been used with excellent results in squamous cell carcinoma of the rectum.[156] A number of head and neck cancer studies are being conducted to evaluate the usefulness of concomitant radiation and *cis*-platinum and/or 5-FU.[157-161] These studies must be considered pilot studies by virtue of their small patient numbers and the lack of randomization, but this therapy certainly deserves more detailed study. The response rates varied from 85 to 100%. Two of the studies showed complete responses of 58 and 70% in patients who had surgery,[159,160] and disease-free survival (DFS) of 56% at 2 years and 9+ months, respectively. Ansfield et al.[162] in a randomized trial showed that the concomitant use of 5-FU with radiation had a survival advantage (35%, 5-year survival) for tongue and tonsil, but not for other sites. In randomized trials, MTX, which radiosensitizes by causing an accumulation of cells in GI, has shown no survival advantage when used in combination with radiation over radiation alone.[163-165] Figure 13 shows a palatal cancer that was treated with radiation and 5-FU as a radiation sensitizer.

2. High Dose Chemotherapy

When drug resistance is secondary to a competitive mechanism such as a carrier mediate transport of a drug (e.g., L-phenylalanine mustard) or inactivation of a vital enzyme by a drug (e.g., MTX), it is possible that high doses of that drug might make a resistant tumor sensitive. High dose MTX has not been shown to be more effective than standard dose MTX for treating oral cancer.

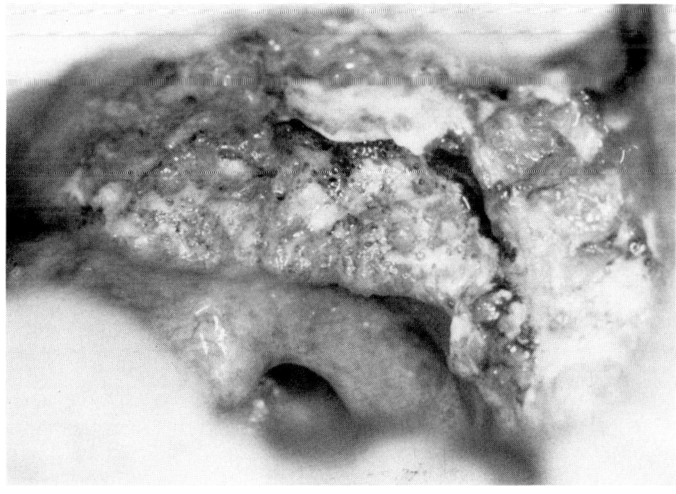

A

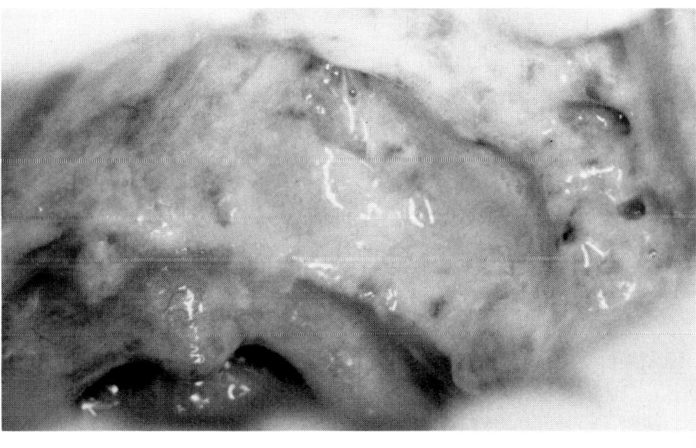

B

FIGURE 13. (A) Carcinoma of the soft palate. (B) Lesion following 1000 rad of radiotherapy using 5-FU as a radiation sensitizer.

Two recent studies have looked at the use of high dose *cis*-platinum.[166,167] In previously treated patients, the response rates were 71 and 43%, but complete responses were rare. Neurotoxicity and myelosuppression were the limiting factors. The use of high dose *cis*-platinum requires further investigation.

3. Biologic Modifiers: Retinoids

The retinoids and carotenoids play a role in the orderly differentiation of various cells. In cell lines deficient in retinoids, keratinization and hyperplasia have been noted.[168] Retinoids have also been shown to reverse keratinization and premalignant changes.[169] In animal studies, a deficiency in retinoids has increased the susceptibility to induced tumors of the lung, colon, and oral cavity.[170] The relationship in humans between a deficiency in retinoids and the propagation of a cancer is more speculative. However, in a number of studies the serum retinoid level has been much lower in patients developing cancers than in controls.[171]

Studies combining chemotherapy and retinoids have been designed, but as yet, no conclusion can be drawn.

4. Pharmacologically Designed Trials

More recently, trials have been designed to take advantage of pharmacologic interactions of various drugs. The two areas that are being investigated are the interaction between 5-FU and MTX and 5-FU and allopurinol. In cell culture, it has been shown that the cytotoxicity of 5-FU plus MTX can be enhanced if the MTX is given prior to the 5-FU. The cytotoxicity is markedly reduced when 5-FU precedes the MTX. Prior treatment with MTX blocks purine synthesis and causes an increase in phosphoribosyl pyrophosphate which converts 5-FU to its active metabolite, 5-dUMP. This activation of 5-FU by MTX has been documented in human tumors.[172] This sequencing of drugs has been of particular interest because of the effectiveness of the drugs individually, but further investigation is needed.[173,174]

The treatment of patients with allopurinol and 5-FU is felt to protect normal cells from the cytotoxic effects of 5-FU by blocking orotic acid phosphoribosyl transferase. Normal cells, but not all tumor cells, rely on this enzyme to activate 5-FU. The use of allopurinol may, therefore, have a protective effect on normal cells without reducing the effect of 5-FU on tumor cells.[175] One study using higher than normal doses of 5-FU and allopurinol as a protectant recorded a 100% response and 50% complete response rate.[176] Toxicity was tolerable.

5. Development of New Drugs

In oncology the hope for the future is always the development of more effective drugs for each disease. For oral cancer, two analogues of platinum carboplatinum, CBCDA and CHIP, are under active investigation. In pretreated patients and those with recurrent disease, a distinctly poor prognosis group, the response rates were 33 to 35%.[177,178] The advantage of these drugs is the lack of renal toxicity.

V. CONCLUSION

Late stage head and neck cancer has a very poor prognosis. Although it is apparent from uncontrolled studies which show high response rates that chemotherapy has a role in the treatment of this disease, the exact nature of this role remains unclear. Many investigators feel that the best way to use chemotherapy is prior to surgery and/or radiation. However, whether this conclusively contributes to an increase in the cure rate or DFS is not known. The role for chemotherapy in stage I or II disease, the role for adjuvant chemotherapy after surgery and/or radiation, and the proper sequencing of the multimodality therapy is unknown. Because of the great variability in head and neck cancer, the only way these questions will be answered will be through methodical, well-designed, large, multiinstitutional, cooperative, randomized studies. Few of these exist at the present time.

REFERENCES

1. **Wile, A. G., Novotny, J., Mason, G. R., Passy, V., and Berns, M. W.,** Photoradiation therapy of head and neck cancer, *Am. J. Clin. Oncol.,* 7, 39, 1984.
2. **Kaplan, I., Gassner, S., and Shindel, Y.,** Carbon dioxide laser in head and neck surgery, *Am. J. Surg.,* 128, 543, 1974.
3. **Byers, R. M., Bland, K. I., Borlase, B., and Luna, M.,** The prognostic and therapeutic value of frozen section determinations in the surgical treatment of squamous carcinoma of the head and neck, *Am. J. Surg.,* 136, 525, 1978.

4. **Baker, S. R. and Swanson, N. A.,** Complete microscopic controlled surgery for head and neck cancer, *Head Neck Surg.,* 6, 914, 1984.

5. **Hirata, R. M., Jaques, D. A., Chambers, R. G., Tuttle, J. R., and Mahoney, W. D.,** Carcinoma of the oral cavity. An analysis of 478 cases, *Ann. Surg.,* 182, 98, 1975.

6. **Shaha, A. R., Spiro, R. H., Shah, J. P., and Strong, E. W.,** Squamous carcinoma of the floor of the mouth, *Am. J. Surg.,* 148, 455, 1984.

7. **Moore, C.,** Cigarette smoking and cancer of the mouth, pharynx, and larynx. A continuing study, *JAMA,* 218, 553, 1971.

8. **Suen, J. Y. and Myers, E. N.,** *Cancer of the Head and Neck,* Churchill Livingstone, New York, 1981, 124.

9. **Bradfield, J. S. and Scruggs, R. P.,** Carcinoma of the mobile tongue: incidence of cervical metastases in early lesions related to method of primary treatment, *Laryngoscope,* 93, 1332, 1983.

10. **Vikram, B., Strong, E. W., Shah, J., and Spiro, R. H.,** Elective postoperative radiation therapy in stages III and IV epidermoid carcinoma of the head and neck, *Am. J. Surg.,* 140, 580, 1980.

11. **Mendenhall, W. M., Million, R. R., and Cassisi, N. J.,** Elective neck irradiation in squamous-cell carcinoma of the head and neck, *Head Neck Surg.,* 3, 15, 1980.

12. **Mantravadi, R., Katz, A., Haas, R., Liebner, E. J., Sabato, D., Skolnik, E., and Applebaum, E. L.,** Radiation therapy for subclinical carcinoma in cervical lymph nodes, *Arch. Otolaryngol.,* 108, 108, 1982.

13. **Rabuzzi, D. D., Chung, C. T., and Sagerman, R. H.,** Prophylactic neck irradiation, *Arch. Otolaryngol.,* 106, 454, 1980.

14. **Beumer, J., Harrison, R., Sanders, B., and Kurrasch, M.,** Osteoradionecrosis: predisposing factors and outcomes of therapy, *Head Neck Surg.,* 6, 819, 1984.

15. **Larson, D. L., Lindberg, R. D., Lane, E., and Goepfert, H.,** Major complications of radiotherapy in cancer of the oral cavity and oropharynx. A 10 year retrospective study, *Am. J. Surg.,* 146, 531, 1983.

16. **Fletcher, G. H.,** The role of irradiation in the management of squamous-cell carcinomas of the mouth and throat, *Head Neck Surg.,* 1, 441, 1979.

17. **Strong, E. W.,** Preoperative radiation and radical neck dissection, *Surg. Clin. North Am.,* 49, 271, 1969.

18. **Fletcher, G. H. and Jesse, R. H.,** Irradiation management of squamous cell carcinomas of the oral cavity in Proc. 7th Natl. Cancer Conf., Am. Cancer Soc., 1973, 137.

19. **Weaver, A., Fleming, S., Ensley, J., Kish, J. A., Jacobs, J., Kinzie, J., Crissman, J., and Al-Sarraf, M.,** Superior clinical response and survival rates with initial bolus of cisplatin and 120 hour infusion of 5-fluorouracil before definitive therapy for locally advanced head and neck cancer, *Am. J. Surg.,* 148, 525, 1984.

20. **Spaulding, M. B., Kahn, A., De Los Santos, R., Klotch, D., and Lore, J. M., Jr.,** Adjuvant chemotherapy in advanced head and neck cancer. An update, *Am. J. Surg.,* 144, 432, 1982.

21. **Davis, R. K., Perry, D. J., and Zajtchuk, J. T.,** Induction chemotherapy with vinblastine, bleomycin, and cis-diamminedichloroplatinum in squamous cell carcinoma of the head and neck, *Otolaryngol. Head Neck Surg.,* 91, 627, 1983.

22. **Hong, W. K. and Bromer, R.,** Chemotherapy in head and neck cancer, *N. Engl. J. Med.,* 308, 75, 1983.

23. **Kies, M. S., Pecaro, B. C., and Gordon, L. I.,** Preoperative combination chemotherapy for advanced stage head and neck cancer. Promising early results, *Am. J. Surg.,* 148, 367, 1984.

24. **Espana, P., Smith, F., Abrams, J., Haidak, D., Veno, W., Woolley, P., and Schein, P.,** Phase-II study of cis-diamminedichloroplatinum (cis-platinum), bleomycin and methotrexate for advanced squamous cell carcinoma of head and neck, *Cancer Chemother. Pharmacol.,* 12, 98, 1984.

25. **Janfaza, P.,** Tattooing in cancer surgery, *Laryngoscope,* 90, 1191, 1980.

26. **Eneroth, C. M.,** Aspiration biopsy of head and neck tumours, *Swed. Dent. J.,* 66, 177, 1973.

27. **Frable, W. J. and Frable, M. A. S.,** Thin-needle aspiration biopsy, *Cancer,* 43, 1541, 1979.

28. **Weymuller, E. A., Jr., Kiviat, N. B., and Duckert, L. G.,** Aspiration cytology: an efficient and cost-effective modality, *Laryngoscope,* 93, 561, 1983.

29. **Nahum, A. M., Bone, R. C., and Davidson, T. M.,** The case for elective prophylactic neck dissection, *Laryngoscope,* 87, 588, 1977.

30. **DeSanto, L., Holt, J. J., Beahrs, O. H., and O'Fallon, W. M.,** Neck dissection: is it worth it?, *Laryngoscope,* 92, 502, 1982.

31. **Byers, R. M.,** Modified neck dissection. A study of 967 cases from 1970 to 1980, *Am. J. Surg.,* 150, 414, 1985.

32. **Bocca, F., Pignataro, O., and Sasaki, C. T.,** Functional neck dissection. A description of operative technique, *Arch. Otolaryngol.,* 106, 524, 1980.

33. **Ariyan, S.,** Functional radical neck dissection, *Plast. Reconstr. Surg.,* 65, 768, 1980.

34. **Calearo, C. V. and Teatini, G.,** Functional neck dissection. Anatomical grounds, surgical technique, clinical observations, *Ann. Otol. Rhinol. Laryngol.,* 92, 215, 1983.

35. **Leipzig, B., Suen, J. Y., English, J. L., Barnes, J., and Hooper, M.,** Functional evaluation of the spinal accessory nerve after neck dissection, *Am. J. Surg.,* 146, 526, 1983.

36. **Short, S. O., Kaplan, J. N., Laramore, G. E., and Cummings, C. W.,** Shoulder pain and function after neck dissection with or without preservation of the spinal accessory nerve, *Am. J. Surg.,* 148, 478, 1984.

37. **Jesse, R. H., Ballantyne, A. J., and Larson, D.,** Radical or modified neck dissection: a therapeutic dilemma, *Am. J. Surg.,* 136, 516, 1978.

38. **Carenfelt, C. and Eliasson, K.,** Cervical metastases following radical neck dissection that preserved the spinal accessory nerve, *Head Neck Surg.,* 2, 181, 1980.

39. **Marks, J. E., Lee, F., Smith, P. G., and Ogura, J. H.,** Floor of mouth cancer: patient selection and treatment results, *Laryngoscope,* 93, 475, 1983.

40. **Copeland, E. M., MacFadyen, B. V., MacComb, W. S., Guillamondegui, O., Jesse, R. H., and Dudrick, S. J.,** Intravenous hyperalimentation in patients with head and neck cancer, *Cancer,* 35, 606, 1975.

41. **Daly, J. M., Dudrick, S. J., and Copeland, E. M., III,** Intravenous hyperalimentation. Effect on delayed cutaneous hypersensitivity in cancer patients, *Ann. Surg.,* 192, 587, 1980.

42. **Daly, J. M., Hearne, B., Dunaj, J., LePorte, B., Vikram, B., Strong, E., Green, M., Muggio, F., Groshen, S., and DeCosse, J. J.,** Nutritional rehabilitation in patients with advanced head and neck cancer receiving radiation therapy, *Am. J. Surg.,* 148, 514, 1984.

43. **Goodwin, W. J., Jr. and Torres, J.,** The value of the prognostic nutritional index in the management of patients with advanced carcinoma of the head and neck, *Head Neck Surg.,* 6, 932, 1984.

44. **Feldman, M., Ucmakli, A., Strong, S., Vaughn, C., Kim, S., and Bylinski, A.,** Applications of carbon dioxide laser surgery and radiation, *Arch. Otolaryngol.,* 109, 240, 1983.

45. **Hendee, W. R.,** *Medical Radiation Physics,* Year Book Medical Publishing, Chicago, 1984.

46. **Hall, E. J.,** *Radiobiology for the Radiologist,* 2nd ed., Harper & Row, Philadelphia, 1973.

47. **Puck, T. T. and Marcus, P. I.,** Action of x-rays on mammalian cells, *J. Exp. Med.,* 103, 653, 1956.

48. **Thames, H. D., Peters, L. J., Withers, H. R., and Fletcher, G. H.,** Accelerated fractionation vs. hyperfractionation: rationales for several treatments per day, *Int. J. Radiat. Oncol. Biol. Phys.,* 9, 127, 1983.

49. **Fowler, J. F.,** The rationale of dose fractionation, *Front. Radiat. Ther. Oncol.,* 3, 6, 1968.

50. **Maor, M. H., Hussey, D. H., Fletcher, G. H., and Jesse, R. H.,** Fast neutron therapy for locally advanced head and neck tumors, *Int. J. Radiat. Oncol. Biol. Phys.,* 7, 155, 1981.

51. **Barkley, H. T., Jr., Fletcher, G. H., Jesse, R. H., and Lindberg, R. D.,** Management of cervical lymph node metastases in squamous cell carcinoma of the tonsillar fossa, base of tongue, supraglottic larynx, and hypopharynx, *Am. J. Surg.,* 124, 462, 1972.

52. **Dische, S., Saunders, M. I., Anderson, P., Stratford, M. R., and Minchinton, A.,** Clinical experience with nitroimidazoles as radiosensitizers, *Int. J. Radiat. Oncol. Biol. Phys.,* 8, 335, 1982.

53. **Emami, B., Marks, J. E., Perez, C. A., Nussbaum, G. H., Leybovich, L., and Von Gerichten, D.,** Interstitial thermoradiotherapy in the treatment of recurrent/residual malignant tumors, *Am. J. Clin. Oncol.,* 7, 699, 1984.

54. **Suit, H. D. and Gerweck, L. E.,** Potential for hyperthermia and radiation therapy, *Cancer Res.,* 39, 2290, 1979.

55. **Bradfield, J. S. and Scruggs, R. P.,** Carcinoma of the mobile tongue: incidence of cervical metastases in early lesions related to method of primary treatment, *Laryngoscope,* 93, 1332, 1983.

56. **Vermund, H., Brennhoud, I., Kaalhus, O., and Poppe, E.,** Incidence and control of occult neck node metastases from squamous cell carcinoma of the anterior two-thirds of the tongue, *Int. J. Radiat. Oncol, Biol. Phys.,* 10, 2025, 1984.

57. **Griffin, T. W., Pajak, T. F., Gillespie, B. W., Davis, L. W., Brady, L. W., Rubin, P., and Marcial, V. A.,** Predicting the response of head and neck cancers to radiation therapy with a multivariate modelling system: an analysis of the RTOG head and neck registry, *Int. J. Radiat. Oncol. Biol. Phys.,* 10, 481, 1984.

58. **Quimby, E. H.,** Dosage table for linear radium sources, *Radiology,* 43, 572, 1944.

59. **Patterson, R. and Parker, H. M.,** A dosage system for interstitial radium therapy, *Br. J. Radiol.,* 11(252), 313, 1938.

60. **Kumar, P. P. and Henschke, U. K.,** Five year's experience with the gold button technique for intraoral interstitial implants with iridium-192 seeds, *Radiology,* 124, 227, 1977.

61. **Vikram, B., Hilaris, B. S., Anderson, L., and Strong, E. W.,** Permanent iodine-125 implants in head and neck cancer, *Cancer,* 51, 1310, 1983.

62. **Aygun, C., Salazar, O. M., Sewchand, W., Amornmarn, R., and Prempree, T.,** Carcinoma of the floor of the mouth: a 20-year experience, *Int. J. Radiat. Oncol. Biol. Phys.,* 10, 619, 1984.

63. **Biggs, P. J. and Wang, C. C.,** An intra-oral cone for an 18 MeV linear accelerator, *Int. J. Radiat. Oncol. Biol. Phys.,* 8, 1251, 1982.

64. **Fayos, J. V. and Lampe, I.,** Radiotherapy of squamous cell carcinoma of the oral portion of the tongue, *Arch. Surg.,* 94, 316, 1967.
65. **Wang, C. C., Doppke, K. P., and Biggs., P. J.,** Intra-oral cone radiation therapy for selected carcinomas of the oral cavity, *Int. J. Radiat. Oncol. Biol. Phys.,* 9, 1185, 1983.
66. **Delclos, L., Lindberg, R. D., and Fletcher, G. H.,** Squamous cell carcinoma of the oral tongue and floor of mouth: evaluation of interstitial radium therapy, *Am. J. Roentgenol.,* 126, 223, 1976.
67. **Fu, K. K., Chan, E. K., Phillips, T. L., and Ray, J. W.,** Time, dose and volume factor in interstitial radium implants of carcinoma of the oral tongue, *Radiology,* 119, 209, 1976.
68. **Gilbert, E. H., Goffinet, D. R., and Bagshaw, M. A.,** Carcinoma of the oral tongue and floor of mouth: fifteen years experience with linear accelerator therapy, *Cancer,* 35, 1517, 1975.
69. **Mendenhall, W. M., Van Cise, W. S., Bova, F. J., and Million, R. R.,** Analysis of time-dose factors in squamous cell carcinoma of the oral tongue and floor of mouth treated with radiation therapy alone, *Int. J. Radiat. Oncol. Biol. Phys.,* 7, 1005, 1981.
70. **Marks, J. E., Lee, F., Freeman, R. B., Zivnuska, F. R., and Ogura, J. H.,** Carcinoma of the oral tongue: a study of patient selection and treatment results, *Laryngoscope,* 91, 1548, 1981.
71. **Ange, D. W., Lindbert, R. D., and Guillamondegui, O. M.,** Management of squamous cell carcinoma of the oral tongue and floor of mouth after excisional biopsy, *Radiology,* 116, 143, 1975.
72. **Fu, K. K., Lichter, A., and Galante, M.,** Carcinoma of the floor of mouth: an analysis of treatment results and the sites and causes of failure, *Int. J. Radiat. Oncol. Biol. Phys.,* 1, 829, 1976.
73. **Marks, J. E., Lee, F., Smith, P. G., and Ogura, J. H.,** Floor of mouth cancer: patient selection and treatment results, *Laryngoscope,* 93, 475, 1983.
74. **Hanks, G. E., Kramer, S., Diamond, J. J., and Herring, D. F.,** Patterns of care outcome survey: national outcome data for six disease sites, *Am. J. Clin. Oncol.,* 5, 349, 1982.
75. **Fletcher, G. H.,** *Textbook of Radiotherapy,* 3rd ed., Lea & Febiger, Philadelphia, 1980.
76. **MacComb, W. S. and Fletcher, G. H.,** *Cancer of the Head and Neck,* Williams & Wilkins, Baltimore, 1967.
77. **Million, R. R. and Cassisi, N. J.,** *Management of Head and Neck Cancer: A Multidisciplinary Approach,* Lippincott, Philadelphia, 1984, 295.
78. **Wang, C. C.,** *Radiation Therapy for Head and Neck Neoplasms: Indications, Techniques, and Results,* John Wright, Bristol, 1983, 102.
79. **Million, R. R. and Cassisi, N. J.,** *Management of Head and Neck Cancer: A Multidisciplinary Approach,* Lippincott, Philadelphia, 1984, 30.
80. **Baker, S. R. and Krause, C. J.,** Carcinoma of the lip, *Laryngoscope,* 90, 19, 1980.
81. **Hong, W. K. and Bromer, R.,** Chemotherapy in head and neck cancer, *N. Engl. J. Med.,* 308, 75, 1983.
82. **Mead, G. M. and Jacobs, C.,** Changing role of chemotherapy in head and neck cancer, *Am. J. Med.,* 73, 582, 1982.
83. **Muggia, F. M., Rozencweig, M. and Louie, A. E.,** Role of chemotherapy in head and neck cancer: systemic use of single agents and combinations in advanced disease, *Head Neck Surg.,* 2, 196, 1980.
84. **Ervin, T. J., Weichselbaum, R. R., Fabian, R. L., Karp, D. D., Posner, M. R., and Miller, D.,** Role of chemotherapy in the multidisciplinary approach to advanced head and neck cancer: potentials and problems, *Ann. Otol.,* 90, 506, 1981.
85. **Wolf, G. T.,** An overview of preoperative chemotherapy: where do we go from here?, *Am. J. Otolaryngol.,* 5, 77, 1984.
86. **Grose, W. E. and Dixon, D. O.,** Distant metastases in patients with head and neck squamous cell carcinoma, in *Proceedings of the american Society of Clinical Oncologists,* Foti, M., Mennite, M. A., and Pusztay, H. M., Eds., Waverly Press, Baltimore, 1985, 148.
87. **Bertino, J. R., Boston, B., and Capizzi, R. L.,** The role of chemotherapy in the management of cancer of the head and neck: a review, *Cancer,* 36, 752, 1975.
88. **Goldsmith, M. A. and Carter, S. K.,** The integration of chemotherapy into a combined modality approach to cancer therapy. V. Squamous cell cancer of the head and neck, *Cancer Treat. Rev.,* 2, 137, 1975.
89. **Jacobs, C.,** The role of cisplatin in the treatment of recurrent head and neck cancer, in *Cisplatin: Current Status and New Developments,* Prestayko, A. W., Crooke, S. T., and Carter, S. K., Eds., Academic Press, New York, 1980, 423.
90. **Elias, E. G., Chretien, P. B., Monnard, E., Khan, T., Bouchelle, W. H., Wiernik, P. H., Lipson, S. D., Hande, K. R., and Zentai, T.,** Chemotherapy prior to local therapy in advanced squamous cell carcinoma of the head and neck: preliminary assessment of an intensive drug regimen, *Cancer,* 43, 1025, 1979.
91. **Livingston, R. B., Einhorn, A. H., Burgess, M. A., and Gotthiel, J. A.,** Sequential combination chemotherapy for advanced, recurrent squamous carcinoma of the head and neck, *Cancer Treat. Rep.,* 60, 103, 1976.
92. **Soper, W. T. and Gott, A. B.,** New Drug Seminar on Bleomycin, National Cancer Institute, Bethesda, Md., 1974.

93. **Amer, M. H., Al-Sarrat, M., and Vaitkevicius, V. K.,** Factors that affect response to chemotherapy and survival of patients with advanced head and neck cancer, *Cancer,* 43, 2202, 1979.

94. **Looney, W. B., Ritenour, E. R., and Hopkins, H. A.,** Solid tumor models for the assessment of different treatment modalities, *Cancer,* 47, 860, 1981.

95. **Fisher, B., Slack, N., Katrych, D., and Wolmark, N.,** Ten year follow-up results of patients with carcinoma of the breast in a cooperative clinical trial evaluating surgical adjuvant chemotherapy, *Surg. Gynecol. Obstet.,* 140, 528, 1975.

96. **Nissen-Meyer, R., Host, H., Kjellgren, K., Mansson, B., and Norin, T.,** Scandinavian trials with a short postoperative course versus a 12 cycle course, recent results, *Cancer Res.,* 96, 48, 1984.

97. **Bonadonna, G. and Valagussa, P.,** Adjuvant systemic therapy for resectable breast cancer, *J. Clin. Oncol.,* 3, 259, 1985.

98. **Rosen, G. and Nirenberg, A.,** Chemotherapy for osteogenic sarcoma: an investigative method, not a recipe, *Cancer Treat. Rep.,* 66, 1687, 1982.

99. **Jacobs, C., Goffinet, D., Fee, W., Goffinet, L., and Hopp, M.,** Chemotherapy as a substitute for surgery in the treatment of advanced operable head and neck cancer: an NCOG pilot, in *Proceedings of the American Society of Clinical Oncologists,* Foti, M., Mennite, M. A., and Pusztay, H. M., Eds., Waverly Press, Baltimore, 1985, 137.

100. **Harris, J. R., Beadle, G. F., and Hellman, S.,** Clinical studies on the use of irradiation therapy as a primary treatment of early breast cancer, *Cancer,* 52, 705, 1984.

101. **Smale, B. F., Mullen, J. L., Buzby, G. P., and Rosato, E. F.,** The efficacy of nutritional assessment and support in cancer surgery, *Cancer,* 47, 2375, 1981.

102. **Jacobs, C., Wolf, G. T., Makuch, R. W., and Vikram, B.,** Adjuvant chemotherapy for head and neck squamous carcinomas, in *Proceedings of the American Society of Clinical Oncologists ,* Foti, M., Mennite, M. A., and Pusztay, H. M., Eds., Waverly Press, Baltimore, 1984, 182.

103. **Rooney, M., Kish, J., Jacobs, J., Kinzie, J., Weaver, A., Crissman, J., and Al-Sarraf, M.,** Improved complete response rate and survival in advanced head and neck cancer after three-course induction chemotherapy with 120-hour 5-FU infusion and cisplatin, *Cancer,* 55, 1123, 1985.

104. **Cairns, J.,** The treatment of disease and the war against cancer, *Sci. Am.,* 253, 51, 1985.

105. **Haas, C., Byhardt, R., Cox, J., Duncavage, J., Grossman, T., Haas, J., Hartz, A., Libnoch, J., Malin, T., Ritch, P., and Toohill, B.,** Randomized study of 5-fluorouracil (f) and cis-platinum (p) as initial therapy of locally advanced squamous carcinoma of the head and neck (laschn): a preliminary analysis, in *Proceedings of the American Society of Clinical Oncology,* Foti, M., Mennite, M. A., and Pusztay, H. M., Eds., Waverly Press, Baltimore, 1985, 143.

106. **Harrison R. C., Brown, B. W., and Gottlieb, J. A.,** Platinum (II) complexes of DNA constituents, *Inorg. Perspect. Biol. Med.,* 1, 261, 1978.

107. **Drewinko, B., Brown, B. W., and Gottlieb, J. A.,** The effect of cis-diamminedichloroplatinum (II) on cultured human lymphoma cells and its therapeutic implications, *Cancer Res.,* 33, 3091, 1973.

108. **Fraval, H. N. A. and Roberts, J. J.,** Effects of cis-platinum (II) diamminedichloride on survival and the rate of DNA synthesis in synchronously growing Chinese hamster V79-379A cells in the absence and presence of caffeine inhibited post-replication repair, evidence for an inducible repair mechanism, *Chem. Biol. Interact.,* 23, 99, 1978.

109. **Zaharko, D. S., Fung, W. -P., and Yang, F. -H.,** Relative biochemical aspects of low and high doses of methotrexate in mice, *Cancer Res.,* 37, 1602, 1977.

110. **Jaffe, N.,** Recent advances in the chemotherapy of metastatic osteogenic sarcoma, *Cancer,* 30, 1627, 1972.

111. **Chien, M., Grollman, A. P., and Horwitz, S. B.,** Bleomycin-DNA interactions: fluorescence and proton magnetic resonance studies, *Biochemistry,* 16, 3641, 1977.

112. **Povirk, L. F., Hogan, M., and Dattagupta, N.,** Binding of bleomycin to DNA: intercalation of the bithiazole rings, *Biochemistry,* 18, 96, 1979.

113. **Lown, J. W. and Sim, S.,** The mechanism of the bleomycin-induced cleavage of DNA, *Biochem, Biophys. Res. Commun.,* 77, 1150, 1157, 1977.

114. **Santi, D. V., McHenry, C. S., and Sommer, A.,** Mechanisms of interactions of thymidylate synthetase with 5-fluorodeoxyuridylate, *Biochemistry,* 13, 471, 1974.

115. **Santelli, G. and Valeriote, F.,** In vivo enhancement of 5-fluorouracil cytotoxicity to AKR leukemia cells by thymidine in mice, *J. Natl. Cancer Inst.,* 61, 843, 1978.

116. **Wilson, L.,** Action of drugs on microtubules, *Life Sci.,* 17, 303, 1975.

117. **Wilson, L., Morse, N. C., and Bryan, J.,** Characterization of acetyl-^{3}H-labelled vinblastine binding to vinblastine-tubulin crystals, *J. Mol. Biol.,* 121, 255, 1978.

118. **Owellen, R. J., Hartke, C. A., Dickerson, R. M., and Hains, F. O.,** Inhibition of tubulin-microtubule polymerization by drugs of the vinca alkaloid class, *Cancer Res.,* 36, 1499, 1976.

119. **Bensch, K. G. and Malawista, S. E.,** Microtubule crystals in mammalian cells, *J. Cell Biol.,* 40, 95, 1969.

120. **DeConti, R. C. Schoenfeld, D.,** A randomized prospective comparison of intermittent methotrexate, methotrexate with leucovorin, and a methotrexate combination in head and neck cancer, *Cancer,* 48, 1061, 1981.
121. **Woods, R. L., Fox, R. M., and Tattersall, M. H. N.,** Methotrexate treatment of squamous cell head and neck cancers: dose-response evaluation, *Br. Med. J.,* 282, 600, 1981.
122. **Kirkwood, J. M. Canellos, G., Pervin, T. J., Pitman, S. W., Weichselbaum, R., and Miller, D.,** Increased therapeutic index using moderate dose methotrexate and leucovorin twice weekly vs. weekly high dose methotrexate-leucovorin in patients with advanced squamous carcinoma of the head and neck. A safe new effective regimen, *Cancer,* 47, 2414, 1981.
123. **Goldin, A., Venditti, J. M., Line, I., and Mantel, M.,** Eradication of leukemic cells (L1210) by methotrexate and methotrexate plus leucovorin factor, *Nature (London),* 212, 1548, 1966.
124. **Vogler, W. R., Jacobs, J., Moffit, S., Velez-Garcia, E., Goldsmith, A., Johnson, L., and Mackay, S.,** Methotrexate therapy with or without citrovorum factor in carcinoma of the head and neck, breast and colon, *Cancer Clin. Trials,* 2, 227, 1979.
125. **Baker, R. R. and Gaertner, R. A.,** Regional arterial infusion of antimetabolites, *J. Surg. Res.,* 5, 132, 1965.
126. **Krakoff, I. H., Cvitkovic, E., Currie, V., Yeh, S., and LaMonte, C.,** Clinical pharmacologic and therapeutic studies of bleomycin given by continuous infusion, *Cancer,* 40, 2027, 1977.
127. **Wittes, R. E., Cvitkovic, E., Shah, J., Gerold, F. P., and Strong, E. W.,** Cis-dichlorodiammineplatinum (II) in the treatment of epidermoid carcinoma of the head and neck, *Cancer Treat. Rep.,* 61, 359, 1977.
128. **Hong, W. K., Shapshay, S. M., Bhutani, R., Craft, M. L., Ucmakli, A., Yamaguchi, K. T., Vaughan, C. W., and Strong, M. S.,** Induction chemotherapy in advanced squamous head and neck carcinoma with high-dose cis-platinum and bleomycin infusion, *Cancer,* 44, 19, 1979.
129. **Wittes, R., Heller, K., Randolph, V., Howard, J., Vallejo, A., Farr, H., Harrold, C., Gerold, F., Shah, J., Spiro, R, and Strong, E.,** cis-Dichlorodiammineplatinum (II)-based chemotherapy as initial treatment of advanced head and neck cancer. *Cancer Treat. Rep.,* 63, 1533, 1979.
130. **Cloughlin, C. T., Grace, M., O'Donnell, J. F., LeMarbre, P. J., Morain, W. D., Geurkink, N. A., and McIntyre, O. R.,** Combined modality approach in management of locally advanced head and neck cancer, *Cancer Treat. Rep.,* 68, 591, 1984.
131. **Baker, S. R., Makuch, R. W., and Wolf, G. T.,** Preoperative cisplatin and bleomycin therapy in head and neck squamous carcinoma, *Arch. Otolaryngol.,* 107, 683, 1981.
132. **Bradfield, J., Scruggs, R., and Mennel, R. G.,** unpublished data, 1981.
133. **Gill, P. G., Hains, J. D., Iyer, P., Rozenbilds, J. G., Ahmad, A., Abbott, R. L., David, D. J., Ward, G. G., Brown, M. W., and Harvey, D. M.,** Chemotherapy of squamous cell cancer of the head and neck, *Med. J. Aust.,* 1, 463, 1983.
134. **Kles, M. S., Pecaro, B. C., Gordon, L. I., Hauck, W. W., Kraut, M. J., Krespi, Y., Ossoff, R. H., Schiff, C., Shetty, R., and Sisson, G. A.,** Preoperative combination chemotherapy for advanced state head and neck cancer, *Am. J. Surg.,* 148, 367, 1984.
135. **Weichselbaum, R. R., Clark, J. R., Miller, D., Posner, M. R., and Ervin, T. J.,** Combined modality treatment of head and neck cancer with cisplatin, bleomycin, methotrexate-leucovorin chemotherapy, *Cancer,* 55, 2149, 1985.
136. **Tannock, I., Cummings, B., Sorrenti, V., and the ENT Group,** Combination chemotherapy used prior to radiation therapy for locally advanced squamous cell carcinoma of the head and neck, *Cancer Treat. Rep.,* 66, 1421, 1982.
137. **Elias, E. G., Chretien, P. B., Monnard, E., Khan, T., Bouchelle, W. H., Wiernik, P. H., Lipson, S. D., Hande, K. R., and Zentai, T.,** Chemotherapy prior to local therapy in advanced squamous cell carcinoma of the head and neck, *Cancer,* 43, 1025, 1979.
138. **Spaulding, M. B., Khan, A., De Los Santos, R., Klotch, D., and Lore, J. M., Jr.,** Adjuvant chemotherapy in advanced head and neck cancer. *Am. J. Surg.,* 144, 432, 1982.
139. **Rosso, R., Merlano, M., Sertoli, M., Campora, E, Scarpati, D., Borasi, F., and Pallestrini, E.,** Multidrug chemotherapy (vincristine, bleomycin, and methotrexate, VBM) with radiotherapy in stage III-IV squamous cell carcinoma of the head and neck, *Cancer Treat. Rep.,* 68, 1019, 1984.
140. **Schuller, D. E., Wilson, H. E., Smith, R. E., Batley, F., and James, A. D.,** Preoperative reduction chemotherapy for locally advanced carcinoma of the oral cavity, oropharynx and hypopharynx, *Cancer,* 51, 15, 1983.
141. **Amrein, P. and Weitzman, S.,** 24-hour infusion cisplatin (CP) and 5-day infusion 5-fluorouracil (FU) in squamous cell carcinoma of the head and neck (SCC H + N) in *Proceedings of the American Society of Clinical Oncologists,* Foti, M., Mennite, M. A., and Pusztay, H. M., Eds., Waverly Press, Baltimore, 1985, 133.

142. **Mukhopadhyay, P., Osman, M. R., Wajima, T., Maxwell, V., Alverson, E., Subramanian, V. P., and Kroening, P. M.,** Combined modality therapy for previously untreated advanced squamous cell carcinoma of the head and neck, in *Proceedings of the American Society for Clinical Oncologists,* Foti, M., Mennite, M. A., and Pusztay, H. M., Eds., Waverly Press, Baltimore, 1985, 135.

143. **Kies, M. S., Lester, E. P., Gordon, L. I., Blough, R. R., Gongol, J., and Taylor, S. G., IV,** Cisplatin and infusion 5-fluorouracil (5-FU) in stage III and IV squamous cancer of the head and neck, in *Proceedings of the American Society of Clinical Oncologists,* Foti, M., Mennite, M. A., and Pusztay, H. M., Eds., Waverly Press, Baltimore, 1985, 139.

144. **Fallon, B., Clark, J., Weichselbaum, R., Miller, D., Norris, C., Fabian, R., Frei, E., and Ervin, T.,** Locoregional control in advanced squamous cell carcinoma of the head and neck (SCCHN) after induction chemotherapy, in *Proceedings of the American Society of Clinical Oncologists,* Foti, M., Mennite, M. A., and Pusztay, H. M., Eds., Waverly Press, Baltimore, 1985, 139.

145. **Acquarelli, M., Feder, R., and Gordon, H.,** Continuous intra-arterial infusion of methotrexate for recurrent squamous cell carcinoma of the head and neck, *Am. Surg.,* 30, 423, 1964.

146. **Muggia, F. M. and Wolf, G. T.,** Intraarterial chemotherapy of head and neck cancer: worth another look?, *Cancer Clin. Trials,* 3, 375, 1980.

147. **Carter, S. K.,** The chemotherapy of head and neck cancer, *Semin. Oncol.,* 4, 413, 1977.

148. **Creagan, E. T., Fleming, T. R., Edmonson, J. H., Ingle, J. N., and Woods, J. E.,** Cyclophosphamide, adriamycin and cis-diamminedichloroplatinum in the treatment of patients with advanced head and neck cancer, *Cancer,* 47, 240, 1981.

149. **Creagan, E. T., Fleming, T. R., Edmonson, J. H., Ingle, J. N., and Woods, J. E.,** Chemotherapy for advanced head and neck cancer with combination adriamycin, cyclophosphamide, and cis-diamminedichloroplatinum (II), preliminary assessment of a one-day vs. three-day drug regimen, *Cancer,* 47, 2549, 1981.

150. **Price, L. A., Hill, B. T., Calvert, A. H., Dalley, M., Levene, A., Busby, E. R., Schachter, M., and Shaw, H. J.,** Improved results in combination chemotherapy of head and neck cancer using a kinetically-based approach: a randomized study with and without adriamycin, *Oncology,* 35, 26, 1978.

151. **Woods, R. L., Stewart, J., Fox, R. M., and Tattersall, M. H. N.,** Combination chemotherapy with vincristine, bleomycin and methotrexate for advanced head and neck cancers, *Cancer Treat. Rep.,* 63, 1997, 1979.

152. **Vogl, S. E. and Kaplan, B. H.,** Chemotherapy of advanced head and neck cancer with methotrexate, bleomycin and cis-diamminedichloroplatinum (11) in an effective out-patient schedule, *Cancer,* 44, 26, 1979.

153. **Dritschilo, A, Piro, A. J., and Kelman, A. D.,** The effect of cis-platinum on the repair of radiation damage in plateau phase Chinese hamster (V-79) cells, *Int. J. Radiat. Oncol. Biol. Phys.,* 5, 1345, 1979.

154. **Byfield, J. E., Sharp, T. R., Frankel, S. S., Tang, S. G. and Callipari, F. B.,** Phase I and II trial of five-day infused 5-fluorouracil and radiation in advanced cancer of the head and neck, *J. Clin. Oncol.,* 2, 406, 1984.

155. **Vietti, T., Eggerding, F., and Valeriote, F.,** Combined effect of x-radiation and 5-fluorouracil on survival of transplanted leukemic cells, *J. Natl. Cancer Inst.,* 47, 865, 1972.

156. **Nigro, N. D., Seydel, H. G., Considine, B., Vaitkevicius, V. K., Leichman, L., and Kinzie, J. J.,** Combined preoperative radiation and chemotherapy for squamous cell carcinoma of the anal canal, *Cancer,* 51, 1826, 1983.

157. **Bloom, E. J., Green, M. D., Cooper, J. S., Cohen, N., and Muggia, F. M.,** Concomitant use of cis-platinum (CDDP) chemotherapy and radiation therapy (RT) in the treatment of advanced head and neck cancer, in *Proceedings of the American Society of Clinical Oncologists,* Foti, M., Mennite, M. A., and Pusztay, H. M., Eds., Waverly Press, Baltimore, 1985, 137.

158. **Miller, B., Yu, A., Tefft, M., and Leone, L.,** Improved response rate in patients with advanced unresectable cancer of the head and neck, in *Proceedings of the American Society of Clinical Oncologists,* Foti, M., Mennite, M. A., and Pusztay, H. M., Eds., Waverly Press, Baltimore, 1985, 142.

159. **Murthy, A. K., Taylor, S. G., Showel, J., Kramer, T., Kiel, K., Caldarelli, D. D., Hutchinson, J. C., Holinger, L. D, and Witt, T. R.,** Improved results with simultaneous chemotherapy and radiation in head and neck cancer, in *Proceedings of the American Society of Clinical Oncologists,* Foti, M., Mennite, M. A., and Pusztay, H. M., Eds., Waverly Press, Baltimore, 1985, 138.

160. **Adelstein, D. J., Sharan, V. M., Earle, A. S., Shah, A. C., Vlastou, C., Haria, C. D., Damm, C., Carter, S. G., and Hines, J. D.,** Combined modality therapy (CMT) with simultaneous 5-fluorouracil (5-FU), cis-platinum (DDP) and radiation therapy (RT) in the treatment of squamous cell cancer of the head and neck, in *Proceedings of the American Society of Clinical Oncologists* Foti, M., Mennite, M. A., and Pusztay, H. M., Eds., Waverly Press, Baltimore, 1985, 142.

161. **Slotman, G. J., Glickman, A. S., Doolittle, C. H., and Cummings, F. J.,** Preliminary experience within pre-operative synchronous cis-platinum (DDP) and radiation therapy (RT) in stage III and IV head and neck cancer, in *Proceedings of the American Society of Clinical Oncologists,* Foti, M., Mennite, M. A., and Pusztay, H. M., Eds., Waverly Press, Baltimore, 1985, 148.

162. **Ansfield, R. J., Ramierez, G., Davis, H. L., Jr., Korbitz, B. C., Vermud, H., and Gollin, F. F.,** Treatment of advanced cancer of the head and neck, *Cancer,* 25, 78, 1970.

163. **Knowlton, A. H., Percarpio, B., Bobrow, S., and Fischer, J. J.,** Methotrexate and radiation therapy in the treatment of advanced head and neck tumors, *Radiology,* 116, 709, 1975.

164. **Fazekas, J. T., Somer, C., and Kramer, S.,** Adjuvant intravenous methotrexate or definitive radiotherapy alone for advanced squamous cancers of the oral cavity, oropharynx, supraglottic larynx or hypopharynx, *Int. J. Radiat. Oncol. Biol. Phys.,* 6, 533, 1980.

165. **Lustig, R. A., Demare, P. A., and Kramer, S.,** Adjuvant methotrexate in the radiotherapeutic management of advanced tumors of the head and neck, *Cancer,* 37, 2703, 1976.

166. **Forastiere, A. A., Wolf, G. T., Medvec, B. R., and Baker, S. R.,** Treatment of head and neck cancer (H&N CA) with high-dose cisplatinum (DDP) in hypertonic saline, in *Proceedings of the American Society of Clinical Oncologists* Foti, M., Mennite, M. A., and Pusztay, H. M., Eds., Waverly Press, Baltimore, 1985, 141.

167. **Myers, J., Kuhn, J., Von Hoff, D., Mattox, D., Messerschmidt, G., Clark, G., Jurzec, K., and Ozois, R.,** High-dose cisplatinum in locally advanced and metastatic head and neck carcinoma, in *Proceedings of the American Society of Clinical Oncologists,* Foti, M., Mennite, M. A., and Pusztay, H. M., Eds., Waverly Press, Baltimore, 1985, 148.

168. **Wolback, S. B. and Howe, P. R.,** Tissue changes following deprivation of fat soluble A vitamin, *J. Exp. Med.,* 42, 753, 1925.

169. **Lasnitski, I.,** Growth pattern of the mouse prostate gland in organ culture and its response to sex hormones, vitamin A and 3-methylcholanthrene, *Natl. Cancer Inst. Monogr.,* 12, 381, 1963.

170. **Rowe, N. A. and Gorlin, R. J.,** The effect of vitamin A deficiency upon experimental oral carcinogenesis, *J. Dent. Res.,* 38, 72, 1959.

171. **Wald, N., Idle, M., Boreham, J., and Bailey, A.,** Low serum-vitamin A and subsequent risk of cancer. Preliminary results of a prospective study, *Lancet,* 2, 813, 1980.

172. **Benz, C. and Cadman, E.,** Modulation of 5-fluorouracil metabolism and cytotoxicity by antimetabolite pretreatment in human colorectal adenocarcinoma HCT-8, *Cancer Res.,* 41, 994, 1981.

173. **Gravenor, D., Panascl, L., Black, M., Frenkiel, S., and Margolese, R.,** Alternation of two active chemotherapies in squamous head and neck carcinoma (HNCA), in *Proceedings of the American Society of Clinical Oncologists,* Foti, M., Mennite, M. A., and Pusztay, H. M., Eds., Waverly Press, Baltimore, 1985, 126.

174. **Ensley, J., Kish, J., Jacobs, J., Weaver, A., Kinzie, J., Crissman, J., and Al-Sarraf, M.,** The use of five course, alternating combination chemotherapy induction regimen in advanced squamous cell cancer of the head and neck (SCC of H&N), in *Proceedings of the American Society of Clinical Oncologists,* Foti, M., Mennite, M. A., and Pusztay, H. M., Eds., Waverly Press, Baltimore, 1985, 143.

175. **Fox, R. M., Woods, R. L., and Tattersall, M. H. N.,** Allopurinol modulation of high-dose fluorouracil toxicity, *Cancer Treat. Rev.,* Suppl. 6, 143, 1979.

176. **Greenberg, B., Ahmann, F., Garewal, H., Koopman, C., Coulthard, S., Berzes, H., and Alberts, D.,** Neoadjuvant therapy for advanced head and neck cancer with allopurinol-modulated high dose 5-fluorouracil (5-FU) and cis-platinum (CP), in *Proceedings of the American Society of Clinical Oncologists,* Foti, M., Mennite, M. A., and Pusztay, H. M., Eds., Waverly Press, Baltimore, 1985, 146.

177. **Hornedo-Muguiro, J., So, M., Spaulding, M. B., Van Echo, D. A., Donehower, R., Ettinger, D., and Aisner, J.,** in *Proceedings of the American Society of Clinical Oncologists,* Foti, M., Mennite, M. A., and Pusztay, H. M., Eds., Waverly Press, Baltimore, 1985, 136.

178. **Kish, J., Ensley, J., Al-Sarraf, M., VonHoff, D., and Schuller, D.,** Activity of CHIP and CBDCA (platinum analogs) in recurrent epidermoid cancer of the head and neck (HNC) — randomized phase II trial of WSU and SWOG, in *Proceedings of the American Society of Clinical Oncologists,* Mennite, M. A., and Pusztay, H. M., Eds., Waverly Press, Baltimore, 1985, 130.

Chapter 7

COMPLICATIONS OF THE TREATMENT OF ORAL CANCER: PREVENTION, DIAGNOSIS, AND MANAGEMENT

John M. Wright, Fritz E. Barton, D. Lamar Byrd, Eugene W. Dahl, John S. Bradfield, and Robert G. Mennel

TABLE OF CONTENTS

I. INTRODUCTION

All therapeutic modalities for oral cancer produce side effects. Some of these are self limiting while others are permanent and produce significant cosmetic and/or functional impairment. An understanding of these side effects allows prevention in some instances and at least palliation or rehabilitation in others.

II. HEAD AND NECK RECONSTRUCTION

The major morbidity associated with the surgical treatment of oral cancer is the anatomic defect resulting from resection. Reconstitution of the oropharynx following head and neck cancer surgery presents one of the greatest challenges to reconstructive surgery, largely because the basic life functions of eating, breathing, and speaking all take place within this common anatomic cavity.

When planning the surgical reconstruction of oropharyngeal defects, one must keep in mind the management priorities. In descending order of importance these are (1) ablative cure, (2) restoration of function, and (3) reconstruction of form.

A. Goals of Reconstruction

The oral cavity and oropharynx represent a water-tight lining surrounded by a myriad of muscles which act in concert. In general, it is not possible to restore the delicate dynamic motions of the oral cavity; rather, reconstructions are crude replacements of static tissues. The surgeon must resist the temptation to become overimaginative in reconstructive attempts. The provision of a water-tight static lining that heals primarily is a practical and achievable goal.

The functional objectives[1] of oropharyngeal reconstruction are to (1) maintain oral continence, (2) enable swallowing, (3) prevent aspiration, (4) preserve speech, (5) protect vital structures, and (6) achieve primary healing.

Oral continence is a function of lip integrity. It requires adequate soft tissue as well as innervated musculature, especially in the lower lip.

Deglutition depends on a structurally intact upper digestive tract through which the food bolus moves from the mouth to the stomach. Resections in the area of the floor of the mouth or tongue may impair the ability of the tongue to propel the food bolus posteriorly into the hypopharynx. In such a case, deglutition can be facilitated by the creation of a funnel from the anterior oral cavity backward toward the hypopharynx.

Aspiration and its attendant pneumonitis is a common sequela of oral cancer resection. It may result from loss of muscular control at the base of the tongue, restriction of the epiglottis in protecting the glottic orifice, lack of suspension of the larynx in an anterior and superior position, or from lack of sensation in the posterior hypopharnyx.

Successful speech depends upon the ability of the larynx to generate sound and the ability of the soft palate, tongue, and lips to shape this sound into words. These sound-shaping structures are dynamic and cannot be replaced. After resections involving the speech musculature, it is important to avoid tethering the dynamic remnants and further compromising speech capability.

Protection of vital structures usually implies protection of either the carotid artery or the mandibular bone, especially if postoperative radiation therapy is to be undertaken.

There is no substitute for uneventful primary healing. Postoperative complications in healing lead to salivary fistulas and carotid artery erosion and delay the institution of postoperative radiation or chemotherapy.

B. Methods of Surgical Reconstruction

As with all reconstructive problems, the alternatives must be considered in hierarchical order, from the simplest to the most complex. The least involved and most direct method that will provide adequate reconstruction is the procedure of choice.

1. Healing by Primary Intention

Primary closure is desirable whenever possible. It is most feasible on the side of the tongue, the buccal mucosa, and the esophagus. Direct approximation assumes that there is adequate laxity of the tissues to bring the edges together without undue tension and without tethering vital dynamic structures.

2. Healing by Secondary Intention

If complete primary closure is not possible due to the dimension of the wound, then healing by secondary intention should be considered. It is an acceptable option if a water-tight seal is not mandatory and if the wound base contains well-vascularized tissue.

3. Skin Grafts

The next echelon of closure is that of skin grafting. A skin graft is amputated tissue that must survive by vascular ingrowth from the recipient bed over a period of several days. In the oropharynx split-thickness skin grafts (STSG) are the usual method of choice. The indication for STSG is the same as for healing by secondary intention, but grafting has the advantages of more rapid healing and less constriction of the wound.

Areas that lend themselves best to STSG are those in the superior part of the oral cavity, i.e., the maxilla. STSG is also useful as a secondary procedure in vestibuloplasty.

When STSG is chosen for defects of the oral cavity, the graft may be harvested with a surgical dermatome, i.e., the Brown, Reese, or Padgett. The desired thickness of the graft usually varies between 15/1000 and 17/1000 of an inch. The usual donor sites are the upper outer thighs since they are a ready source of thick dermis.

In applying the graft, it is important to avoid any dead space beneath the graft surface. Adherence to the bed may be enhanced either by quilting sutures which penetrate the graft into the depth of the recipient bed or by applying pressure through a bolus dressing left in place for approximately 1 week.

4. Skin Flaps

Unlike skin grafts, skin flaps refer to sections of skin that are transferred to a new location while maintaining their own nutrient blood flow. Flap closure is the most complicated of the reconstructive methods and is indicated in the following:

1. For preservation of mobility. There are four points of critical mobility within the oropharynx: the tongue, the soft palate, mandible at the retromolar trigone, and the larynx. It is critical to avoid restriction in these areas. Skin flaps bring pliable tissue capable of stretching to allow full range of motion.
2. Inadequate vascularity of the recipient site. Exposed bone or cartilage does not provide a suitable bed for healing either by secondary intention or by skin grafting. Flap tissue carrying its own vasculature is indicated.
3. Water-tight seal. When a floor-of-mouth resection is carried out in continuity with a radical neck dissection, the salivary pool must be isolated from the vasculature and soft tissue space in the neck. If primary closure is not possible, then flap tissue is usually required.
4. To protect vital structures. In patients with extensive lesions in the oral cavity, the curative effort of surgical resection may be supplemented with radiotherapy. A sturdy soft tissue cover over vital structures, i e,, the mandible or carotid artery, is of benefit in preventing secondary wound breakdown due to the radiation.

Table 1
SKIN FLAPS USED IN HEAD AND NECK RECONSTRUCTION

Pedicle	Flap	Application
Random (dermal)	Nasolabial	Anterior floor of mouth, palate
Axial (direct cutaneous)	Temporal forehead	Oral cavity down to level of larynx
	Deltopectoral	Oral cavity up to level of maxilla
Myocutaneous	Tongue	Small defects of lateral oral cavity and cheek
	Latissimus dorsi	Oral cavity and esophagus
	Pectoralis major	Oral cavity and esophagus
	Trapezius	Cheek, mandible
Free microvascular	Dorsalis pedis	Floor of mouth
	Jejunal	Esophagus
	Iliac	Mandible

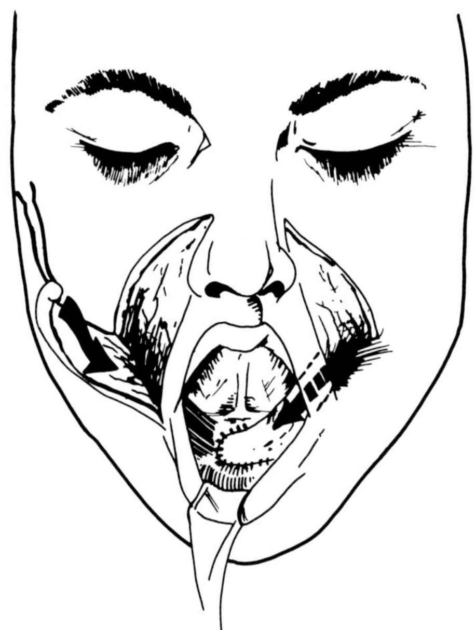

FIGURE 1. Nasolabial flap.

A large variety of flaps have been described for use in the head and neck. Based upon their pattern of blood supply, the more common flaps applicable to oropharyngeal reconstruction are summarized in Table 1.

Tongue flaps — Tongue flaps are usually constructed longitudinally from the lateral 20 to 40% of the tongue, based posteriorly on a branch of the lingual artery. They are most helpful for defects of the retromolar trigone or tonsillar area.

Nasolabial flaps — Nasolabial flaps are usually based inferiorly, where they are supplied by branches of the angular artery from the anterior facial artery. The flap is tunneled through the cheek into the anterior floor of the mouth, and may be elevated bilaterally when necessary. The flap pedicle is secondarily divided and inset (Figures 1 and 2).

Temporal forehead flaps — Based on the superficial temporal artery, the temporal forehead flap has been a mainstay of oropharyngeal reconstruction throughout its history. The flap may be designed to extend across the midline almost to the opposite temporal area. It is folded internally to be delivered into the oral cavity through a buccal penetration. Secondary division and inset of the pedicle are necessary. Temporal forehead flaps are useful in defects throughout the entire oral cavity. The lowermost limit of flap excursion is at a point just above the larynx.

Deltopectoral flap — The deltopectoral flap is based on the perforating branches of the internal mammary artery, primarily from the second and third interspaces. This direct cutaneous flap can be extended over the deltoid area without delay and used for reconstruction of the esophagus and lower oral cavity. A secondary division and inset of the pedicle is usually required.

Latissimus dorsi flap — The latissimus dorsi island myocutaneous flap is taken from the middle third of the lateral border of the latissimus dorsi muscle when intended for head and neck reconstruction. The flap is tunneled through the axilla and into the neck, where it can be used for reconstruction of the pharynx or the entire oral cavity. Since blood supply to the skin is supplied from the muscle beneath, the cutaneous island may be inset in a single stage without the need for secondary division of the pedicle.

Pectoralis major flap — Based upon the thoracoacromial artery, the pectoralis major myocutaneous flap can transfer an island of parasternal skin into the neck or oral cavity in a single operative stage.

Trapezius flap — Based on either the superior or inferior portion of the trapezius muscle, a cutaneous island can be transferred on the transverse cervical artery. This flap is most helpful in lateral defects of the cheek or oral cavity, but can be modified to carry the spine of the scapula for reconstruction of the mandible as well.

Jejunal free flap — A segment of jejunum, based on the mesenteric vessels, can be transferred from the abdomen into the neck by microvascular anastomoses. It is especially useful for segmental esophageal reconstruction.

Deep circumflex iliac osteocutaneous flap — The deep circumflex iliac osteocutaneous flap can be mobilized on the vascular branch for which it is named. A hemimandible can be carved from the iliac wing and transferred by microvascular anastomoses to preserve nutrient blood flow.

Dorsalis pedis free flap — The dorsalis pedis free flap can be used on its named artery to provide soft, thin, and mobile tissue from the dorsum of the foot for the floor of the mouth.

C. Mandibular Reconstruction

Because of the proximity of the jaws to sites prone to develop oral malignancy, invasion of the tumor often involves the periosteum and bone. Once bone invasion occurs, radiation therapy offers little hope for cure, and the involved bone must be removed surgically. Depending on the extent of involvement, the surgical procedure may range from a small, marginal resection with little morbidity to hemimandibulectomy which results in a major discontinuity defect. Primary squamous carcinomas of the maxillary gingiva and palatal mucosa are rare. Involvement of the maxilla by tumor usually requires hemimaxillectomy or maxillectomy, and the resulting defect is managed prosthodontically, not surgically.

Minimal bone involvement can often be managed by marginal mandibular resection of the inner and outer cortical plates. This procedure spares the inferior border of the mandible and maintains mandibular continuity, which significantly decreases morbidity. Stabilization of the partially resected mandible will aid in healing of the soft tissues and bone, maintain facial symmetry, maintain mandibular position for immediate or delayed reconstruction, retain laryngeal suspension to maintain swallowing, and reduce functional and cosmetic disability.

Stabilization of the mandible for dentulous patients can be accomplished by osteotomy of the mandible followed by intraoral wire or arch bar fixation (Figure 3), or bone plates and extraoral skeletal fixation. The edentulous mandible may be stabilized with a Gunning's splint constructed like new dentures (Figure 4) or modified from the patient's existing dentures (Figure 5).

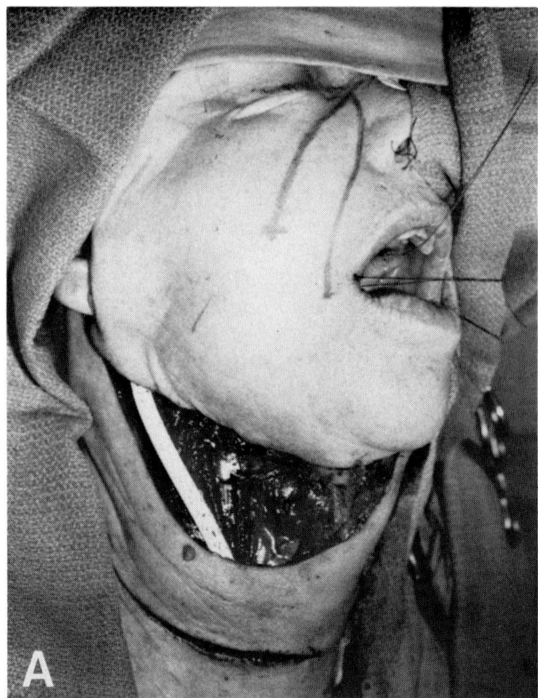

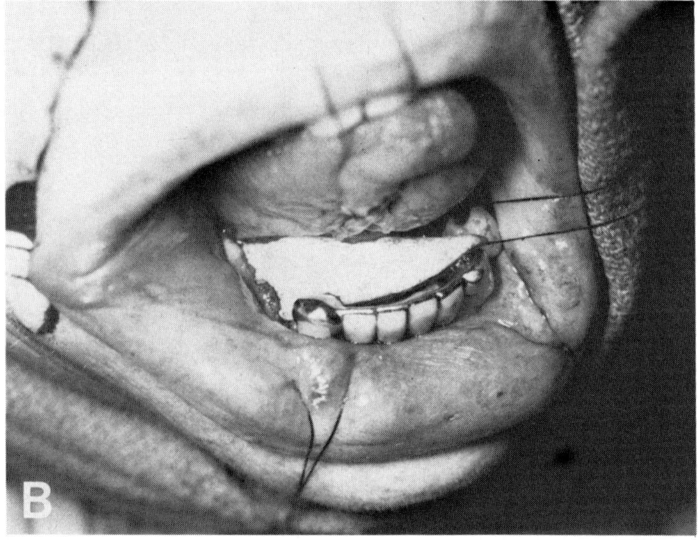

FIGURE 2.   (A) Design of nasolabial flap. (B) Flap inset in the floor of the mouth. (C) Postoperative result at 4 months.

Attempts at reconstruction of the mandible have been remarkable for their diversity and ingenuity. Among the nonvascularized tissue approaches are single-block cortical-cancellous carved mandibles from the ipsilateral ilium,[2] cancellous bone chips seated in an alloplastic tray form,[3,4] freeze-dried autogenous mandible,[5] homologous mandibular tray with autogenous bone chips,[6] allogeneic rib,[7] autoclaved mandible,[8] and irradiated mandible.[9]

In addition, vascularized bone has been transferred based on the periosteal blood supply

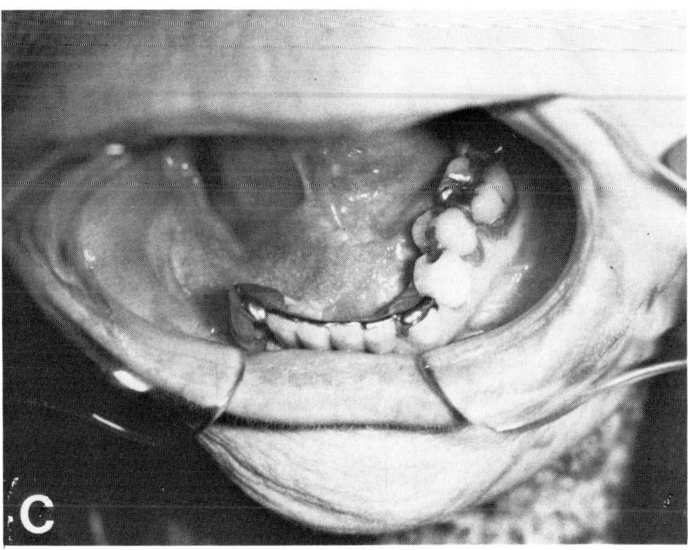

FIGURE 2C.

of the sternocleidomastoid,[10] pectoralis major,[11] latissimus dorsi,[12,13] and trapezius muscles,[14,15] as well as via the direct nutrient circulation from the deep circumflex iliac artery, primarily to the iliac wing.[16,17]

Short segments of the mandible, lost from either trauma or benign tumor resection, present little reconstructive problems by any method. The long mandibular segment defects in patients with extensive resections of bone and oral lining for malignant disease constitute the extreme challenge.

D. Maxillofacial Prosthodontics

Dental consultation should be a routine part of the clinical evaluation for patients about to undergo treatment for cancer of the head and neck region. A thorough dental examination, routine radiographs, and impressions of the teeth and adjacent soft tissue should be made. Dentulous patients should be educated about oral hygiene regimens, and a routine oral prophylaxis should be performed. Patients with active oral infections should be controlled prior to receiving their definitive cancer therapy. The decision to extract or retain existing teeth should also be made (see Section III.B.6).

Following ablative surgery, reconstruction often utilizes the patient's own tissue for repair of the defect. There are many limitations to these procedures because of the lack of available tissue and the need to monitor the surgical site for recurrent disease. The prosthetic restoration of the defect becomes a viable option in many cases. In order to achieve optimal rehabilitation, careful preoperative planning between the surgeon and the maxillofacial prosthodontist is essential. Consultation between the surgeon and prosthodontist prior to treatment allows the patient the greatest chance for successful prosthetic reconstruction.

1. Intraoral Prostheses

a. Maxillary Defects

Surgical resection of a portion of the maxilla and adjacent soft tissue results in anatomic and functional defects of the oral cavity and oropharynx. These defects result in a communication between the oral and nasal cavities and cause unintelligible speech and nasal reflux of liquid and solid food. The resulting disabilities affect the patient's nutritional status, and normal communication is lost.

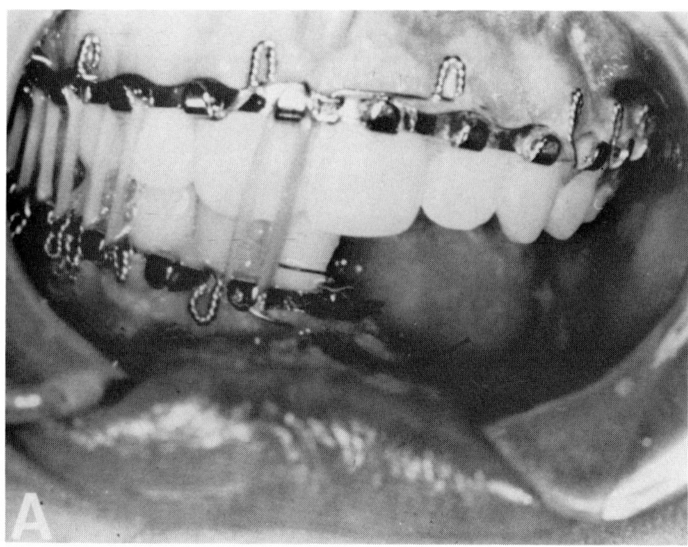

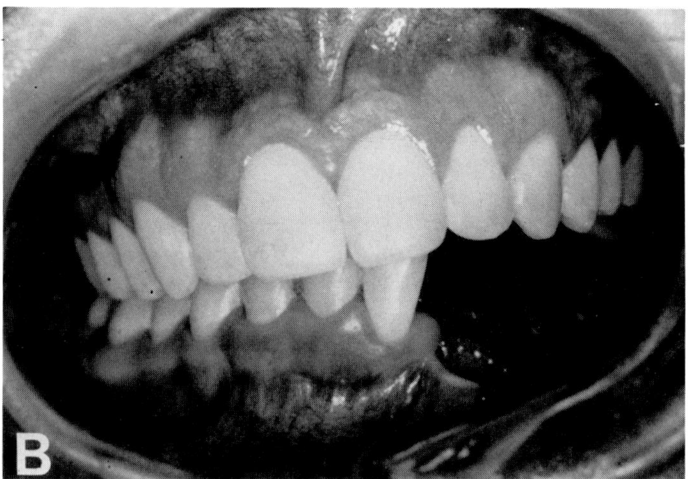

FIGURE 3. (A) Stabilization of the mandible following surgical resection for an oral malignancy. (B) Stabilization maintaining occlusion and facial symmetry and reducing functional and cosmetic disability.

When a maxillectomy is planned, presurgical impressions are taken and stone casts are made. The surgical area is removed on the cast, and an obturator prothesis is then fabricated using the remaining teeth with circumdental wires for retention.[18] For edentulous patients, the remaining residual alveolar ridge is used to support the prosthesis, and a bone screw secures it during the healing phase. The obturator is inserted at surgery using a soft denture liner to allow adaption to the resultant oral defect. The artificial palate enables the patient to take food orally, which eliminates the need for a nasogastric tube. Speech is virtually unaffected, wound hygiene is improved, and the soft liner acts as a pressure stent against the skin graft to decrease wound oozing and possible hematoma formation. In 6 to 7 days the surgical obturator and soft liner packing are removed. Utilizing the obturator platform, a soft denture liner is adapted to the maxillary defect to obtain a seal.

As the healing progresses an interim obturator is fabricated once the wound margins

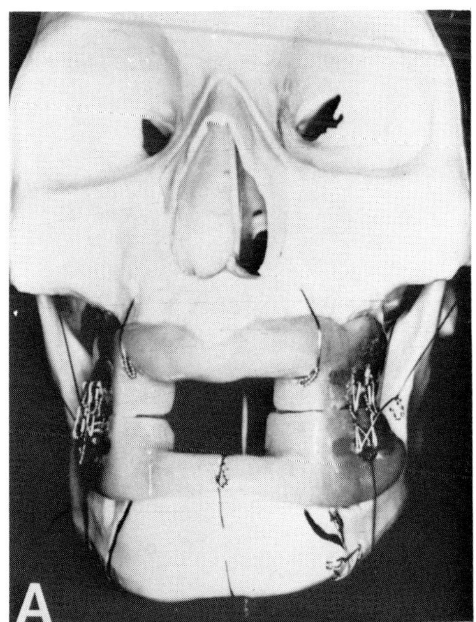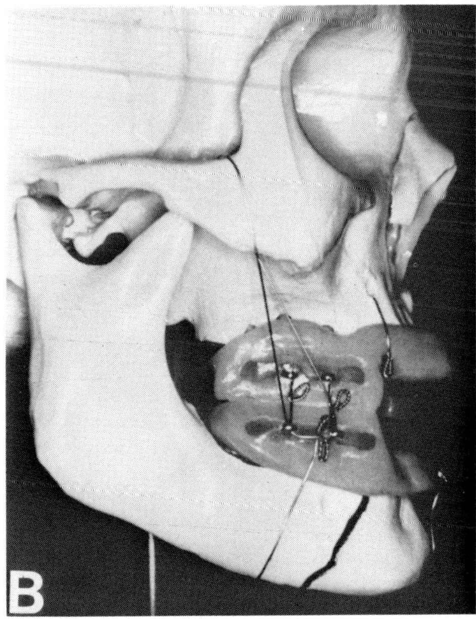

FIGURE 4.   (A) and (B) Gunning's splint stabilization of the mandible for edentulous patients.

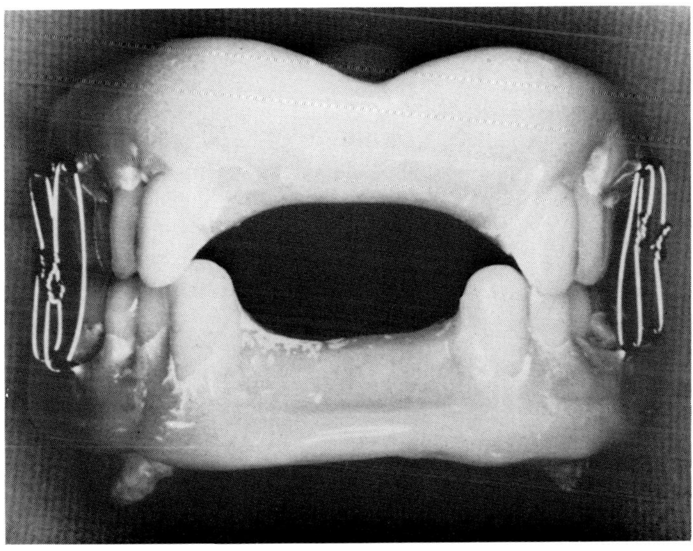

FIGURE 5.   Stabilization of resected mandible utilizing patients' existing dentures.

stabilize. This prosthesis is made from methylmethacrylate resin for easy cleaning. The obturator bulb is hollowed to decrease the weight of the prosthesis. Once the defect has healed, a definitive obturator can be fabricated with a chromium framework that is supported by restored and prepared teeth or a well-healed edentulous alveolar ridge utilizing sound prosthodontic principles of maximum extension for support, stability, and retention (Figure 6).

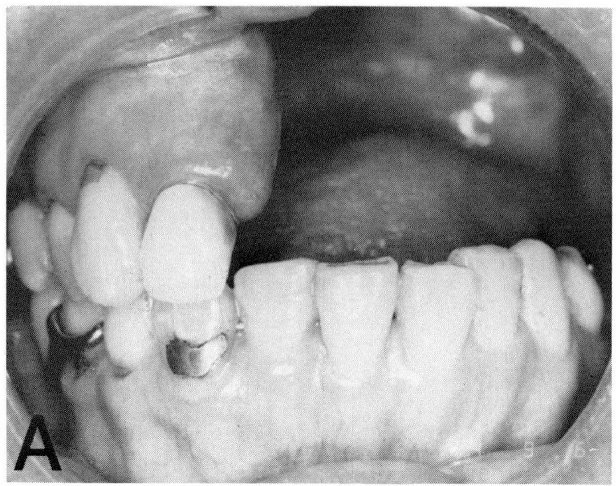

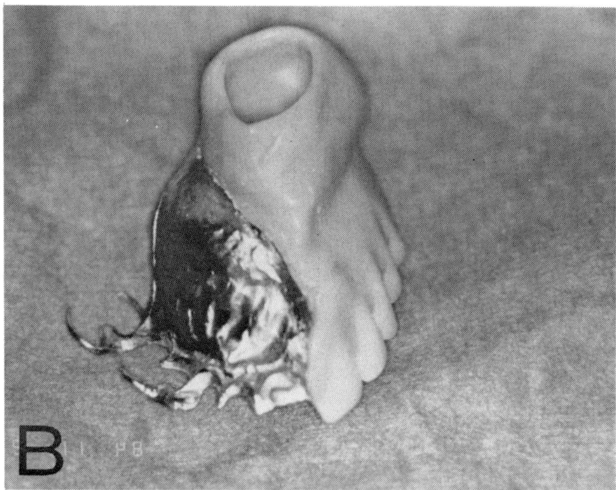

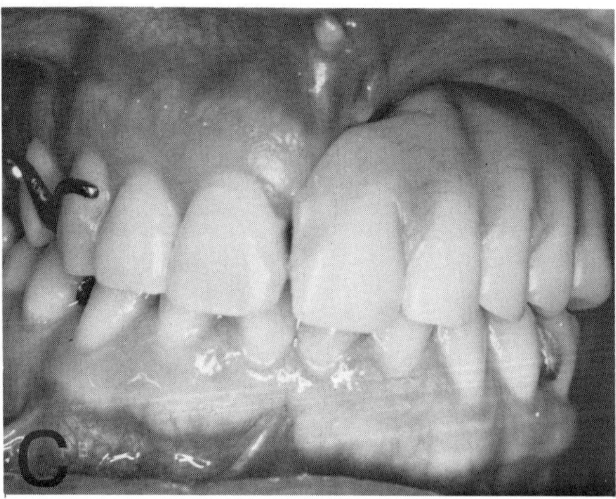

FIGURE 6. (A) Healed defect following maxillectomy for oral cancer. (B) Final prosthesis containing hollow obturator. (C) Prosthesis restoring aesthetics and function.

b. Mandibular Defects

Surgical resection of the mandible results in one of the greatest challenges in patient rehabilitation. Prosthodontic treatment for the hemimandibulectomy patient is a difficult task because of the lack of bony support, restricted tongue movement, limited opening, and mandibular deviation upon opening.[19] Mandibular deviation following surgery in some patients can be decreased by intermaxillary fixation. Although the maxillary denture is readily accepted by most patients, patient acceptance of a mandibular denture after a partial mandibular resection is variable. A functionally developed mandibular prosthesis is more successful and generally better tolerated than a denture fabricated using conventional denture techniques. The mandibular deviation during closing dictates that the occlusal scheme be developed using a functionally generated path technique to capture the dynamic movements of the mandible.[20] In most cases a mandibular resection prosthesis can be successfully worn by the patient if adequate time to adjust is allowed and encouragement is given.

2. Extraoral Prostheses

Resection of some oral cancers results in facial defects, and the fabrication of a facial prosthesis can in many instances successfully restore facial appearance and the self-image of the patient.[21] The psychological status of the patient may hinder prosthetic replacement because in some instances the patient cannot accept the prosthesis as a replacement.

A successful facial prosthesis depends upon careful preparation of the surgical defect. Retention and hygiene of the prosthesis are more dependent on the nature of the defect than on the materials and skills of the clinician.

Once the surgical defect is healed, a facial prosthesis can be fabricated using silicone, acrylic resin, or a combination of the two materials.[22] The prosthesis is processed in a custom-made mold after facial impressions are obtained using an elastomeric impression material. The degree of resiliency of the prosthesis can be controlled by blending different silicone materials together and custom coloration applied to give a lifelike appearance. The margins of the prosthesis can be camouflaged by using hair, eye glasses, make-up, or a transparent polyurethane film to blend the prosthesis with the natural facial contours (Figure 7). In some instances with combined defects involving the oral cavity and facial structures, the prostheses are fabricated and joined to each other utilizing special attachment systems to gain additional retention and stability.

The fabrication of intra- and extraoral prostheses can satisfy the functional and aesthetic needs of the patient and permit observation of the area by the surgeon. It is necessary for the prosthodontist to become part of the oncologic team and participate in the treatment planning for comprehensive management and quality care. The prosthodontist can contribute to the overall rehabilitation of the head and neck cancer patient by permitting a potentially handicapped person normal participation in everyday social interactions.

III. COMPLICATIONS OF RADIOTHERAPY FOR ORAL CANCER

The complications of high dose radiotherapy for the treatment of squamous cell carcinoma of the oral cavity may be divided into the acute side effects which are self-limiting and the chronic irreversible complications which may become more severe with time.

The primary manifestation of the acute effects of radiation to the oral cavity is a painful mucositis which develops because radiation destroys the rapidly dividing epithelial cells of the oral mucosa and results in the formation of a membrane of dead epithelial cells over the denuded submucosa. This mucositis heals within 2 to 3 weeks of the completion of radiotherapy.

The chronic effects or complications of high dose radiotherapy to the oral cavity are due to direct injury to the microvascular or parenchymal cells and result in atrophy of these tissues. Chronic complications which include xerostomia, dysgeusia, hypogeusia, acceler-

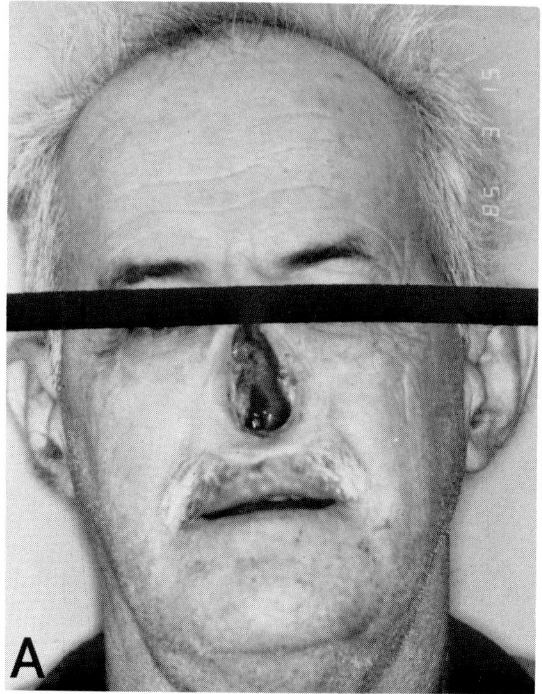

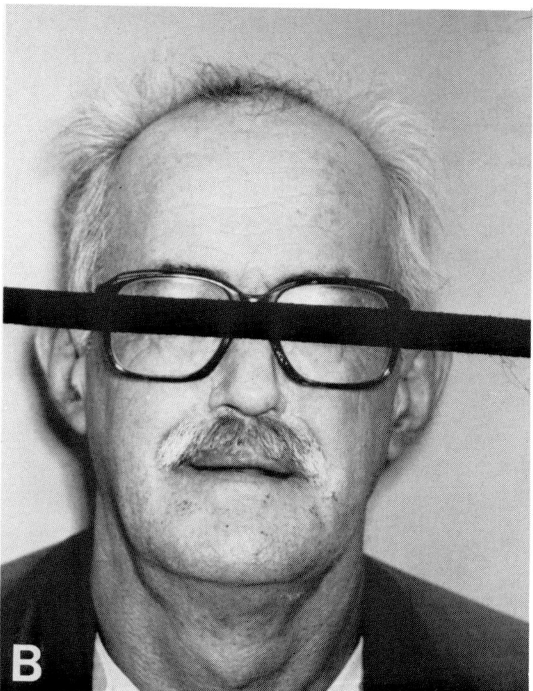

FIGURE 7.   (A) Healed facial defect lined with a skin graft.
(B) Silicone nasal prosthesis.

ation of dental caries, and on occasion, osteoradionecrosis are most distressing to the patient as they are progressive and for the most part irreversible complications of treatment.

A. Acute Effects of Radiotherapy on the Oral Cavity

The acute effects of radiotherapy on the oral cavity follow a predictable course when patients are treated with conventional fractionated radiotherapy (200 rad/day, 5 days/week) and may be outlined as follows.[23,24]

Week 1 — Approximately 5% of patients will experience a transient, occasionally painful, swelling of one or more salivary glands within 12 hr of the first treatment which resolves within 48 to 72 hr. There may be a transient rise in the serum amylase. Some prominence of the circumvallate papillae may be the only oral physical finding at this early stage, although occasional patients will develop an erythema as well.

Week 2 — The patient begins to complain of soreness, pain on swallowing, and dryness of the mouth. Examination reveals a definite erythema and an early patchy mucositis especially on the palate and uvula. This mucositis consists of a pseudomembrane consisting of dead epithelial cells, fibrin, and polymorphonuclear leukocytes. An early reaction on and adjacent to the tumor is called a "tumoritis" and is an indication to the radiation therapist of the adequecy of the treatment field (see Chapter 6).

Week 3 — Eating becomes more difficult and pain increases. Although some patients may complain of a bitter taste (dysgeusia) and diminished taste (hypogeusia) early in the course of therapy, definite impairment of taste detection and recognition thresholds are observed at this time.[25] Bitter and salt perception show the earliest and greatest impairment, while sweetness shows the least impairment. The saliva becomes thickened and tenacious, and the patchy mucositis which began on the palate and uvula extends onto the tonsillar pillars and posterior pharyngeal wall.

Week 4 — The intensity of these complaints increases, and the mucositis becomes confluent, extending onto the buccal mucosa. Patients with metallic restorations will develop a more pronounced mucosal reaction adjacent to these restorations as a result of back-scattered, low energy electrons. This problem can be minimized by placing a thin paraffin wedge between the mucosa and teeth at the time of treatment.

Week 5 — The patient's oral intake may become limited, and oral analgesics are required to keep the patient comfortable. The mucositis extends to the lateral surface of the tongue which is the last site to become affected.

Week 6 — Symptoms may plateau and even abate. However, superficial ulceration may appear particularly where the confluent mucositis or pseudomembrane has been removed.

Following completion of the course of radiotherapy the mucositis will persist for approximately 2 to 3 weeks and then rapidly improve over a 2- to 3-day period. Most patients have complete healing of their mucosa and are asymptomatic 1 month after treatment.

A confluent mucositis may also be seen approximately 2 weeks after the removal of an interstitial implant (Figure 8). Healing is complete by 4 to 6 weeks, but patients generally require oral analgesics during the period of mucositis.

Control of the patient's symptoms during the phase of acute radiation mucositis depends on good oral hygiene. Prior to radiotherapy the patient's dental condition must be assessed and plaque removed, teeth repaired or extracted, and gingival disease controlled. The patient must maintain exemplary oral hygiene by frequent brushing with a soft toothbrush and frequent use of dental floss. To minimize the pain and extent of mucositis, a dilute saline mouthwash consisting of 1 level teaspoon of table salt and 1 level teaspoon of baking soda in 1 qt of water can be made by the patient. Rinsing the mouth with this solution should begin with the 1st treatment day and vary from every 1 to 2 hr during the early weeks to every $1/2$ hr as the mucositis becomes more intense in the 3rd and 4th week of treatment.

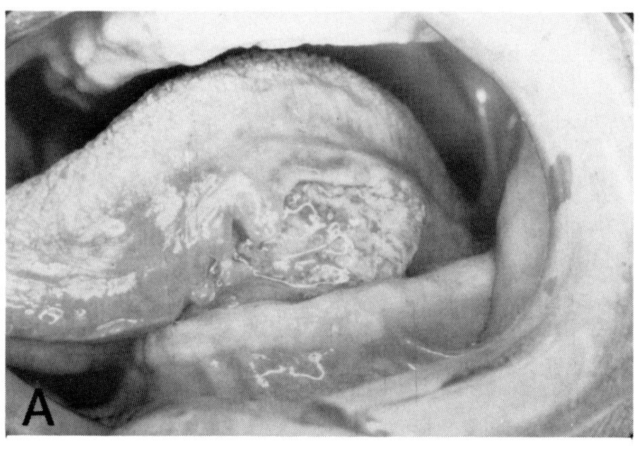

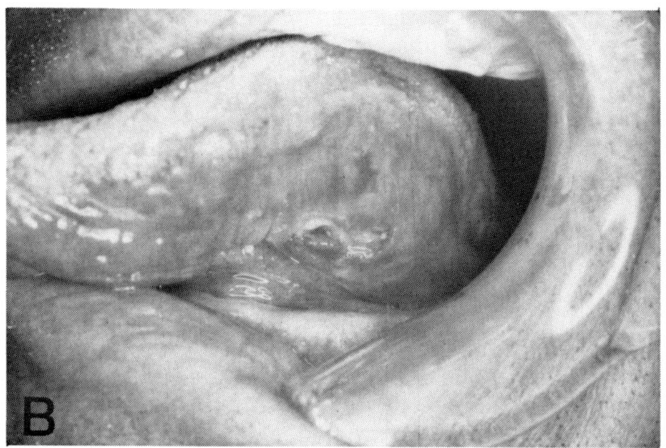

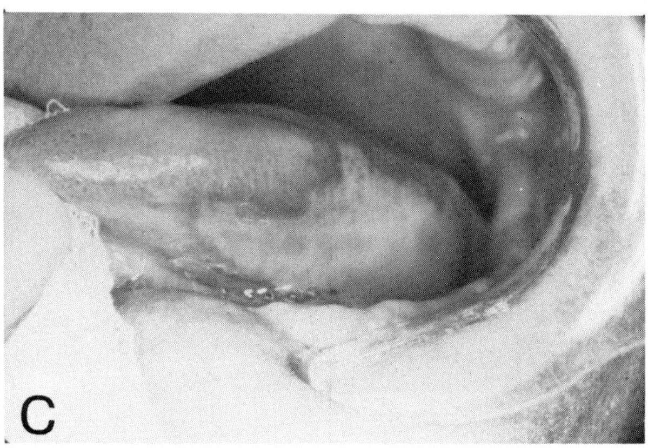

FIGURE 8.   (A) T2N0 carcinoma of mobile tongue. (B) Lesion after 1800 rad external radiotherapy. (C) Confluent mucositis 2 weeks following removal of implant.

B. Late Effects of Radiotherapy on the Oral Cavity

1. Xerostomia

Possibly the most devastating late effect or complication of high dose radiation to the oral cavity is xerostomia. Severe dryness of the oral cavity is incapacitating and also contributes to other complications, i.e., loss of taste acuity, acceleration of dental caries, bone and soft tissue necrosis, and mucosal colonization by *Candida* species.

Loss of salivary gland function is dependent on both the volume of salivary gland tissue irradiated and the radiation dose. For most cases of cancer of the oral cavity all submandibular and sublingual salivary gland tissue is included in the treatment field and approximately 25 to 30% of the parotid salivary glands.[26] Fields of this size are necessary to include both the primary site and potential or actual lymphatic metastases in the submandibular and upper cervical nodes. To avoid severe dryness greater than 50% of the parotids must be excluded from the treatment volume.[27] Patients exhibit great variability in the location of their parotid glands, so that without sialography it is difficult to determine the volume of parotid tissue irradiated and thus predict the extent of xerostomia.[26]

The residual function of the parotid salivary glands is dependent on the dose of radiation received during radiotherapy. Above 6000 rad no measurable saliva can be detected. Only one fifth of parotid glands receiving 4000 to 6000 rad have measurable saliva, while one half of glands receiving an average of 950 rad have salivary flow reduced to one half of normal when measured 2 years after radiotherapy.[28] This latter circumstance is encountered in patients who are treated unilaterally with a mixed photon and electron beam. While the ipsilateral gland is irradiated to greater than 6000 rad, the contralateral gland receives approximately 1000 rad. Many of these patients, despite significant, measurable loss of salivary gland function, do not complain of dry mouth.

Patients may develop a chronic sialadenitis after radiotherapy. A symmetrical, bilateral swelling of the submandibular salivary glands, though usually painless, will give cause for concern to the patient and physician. The symmetry and bilaterality of the glands suggest sialadenitis rather than metastatic carcinoma.[29]

In addition to reduced salivary flow the pH, electrolytes, and secretory IgA of saliva are altered by radiotherapy.[28] Reduction of pH to acidic levels is attributed to a reduction in bicarbonate levels and contributes to altered oral microflora.[30] The reduction of secretory IgA is best explained by progressive destruction of plasma cells by irradiation.

Patients radiated for head and neck cancer have a significantly increased incidence of intraoral opportunistic yeast infections with *Candida* species.[31] Although many healthy people "carry" *C. albicans* asymptomatically as a commensal in their oral flora, radiation-induced salivary changes promote overgrowth of the fungus. This may result in chronic atrophic candidosis which is characterized clinically by a painful, erythematous mucosa (signs and symptoms that are at times difficult to distinguish from radiation mucositis). The infection may include the characteristic white plaques and often extends into the commissures to produce angular cheilitis. The problem of yeast overgrowth is further enhanced by edentulous patients who also wear dentures. The infection is responsive to antifungal medications, but patients are prone to recurrences.

2. Effects on Teeth

Quantitative and qualitative changes in the saliva are responsible for rapid progression of dental caries in the irradiated patient. These changes occur whether the teeth are inside or outside the radiated field and, therefore, are not the direct result of radiation injury to the teeth.[32] Additionally, there is a significant shift in the oral flora of irradiated patients to a more cariogenic, acidogenic bacterial population.[30]

Dental caries commence with the onset of xerostomia and differ from ordinary dental caries in distribution. The buccofacial surfaces of the teeth are primarily affected. These

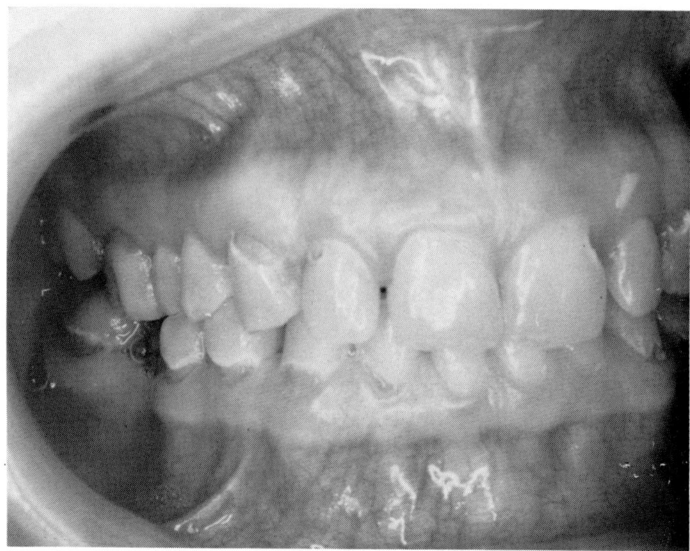

FIGURE 9.   Extensive cervical caries in a patient with xerostomia secondary to radiation for an intraoral carcinoma. (Courtesy of Dr. D. Lamar Byrd.)

surfaces are normally bathed by saliva and are more resistant to caries in the unirradiated mouth. Without treatment, the carious process continues around the exposed cervical portion of the tooth (Figure 9) and may result in amputation of the tooth crown.[32] The incidence of radiation caries can be significantly reduced with meticulous oral hygiene and the daily application of topical fluoride. The root sensitivity experienced by some patients following radiation therapy is not necessarily related to the carious process, and often the cause is unknown.

If radiation therapy is given prior to the age of 20; the developing tooth buds are markedly affected and result in agenesis or defective teeth. However, oral cancer in this age group is rare.

3. Taste Impairment

Many patients with cancer of the oral cavity will have measurable impairment of taste acuity without subjective complaints of alteration in taste prior to any treatment. This may be due to the gradual loss of taste as a result of aging and the slow growth of an intraoral tumor. With the onset of radiation, taste acuity rapidly decreases further so that by the end of the 3rd week of treatment subjective complaints of impairment are seen in the majority of patients.[25] Partial recovery of taste occurs in most patients 2 to 4 months following completion of radiotherapy. In an uncontrolled clinical study zinc supplements improved taste acuity in patients with persistent taste impairment 1 year or more after radiotherapy.[25]

4. Trismus

Radiation fibrosis of the muscles of mastication and the temporomandibular joint may be seen in patients who receive high doses (greater than 7000 rad) via opposed 4 to 6 MeV X-ray beams. This is particularly true when tumor involves the masticatory muscles or the temporomandibular joint. The risk of severe trismus as a result of these complications is also greater in patients who are treated with both surgery and radiation. As there is no simple treatment for severe trismus, the best approach is avoidance of the problem by careful treatment planning and minimizing the dose to the temporomandibular joint and the pterygoid and buccinator muscles. Some relief of trismus can be obtained by using dynamic bite openers.

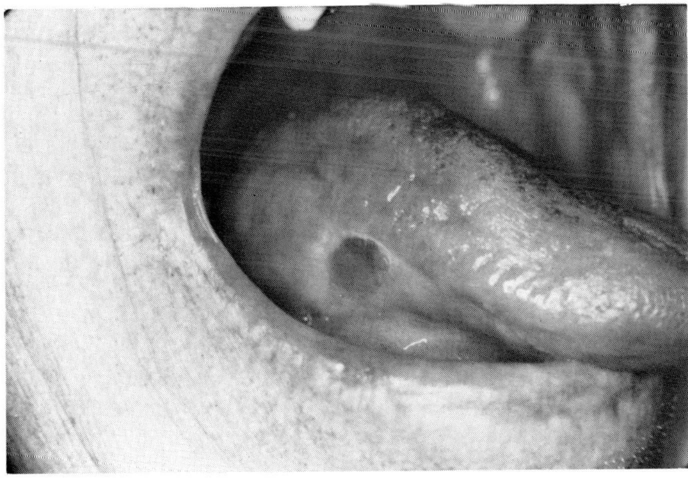

FIGURE 10. Soft tissue necrosis of lateral border of the tongue secondary to external radiotherapy.

5. Soft Tissue Necrosis

Necrosis of soft tissues in the oral cavity secondary to radiation is due to atrophy of the mucosa and reduced tissue vascularity. The majority of soft tissue necroses occur within 2 years of treatment and heal with conservative management (Figure 10).

Soft tissue ulceration can occur in association with dentures. While most radiated patients can wear dentures without a significant risk of soft tissue or bone necrosis, the fabrication of dentures should be delayed about 1 year following radiotherapy. Beumer and colleagues[33] recently published an excellent review of dental and prosthodontic considerations for oral cancer patients treated with radiation.

6. Osteoradionecrosis

The most serious late complication of radiotherapy to the oral cavity is osteoradionecrosis. Bone, like most tissues, is irreversibly damaged by therapeutic doses of radiation and, because of its density, often receives a greater radiation dose than the adjacent tumor. The bone marrow becomes relatively avascular with fibrosis and fatty degeneration, and there is a concomitant depletion of bone cells. These cellular changes significantly compromise the ability of bone to respond to trauma and infection, although it has recently been speculated that infection plays a lesser role in the pathogenesis of osteonecrosis; rather, the basic pathophysiologic defect is one of altered wound healing.[34] Areas of exposed bone, such as frequently occur following combination external radiotherapy and interstitial radiotherapy for carcinoma of the tongue or floor of the mouth, may remain small and heal within a few months with conservative management. Other patients experience persistent, progressive bone necrosis which results in intractable pain and may require surgical resection for control (Figure 11). Areas of devitalized bone tend to sequestrate,[35] and the extent of bony necrosis radiographically is often greater than the area of exposed bone clinically (Figure 12).

Osteoradionecrosis occurs almost exclusively in the mandible because of its density and decreased vascularity. Although the reported incidence of osteoradionecrosis varies widely, the risk of this complication has been studied thoroughly by Daley and Drane,[36] Daly et al.,[37] and Murray et al.[38,39] and may be related to the following factors: (1) anatomic site of the primary tumor, (2) radiation dose, and (3) dental status of the patient. The greatest risk of osteoradionecrosis is seen in patients whose primary tumor is intimately related to bone. In the series of Murray et al.[38] 56% of patients whose lesions arose on the hard palate

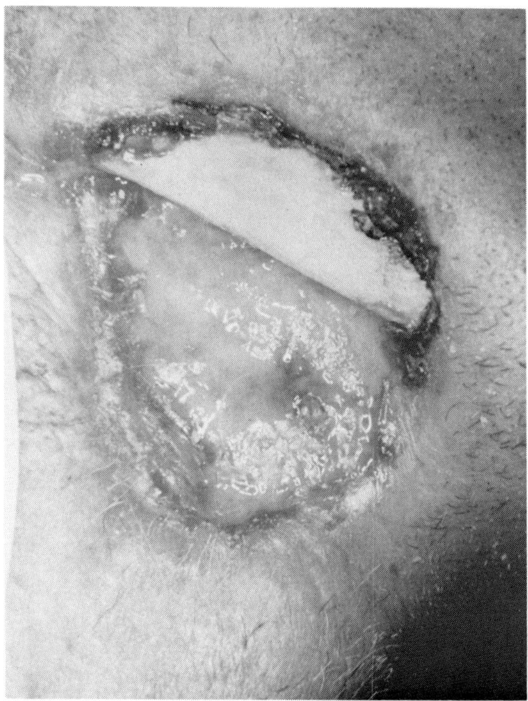

FIGURE 11.   Osteoradionecrosis with exposure of the mandible. (Courtesy of Dr. D. Lamar Byrd.)

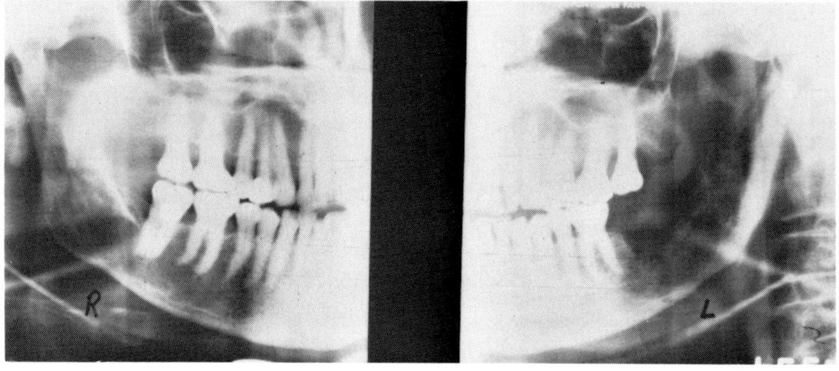

FIGURE 12.   Extensive osteonecrosis of left mandibular body and ramus. (Courtesy of Dr. Robert P. Langlais, The University of Texas Health Science Center, Dental Diagnostic Science, San Antonio.)

or gingiva experienced bone necrosis. A 29% incidence of necrosis was seen in patients with carcinomas adjacent to bone and teeth, i.e., carcinomas of the floor of mouth and retromolar trigone. The least risk of necrosis was observed in patients whose primary tumor was away from bone, i.e., carcinomas of the anterior two thirds of the tongue and buccal mucosa. In this instance the risk of osteoradionecrosis was 21%.

The frequency of osteoradionecrosis is least in patients treated with external radiation alone, intermediate with combinations of external radiation and interstitial therapy, and greatest when interstitial therapy is used alone. However, if bone necrosis develops in a patient treated with a combination of external and interstitial therapy, the size of the defect is likely to be larger than if the patient was treated with interstitial alone.

To some extent, the anatomic site of the tumor determines the amount of radiation received by the bone, and the risk of osteonecrosis correlates closely with bone dosage. Silverman[40] recently reported an 85% incidence of osteoradionecrosis in dentulous patients receiving over 7500 rad to the bone. None of the patients receiving less than 6500 rad to their jaws developed bone necrosis within an average of 24 months follow-up.

A patient with all of the high risk factors will have approximately 18 times the risk of osteoradionecrosis than the patient with none of the high risk factors.[38] Although most necroses occur in a 3- to 12-month period after radiation, the susceptibility of bone to necrosis remains for the life of the patient, and the incidence will increase in patients followed for up to 10 years.[39,41]

The risk of osteoradionecrosis in patients with teeth is approximately twice that of edentulous patients.[40] However, the management of the dentulous patient prior to radiotherapy has been controversial. In the classic studies of Daly and Drane[36] and Daly et al.[37] the incidence of osteoradionecrosis was 35% in dentulous patients treated with radiation at a time when a policy of extraction of all teeth in the proposed radiation field was followed. A more conservative nonextraction policy was adopted in 1969. With the use of fluoride gel applicators and removing only those teeth not salvageable by restorations, the incidence of osteoradionecrosis was reduced to 24.5%. As a more meticulous dental evaluation leads to a more aggressive preradiation extraction policy, the incidence of osteonecrosis can be lowered below 10%.[42] Silverman[40] reported a 16% incidence of osteonecrosis in patients with preradiation tooth extraction and a 61% incidence of osteonecrosis in patients whose teeth were extracted following radiation therapy. The following modified criteria were suggested by Hayward et al.[43] for selecting teeth to be removed prior to radiotherapy: (1) extensive caries, with pulpal involvement; (2) moderate to advanced periodontal disease, especially teeth with furcation involvement; (3) partial impaction or incomplete eruption; and (4) radiographic evidence of periapical pathology. We allow a minimum of 10 days after extractions before beginning radiotherapy. The decision not to extract sound teeth within the radiation field should be based in part on the patient's willingness to accept the responsibility for preventing future dental infections.

Conservative nonsurgical management of osteoradionecrosis is the best initial step and will result in clinical resolution in most cases. Small protruding or rough areas of bone can be filed down by the oral surgeon. Although many patients have little or no pain, this symptom can be controlled with oral analgesics or by the topical application of viscous lidocaine. An occasional patient will benefit from a 2- to 3-week course of antibiotics. Small sequestra will eventually spontaneously extrude or can be gently lifted out as an office procedure. Hyperbaric oxygen has been reported to increase the rate of healing in patients with more severe areas of necrosis.[44] The indications for intraoral curettement or excision of bone are intractable pain, recurrent or severe infections, and trismus. Approximately 20% of patients with osteoradionecrosis will fail conservative treatment and require surgery.[39]

IV. COMPLICATIONS OF CHEMOTHERAPEUTIC AGENTS USED TO TREAT SQUAMOUS CELL CARCINOMA OF THE HEAD AND NECK

All chemotherapeutic agents display toxicity and adverse side effects, and it is often the side effects of the various drugs that determine their dosage. Side effects are generally due to (1) the cytotoxic effect of the drug on DNA, (2) the effect of the drug on the chemoreceptor trigger zone (CTZ) in the CNS, and (3) the chemical or physical properties of the individual drugs.

A. Toxicity Secondary to the Cytotoxic Effect of the Drug on DNA

Most chemotherapeutic agents cause tumor cell death by altering the structure or function of cellular DNA. Unfortunately, the effects of chemotherapeutic agents are not specific for tumor cell DNA, but also affect normal cell DNA. The more rapidly a normal cell or tumor cell divides, the greater is the likelihood that it will divide while under the influence of the cytotoxic agent and suffer the cytotoxic consequence of cell death. The normal organ systems in the body that suffer the greatest cytotoxic side effects of chemotherapy because of their rapid cellular turnover are the skin and its appendages, the GI tract, the bone marrow, and the gonads.

The major side effect related to the skin is hair loss. This may begin about 3 weeks after the initiation of chemotherapy, but is temporary. The hair regrows when the chemotherapy is stopped.

The major side effects related to the GI tract are stomatitis and diarrhea.[45,46] Both symptoms begin approximately 1 week after starting the chemotherapy. The stomatitis is painful and may contribute to the malnutrition that many patients already experience. This may be sufficiently severe to require hyperalimentation. The drugs that most commonly cause stomatitis are methotrexate (MTX) and 5-fluorouracil (5-FU). The stomatitis seen with MTX is much more common with high doses. These symptoms, stomatitis and diarrhea, as well as bone marrow suppression can be prevented or ameliorated if the patient is rescued with leukovorin or thymidine.

The stomatitis can be treated symptomatically with topical local anesthetics, i.e., viscous xylocaine or Benadryl® elixir mixed with equal parts of Kaopectate®. Secondary infections with a herpesvirus or *Candida albicans* may occur and require therapy with antiviral agents, i.e., acyclovir or antifungal agents, respectively. Stomatitis may last a few days to 2 weeks. Diarrhea also occurs approximately 1 week after beginning chemotherapy. However, it is relatively easy to control with such agents as diphenoxylate hydrochloride, atropine sulfate, loperamide hydrochloride, paregoric, or tincture of opium. MTX has a greater potential than other agents to cause GI toxicity, possibly because GI epithelium accumulates and retains the drug more avidly than other tissues.[47]

Another inevitable side effect of chemotherapy is myelosuppression. The bone marrow produces RBCs, WBCs, and platelets, and its suppression results in anemia, leukopenia (with the possibility of sepsis), and thrombocytopenia (with the chance of hemorrhage). The most common problem is leukopenia, which is potentially serious approximately 15% of the time. This usually starts 7 to 10 days after beginning chemotherapy and may last anywhere from a few days to 10 days. Even though a striking increase in sepsis has been documented when the neutrophil count drops below $1000/mm^3$, this is of greater concern if the patient runs a fever. The leukopenic patient with a fever greater than 101.5°F probably has a bacterial infection.[48] Although cancer patients often have very unusual infections with viruses, fungi, or parasites, the initial infection in leukopenic patients is usually bacterial.[49] Approximately 75% of these infections are due to Gram-negative organisms which the patient is harboring in his GI tract. Of major concern are infections with pseudomonas. For an untreated leukopenic patient with pseudomonas sepsis, the median survival is only 48 hr. This is the normal time required for blood culture confirmation. When a leukopenic patient becomes febrile, mortality and morbidity can be markedly decreased by taking the appropriate cultures and immediately treating with broad spectrum coverage, i.e., an aminoglycoside and synthetic penicillin (which covers pseudomonas) or a second generation cephalosporin.[50] Antibiotic coverage can then be altered once the results of cultures become available.

The incidence of thrombocytopenia secondary to chemotherapy is much less than the incidence of leukopenia from the same cause. Spontaneous and serious bleeding is rarely a problem until the platelet count has fallen below 20,000 plateletes per cubic millimeter.[51] The platelets decline 7 to 10 days after the chemotherapy has been administered and remain low for 2 to 10 days. If the platelet count is less than 20,000 per cubic millimeter, it is advisable to transfuse platelets to prevent bleeding until the bone marrow resumes its own production.

Anemia is not an acute problem following the administration of chemotherapy since the life span of the RBC is 120 days. However, with repetitive courses of chemotherapy, the production of RBCs decreases, and new RBCs are not generated to replace the older RBCs that are cleared from the circulation. Therefore, the anemia that develops from the effects of chemotherapy on DNA is a late sequela.

Decreased spermatogenesis and amenorrhea may also develop from chemotherapy and lead to infertility. This is not usually a problem for patients with oral cancer since most of these patients are beyond the child-bearing age. This complication is also less common with the chemotherapeutic agents used for head and neck cancer.

A major concern to the medical oncologist is the possibility of inducing a second malignancy in a patient that he has cured with chemotherapy. This is a particular concern in the use of adjuvant chemotherapy where the purpose is to prevent the recurrence of a malignancy in a high risk patient who has no evidence of the malignancy after his primary therapy. The risk of inducing second malignancies in patients with oral cancer is fairly low since the duration of chemotherapy is relatively short and the drugs used to treat oral cancer have not been strongly associated with the induction of a second malignancy. The alkylating agents, especially cyclophosphamide, L-phenylalanine mustard, thiotepa, nitrogen mustard, chlorambucil, and the nitrosoureas are the chemotherapeutic agents that have been shown to induce second malignancies,[52-57] but these drugs are not commonly used to treat head and neck disease. The prevention of cytotoxic drug-induced second malignancies can only be done by reducing the dose of the chemotherapeutic agents. This is probably not practical since the therapeutic effect of the drug on the tumor may be reduced by decreasing the dose. The fine balance between the therapeutic effect and the dose of the drug has been demonstrated in head and neck cancer.[58]

B. Toxicity Secondary to the Effect of the Drug on the Chemoreceptor Trigger Zone (CTZ)

Nausea and vomiting are major problems in the treatment of oral cancer. cis-Platinum (CDDP) which is one of the most active agents in oral cancer is also one of the most potent emetics that exists. Although the exact chemical reaction is unknown, chemotherapy is thought to induce nausea and vomiting by a reaction with the CTZ which is located in the floor of the fourth ventricle.[59] The CTZ in turn stimulates the vomiting center located in the lateral reticular formation of the medulla oblongata.[60] The vomiting center then stimulates emesis through impulses to the stomach, diaphragm, and abdominal muscles conducted along visceral, phrenic, and spinal nerves, respectively. The start of vomiting may be immediate as with nitrogen mustard or quite late, 1 to 12 hr after drug administration, as with CDDP and cyclophosphamide.

The effective management of nausea and vomiting associated with chemotherapy depends on the control of other causes of nausea and the use of drugs which suppress the CTZ or vomiting center of the medulla.

There are many factors in a patient with cancer, other than chemotherapy, which can induce vomiting. Psychological factors, e.g., stress, and physical factors, e.g., smells, can induce nausea and vomiting. Anticipatory vomiting, which can become a conditioned response, is a major problem in cancer treatment, and patients who expect to be ill from chemotherapy often become nauseated before the chemotherapy is given. This is difficult to control, but measures which may be helpful include (1) the prophylactic use of antiemetics before nausea begins, (2) the administration of chemotherapy in surroundings devoid of odors, strong colors, and noises which can be associated with the chemotherapy and subsequently induce nausea; and (3) the prudent use of sedatives in the very anxious patient.

The mainstay of antiemetic therapy in cancer patients is pharmacologic agents which include phenothiazines (prochlorperazine, thiethylperazine); butyrophenones (droperiodol, haloperidol); cannabinoids (delta-9 tetrahydro-cannabinol, nabilone); antihistamines (dimenhydrinate); and miscellaneous agents (dexamethasone, metaclopramide, and scopolamine).

The exact mechanism of action of these drugs is not known, but there is evidence that they act centrally on the CTZ or vomiting center.[61-63] The cannabinoids have been effective in suppressing nausea from a number of chemotherapeutic drugs,[63] but have not been particularly effective with adriamycin, cytoxan, or CDDP.[64] Dexamethasone, a glucocorticoid, has a good antiemetic effect when used in conjunction with other antiemetics, but is not particularly effective when used alone. The use of metaclopramide in high doses, (2 mg/kg) has a good effect on the severe emesis associated with CDDP.[65]

Different antiemetics have different effects on the nausea and vomiting from different chemotherapeutic drugs. The physician who learns to use the proper antiemetic for each chemotherapeutic agent at proper doses and in a prophylactic fashion before vomiting ensues will help his patients immensely.

C. Toxicity Secondary to the Chemical or Physical Properties of the Individual Drugs

All drugs have side effects related to their chemical or physical properties. These side effects tend to be drug specific.

1. cis-Platinum (CDDP)

Toxicities of CDDP which are related to its chemical properties include renal toxicity, ototoxicity, neurotoxicity, magnesium wasting, and hypersensitivity reactions.

Renal toxicity is the major life-threatening side effect of CDDP. In animal studies, CDDP produces a proximal tubular necrosis,[66] while in a human study the major finding was coagulation necrosis of the endothelium of the distal tubules and collecting ducts.[67] Although there are similarities between the nephrotoxicity of CDDP and other heavy metals, there are differences, i.e., the lack of renal tubular acidosis and proteinuria.[68,69] Since the exact mechanism by which platinum causes renal toxicity is not known, it is difficult to develop an antidote to reverse renal toxicity. Hydration with mannitol diuresis clearly decreases the renal toxicity.[68,70]

Ototoxicity with high frequency hearing loss, but sparing of vestibular function is a problem with CDDP.[71] Hearing loss is age related and occurs most frequently in older patients.

Neurotoxicity presenting primarily as a distal sensory loss has been described with CDDP.[72] This is common and the major therapy-limiting problem with high dose CDDP[73] and may result from segmental demyelination of the peripheral nerves.[74]

Asymptomatic hypomagnesemia is common in CDDP chemotherapy,[75] because CDDP may interfere with the tubular transport of magnesium.[67]

Allergic reactions to CDDP, as with any drug, have been reported.[76,77] These have ranged from atopic dermatitis to anaphylaxis. Patients who have reacted to CDDP with less severe reactions can usually be treated concurrently with an antihistamine to prevent the reaction.

CDDP is probably the most emesis-producing agent used in cancer chemotherapy, and very aggressive antiemetic therapy is required. On the other hand, CDDP by itself produces little myelosuppression.

2. Methotrexate (MTX)

The toxicities of MTX that are independent of its cytotoxic effect and probably related to its physical and chemical properties include (1) renal failure, (2) liver damage, (3) pneumonitis, and (4) sensitivity reactions.

The renal failure is caused by a precipitation of MTX or its metabolites in the kidney.[78]

This toxicity virtually never occurs with standard doses, but is seen with high dose MTX and in patients with impaired renal function. The MTX is soluble in an alkaline urine, and vigorous hydration (3 $\ell/m^2/24$ hr) and alkalinization of the urine (pH ≥ 7) will greatly reduce the renal failure secondary to high dose MTX.

MTX also can cause acute and chronic hepatic toxicity. With the use of high dose MTX, a reversible rise in the bilirubin, SGOT and LDH are seen. Speculation on the mechanism of the damage of MTX to the liver is that it interferes with choline synthesis.[79]

MTX has also been associated with self-limiting acute pneumonitis.[80] This usually presents as a pulmonary infiltrate with cough and fever. Hypersensitivity with anaphylaxis is very rare with MTX.

3. Bleomycin (BLM)

BLM can cause (1) pulmonary toxicity, (2) dermatitis, and (3) fever. BLM is the classic example of drug-induced pulmonary toxicity, and the pulmonary changes are the limiting factors affecting delivery of the drug. When patients receive greater than 450 mg/m² of BLM, the incidence of pulmonary toxicity approaches 10%.[81] Older patients who receive single doses greater than 25 mg/m² or who have underlying lung disease are much more susceptible to the lung toxicity of BLM.[82] This is of particular importance for patients with oral cancer since as a group, they are older and many are smokers with some evidence of lung disease. The pulmonary toxicity is irreversible and slowly progressive with repeated doses of drug. It is characterized by a cough, dyspnea, bilateral pulmonary fibrosis, and hypoxia. There is no effective therapy.

Although the initial pulmonary abnormality is in the arterioles and veins,[83,84] the progressive changes result in fibrosis. BLM increases the production of collagen,[85] and in animal and organ culture studies, the use of dehydroproline, which inhibits collagen synthesis, protects against the pulmonary toxicity of BLM.[86] Hopefully, this will turn out to be of benefit to patients who are to receive treatment with BLM.

BLM is also associated with a high incidence of dermatitis.[81] Hyperpigmentation is very common and erythema, keratosis, and frank dermal ulceration occur. Of patients receiving BLM, 25% will experience fever within the first 2 days of therapy. The fever abates on its own. Hypersensitivity has also been reported with BLM.

One of the major advantages of BLM is that it has virtually no bone marrow toxicity.

4. 5-Fluorouracil (5-FU)

The toxicities of 5-FU which are independent of its cytotoxicity include (1) acute neurologic symptoms and (2) conjunctivitis.

The acute neurologic symptoms seen with 5-FU include lethargy and cerebellar symptoms. These are very unusual and are felt to be secondary to fluorocitrate, which is a metabolic product of 5-FU that is toxic to the CNS.[87]

Conjunctivitis has also been reported with prolonged use of 5-FU. This can progress to stenosis of the tear ducts.[88] The conjunctivitis is reversible if the 5-FU is stopped.

5. Vinblastine and Vincristine

Even though vinblastine and vincristine differ structurally only in a single substitution, their toxicities are different. The toxicities of vinblastine are related to its cytotoxic effect, i.e., myelosuppression and thrombocytopenia, whereas vincristine causes very little myelosuppression and thrombocytopenia except in very high doses. The major toxicity of vincristine is a neuropathy and inappropriate secretion of antidiuretic hormone.

The neurotoxicity from vincristine is manifested by paresthesias and decreased distal deep tendon reflexes.[89] If the drug is not stopped, the neuropathy will become progressive and will lead to severe motor and sensory disturbances. The only way to correct this is to stop application of the drug.

V. CONCLUSION

The management of the side effects of chemotherapeutic drugs is different for each drug and individual patient. The side effects that are secondary to the cytotoxic effect of the drugs on DNA can be managed by reducing the dose. However, reducing the dose of the drug may also reduce the effectiveness of the drug on the tumor. Therefore, the toxicity is usually endured and treated symptomatically. The nausea and vomiting which start because of the effect of the drug on the CTZ are best managed by the prophylactic use of the proper antiemetic and behavior modification. The toxicities associated with the chemical or physical properties of a drug can usually be prevented by either prophylactic measures, i.e., vigorous hydration (CDDP and MTX), alkalinization of the urine (MTX), or close observation of the patient so that the drug can be withdrawn before irreparable damage occurs.

REFERENCES

1. **Jabaley, M. E.,** Reconstruction in patients with oral and pharyngeal cancer, *Curr. Probl. Surg.,* 14, 5, 1977.
2. **Manchester, W. M.,** Immediate reconstruction of the mandible and temporomandibular joint, *Br. J. Plast. Surg.,* 18, 291, 1965.
3. **Boyne, P. J. and Zarem, H.,** Osseous reconstruction of the resected mandible, *Am. J. Surg.,* 132, 49, 1976.
4. **Schwartz, H. C.,** Mandibular reconstruction using the dacron-urethane prosthesis and autogenic cancellous bone: review of 32 cases, *Plast. Reconstr. Surg.,* 73, 387, 1984.
5. **Cummings, C. W. and Leipzig, B.,** Replacement of tumor-involved mandible by cryosurgically devitalized autograft, human experience, *Arch. Otolaryngol.,* 106, 252, 1980.
6. **deFries, H. O.,** Reconstruction of the mandible: use of combined homologous mandible and autologous bone, *Otolaryngol. Head Neck Surg.,* 89, 694, 1981.
7. **Zhe, C. and Tingchun, W.,** Reconstruction of mandibular defects with composite autologous iliac bone and freeze-treated allogeneic rib grafts, *J. Oral Maxillofac. Surg.,* 40, 29, 1982.
8. **Harding, R. L.,** Replantation of the mandible in cancer surgery, *Plast. Reconstr. Surg.,* 19, 373, 1957.
9. **Hamaker, R. C.,** Irradiated autogenous mandibular grafts in primary reconstructions, *Laryngoscope,* 91, 1031, 1981.
10. **Siemssen, S. O., Kirkby, B., and O'Connor, T. P. F.,** Immediate reconstruction of a resected segment of the lower jaw, using a compound flap of clavicle and sternomastoid muscle, *Plast. Reconstr. Surg.,* 61, 724, 1978.
11. **Cuono, C. B. and Ariyan, S.,** Immediate reconstruction of a composite mandibular defect with a regional osteomusculocutaneous flap, *Plast. Reconstr. Surg.,* 65, 477, 1980.
12. **Schlenker, J. D., Robson, M. C., and Parsons, R. W.,** Methods and results of reconstruction with free flaps following resection of squamous cell carcinoma of the head and neck, *Ann. Plast. Surg.,* 6, 362, 1981.
13. **Schmidt, D. R. and Robson, M. C.,** One-stage composite reconstruction using the latissimus myoosteo-cutaneous free flap, *Am. J. Surg.,* 144, 470, 1982.
14. **Bertotti, J. A.,** Trapezius-musculocutaneous island flap in the repair of major head and neck cancer, *Plast. Reconstr. Surg.,* 65, 16, 1980.
15. **Guillamondegui, O. M. and Larson, D. L.,** The lateral trapezius musculocutaneous flap: its use in head and neck reconstruction, *Plast. Reconstr. Surg.,* 67, 143, 1981.
16. **Taylor, G. I., Townsend, P., and Corlett, R.,** Superiority of the deep circumflex iliac vessels as the supply for free groin flaps. Experimental work, *Plast. Reconstr. Surg.,* 64, 595, 1979.
17. **Taylor, G. I., Townsend, P., and Corlett, R.,** Superiority of the deep circumflex iliac vessels as the supply for free groin flaps. Clinical work, *Plast. Reconstr. Surg.,* 64, 745, 1979.
18. **Zarb, G. A.,** The maxillary resection and its prosthetic replacement, *J. Prosthet. Dent.,* 18, 268, 1967.
19. **Cantor, R. and Curtis, T. A.,** Prosthetic management of edentulous mandibulectomy patients. I. Anatomic, physiologic and psychologic considerations, *J. Prosthet. Dent.,* 25, 446, 1971.
20. **Desjardins, R. and Ronald, P.,** Occlusal considerations for the partial mandibulectomy patient, *J. Prosthet. Dent.,* 41, 308, 1979.

21. **Cobb, A. B.**, Medical and psychological problems in the rehabilitation of the cancer patient, in *Counseling and Rehabilitating the Cancer Patient*, Handy, R. E. and Cull, J. C., Eds., Charles C Thomas, Springfield, Ill., 1975, 32.

22. **Chalian, V. A.**, *Extra-Oral Prosthetics in Maxillofacial Prosthetics*, Chalian, V. A., Drane, J. B., and Standish, S. M., Eds., Williams & Wilkins, Baltimore, 1971, 65.

23. **Million, R. R. and Cassisi, N. J.**, *Management of Head and Neck Cancer: A Multidisciplinary Approach*, Lippincott, Philadelphia, 1984, chap. 14.

24. **Rubin, P. and Casarett, G. W.**, *Clinical Radiation Pathology*, Vol. 1, W. B. Saunders, Philadelphia, 1968, chap. 4.

25. **Mossman, K. L. and Henkin, R. I.**, Radiation-induced changes in taste acuity in cancer patients, *Int. J. Radiat. Oncol. Biol. Phys.*, 4, 663, 1978.

26. **Cheng, V. S. R., Downs, J., Herber, D., and Aramany, M.**, The function of the parotid gland following radiation therapy for head and neck cancer, *Int. J. Radiat. Oncol. Biol. Phys.*, 7, 253, 1981.

27. **Mira, J. G., Wescott, W. B., Starcke, E. N., and Shannon, I. L.**, Some factors influencing salivary function when treating with radiotherapy, *Int. J. Radiat. Oncol. Biol. Phys.*, 7, 535, 1981.

28. **Marks, J. E., Davis, C. C., Gottsman, V. L., Purdy, J. E., and Lee, F.**, The effects of radiation on parotid salivary function, *Int. J. Radiat. Oncol. Biol. Phys.*, 7, 1013, 1981.

29. **Evans, J. C. and Ackerman, L. V.**, Irradiated and obstructed submaxillary salivary glands simulating cervical lymph node metastasis, *Radiology*, 62, 550, 1954.

30. **Brown, L. R., Dreizen, S., Handler, S., and Johnston, D. A.**, Effect of radiation-induced xerostomia on human oral microflora, *J. Dent. Res.*, 54, 740, 1975.

31. **Silverman, S., Jr., Luangjarmekorn, L., and Greenspan, D.**, Occurrence of oral candida in irradiated head and neck cancer patients, *J. Oral Med.*, 39, 194, 1984.

32. **Frank, R. M., Herdly, J., and Philippe, E.**, Acquired dental defects and salivary gland lesions after irradiation for carcinoma, *J. Am. Dent. Assoc.*, 70, 868, 1965.

33. **Beumer, J., Curtis, T., and Harrison, R. E.**, Radiation therapy of the oral cavity: sequelae and management. II., *Head Neck Surg.*, 1, 392, 1979.

34. **Marx, R. E.**, Osteoradionecrosis: a new concept of its pathophysiology, *J. Oral Maxillofac. Surg.*, 41, 283, 1983.

35. **Morrish, R. B., Chan, E., Silverman, S., Meyer, J., Fu, K., and Greenspan, D.**, Osteonecrosis in patients irradiated for head and neck carcinoma, *Cancer*, 47, 1980, 1981.

36. **Daly, T. E. and Drane, J. B.**, Osteoradionecrosis of the jaws, *Cancer Bull.*, 24, 86, 1972.

37. **Daly, T. E., Drane, J. B., and MacComb, W. S.**, Management of problems of the teeth and jaw in patients undergoing irradiation, *Am. J. Surg.*, 124, 539, 1972.

38. **Murray, C. G., Herson, J., Daly, T. E., and Zimmerman, S.**, Radiation necrosis of the mandible: a 10 year study. I. Factors influencing the onset of necrosis, *Int. J. Radiat. Oncol. Biol. Phys.*, 6, 543, 1980.

39. **Murray, C. G., Herson, J., Daly, T. E., and Zimmerman, S.**, Radiation necrosis of the mandible: a 10 year study. II. Dental factors: onset, duration and management of necrosis, *Int. J. Radiat. Oncol. Biol. Phys.*, 6, 549, 1980.

40. **Silverman, S.**, Radiation effects, in *Oral Cancer*, Silverman, S., Ed., American Cancer Society, New York, 1985, 75.

41. **Larson, D. L., Lindberg, R. D., Lane, E., and Goepfert, H.**, Major complications of radiotherapy in cancer of the oral cavity and oropharynx: a 10 year retrospective study, *Am. J. Surg.*, 146, 531, 1983.

42. **Beumer, J., Harrison, R., Sanders, B., and Kurrasch, M.**, Preradiation dental extractions and the incidence of bone necrosis, *Head Neck Surg.*, 5, 514, 1983.

43. **Hayward, J. R., Kerr, D. A., Jesse, R. H., Castighiano, S. G., Lampe, I., and Ingle, J. I.**, The management of teeth related to the treatment of oral cancer, in *Oral Care for Oral Cancer Patient*, U.S. Department of Health, Education and Welfare Public Health Service Publ. No. 1958, DHEW, Washington, D.C., 1968, 1.

44. **Davis, J. C., Dunn, J. M., Gates, G. A., and Heimbach, R. D.**, Hyperbaric oxygen: a new adjunct in the management of radiation necrosis, *Arch. Otolaryngol.*, 105, 58, 1979.

45. **Guggenheimer, J., Verbin, R. S., Appel, B. N., and Schmutz, J.**, Clinicopathologic effects of cancer chemotherapeutic agents on human buccal mucosa, *Oral Surg.*, 44, 58, 1977.

46. **Lockhart, P. B. and Sonis, S. T.**, Alterations in the oral mucosa caused by chemotherapeutic agents, *J. Dermatol. Surg. Oncol.*, 7, 1019, 1981.

47. **Sirotnak, F. and Moccio, D. M.**, Pharmacokinetic basis for differences in methotrexate sensitivity of normal proliferative tissues in the mouse, *Cancer Res.*, 40, 1230, 1980.

48. **Bodey, G. P., Buckley, M., and Sathe, Y. S.**, Quantitative relationships between circulating leukocytes and infection in patients with acute leukemia, *Ann. Intern. Med.*, 64, 328, 1966.

49. **Bodey, G. P., Bolivar, R., and Fainstain, V.**, Infectious complications in leukemia patients, *Semin. Hematol.*, 19, 193, 1982.

50. **Bodey, G. P. and Jodeja, L.,** Pseudomonas bacteremia retrospective analysis of 410 episodes, *Arch. Intern. Med.,* 145, 1621, 1985.

51. **Bodey, G. P., Freireich, E. J., and Mantel, N.,** The quantitative relation between platelet count and hemorrhage in patients with acute leukemia, *N. Engl. J. Med.,* 266, 905, 1962.

52. **Casciato, D. A. and Scott, J. L.,** Acute leukemia following prolonged cytotoxic agent therapy, *Medicine,* 58, 32, 1979.

53. **Bloomfield, C. D. and Brunning, R. D.,** Acute leukemia as a terminal event in nonleukemic hematopoietic disorders, *Semin. Oncol.,* 3, 297, 1976.

54. **Bergsagel, D. E., Bailey, A. J., Langley, G. R., MacDonald, R. N., White, D. F., and Miller, A. B.,** The chemotherapy of plasma-cell myeloma and the incidence of acute leukemia, *N. Engl. J. Med.,* 301, 743, 1979.

55. **Coleman, C. N., Williams, C. J., Flint, A., Glatstein, E. J., Rosenberg, S. A., and Kaplan, H. S.,** Hematologic neoplasia in patients treated for Hodgkin's disease, *N. Engl. J. Med.,* 297, 1249, 1977.

56. **Wall, R. L. and Clausen, K. P.,** Carcinoma of the urinary bladder in patients receiving cyclophosphamide, *N. Engl. J. Med.,* 293, 271, 1975.

57. **Pearson, R. M. and Soloway, M. S.,** Does cyclophosphamide induce bladder cancer?, *Urology,* 11, 437, 1978.

58. **Rooney, M., Kish, J., Jacobs, J., Kinzie, J., Weaver, A., Crissman, J., and Al-Sarraf, M.,** Improved complete response rate and survival in advanced head and neck cancer after three-course induction therapy with 120-hour 5-FU infusion and cisplatin, *Cancer,* 55, 1123, 1985.

59. **Wang, S. C.,** Emetic and antiemetic drugs, in *Physiological Pharmacology,* Vol. 2, Root, W. S. and Hofman, F. E., Eds., Academic Press, New York, 1965, 255.

60. **Wang, S. C. and Borison, H. L.,** A new concept of organization of the central emetic mechanism: recent studies on the sites of action of apomorphine, copper sulfate, and cardiac glycosides, *Gastroenterology,* 22, 1, 1952.

61. **Baldessarini, R. J.,** Drugs and the treatment of psychiatric disorders, in *The Pharmacologic Basis of Therapeutics,* 6th ed., Goodman, A. G., Goodman, L. S., and Gilman, A., Eds., Macmillan, New York, 1980, 391.

62. **Sawicka, J. and Sallan, S. E.,** Transdermal therapeutic system scopolamine: prevention of vomiting associated with cancer chemotherapy, in *Proc. Am. Soc. Clin. Oncol.,* Weinhouse, S., Foti, M., and Bergbauer, P. A., Eds., Williams & Wilkins, Baltimore, 1977, 302.

63. **Lamb, H. C. and Cox, F. M.,** Clinical use of droperidol in patients with chemotherapy-induced nausea and vomiting, *Oncol. Nurs. Forum,* 9, 23, 1982.

64. **Chang, A. E., Shilling, D. J., Stillman, R. C., Goldberg, N. H., Seipp, C. A., Barofsky, I., and Rosenberg, S. A.,** A prospective evaluation of delta-9-tetrahydrocanabinol as an antiemetic in patients receiving adriamycin and cytoxan chemotherapy, *Cancer,* 47, 1746, 1981.

65. **Gralla, R. J., Itri, L. M., Pisko, S. E., Squillante, A. E., Kelsen, D. P., Braun, D. W., Jr., Bordin, L. A., Braun, T. J., and Young, C. W.,** Antiemetic efficacy of high-dose metoclopramide: randomized trials with placebo and prochlorperazine in patients with chemotherapy induced nausea and vomiting, *N. Engl. J. Med.,* 305, 905, 1981.

66. **Ward, J. M. and Fauvie, K. A.,** The nephrotoxic effects of cis-dichloroplatinum (II) in male F344 rats, *Toxicol. Appl. Pharmacol.,* 38, 535, 1976.

67. **Gonzales-Vitale, J. C., Hayes, D. M., Cvitkovic, E., and Sternberg, S. S.,** The renal pathology in clinical trials of cis-platinum (II) diamminedichloride, *Cancer,* 39, 1362, 1977.

68. **Madias, N. E. and Harrington, J. T.,** Plantinum nephrotoxicity, *Am. J. Med.,* 65, 307, 1978.

69. **Dentino, M., Luft, F. L., Yum, M. N., Williams, S. D., and Einhorn, L. H.,** Long-term effect of cis-diamminedichloride platinum (CDDP) on renal function and structure in man, *Cancer,* 41, 1274, 1978.

70. **Chary, K. K., Higby, D. J., Henderson, E. S., and Swinerton, K. D.,** Phase I study of high-dose cis-dichlorodiammineplatinum (II) with forced diversis, *Cancer Treat. Rep.,* 61, 367, 1977.

71. **Stadnicki, S. W., Fleischman, R. W., Schaeppi, U., et al.,** Cis-dichlorodiammineplatinum (II) (NSC-119875): hearing loss and other toxic effects in rhesus monkeys, *Cancer Chemother. Rep.,* 59, 467, 1975.

72. **Kedar, A., Cohen, M. E., and Freeman, A. J.,** Peripheral neuropathy as a complication of cis-dichlorodiammineplatinum (II) treatment: a case report, *Cancer Treat. Rep.,* 62, 819, 1978.

73. **Forastiere, A. A., Wolf, G. T., Medvec, B. R., and Baker, S. R.,** Treatment of head and neck cancer (H&N CA) with high-dose cisplatin (DDP) in hypertonic saline, in *Proceedings of the American Society of Clinical Oncologists,* Foti, M., Mennite, M. A., and Pusztay, H. M., Eds., Waverly Press, Baltimore, 1985, 141.

74. **Von Hoff, D. D., Reichert, C. M., Cuneo, R., Reddick, R., Gallagher, M., and Rozencweig, M.,** Demyelination of peripheral nerves associated with cis-diamminedichloroplatinum (II), in *Proceedings of the American Association of Cancer Researchers,* Weinhouse, S., Foti, M., and Bergbauer, P. A., Eds., Waverly Press, Baltimore, 1979, 91.

75. **Schilsky, R. L. and Anderson, T.,** Hypomagnesemia and renal magnesium wasting in patients receiving cisplatin, *Ann. Intern. Med.,* 90, 929, 1979.
76. **Khan, A., Hill, J. M., Grater, W., Loeb, E., MacLellan, A., and Hill, N.,** Atopic hypersensitivity to cis-dichlorodiammineplatinum (II) and other platinum complexes, *Cancer Res.,* 35, 2766, 1975.
77. **Von Hoff, D. D., Slavik, M., and Muggia, F. M.,** Allergic reactions to cis-platinum, *Lancet,* 1, 90, 1976.
78. **Jacobs, S. A., Stoller, R. G., Chabner, B. A., and Johns, D. G.,** 7-Hydroxymethotrexate as a urinary metabolite in human subjects and rhesus monkeys receiving high-dose methotrexate, *J. Clin. Invest.,* 57, 534, 1976.
79. **Tuma, D. J., Barak, A. J., and Sorrell, M. F.,** Interaction of methotrexate with lipotropic factors in rat liver, *Biochem. Pharmacol.,* 24, 1327, 1975.
80. **Sostman, H. D., Matthay, R. A., Putman, C., and Smith, G. J. W.,** Methotrexate-induced pneumonitis, *Medicine,* 55, 371, 1976.
81. **Blum, R. H., Carter, S. K., and Agre, K.,** A clinical review of bleomycin a new antineoplastic agent, *Cancer,* 31, 903, 1973.
82. **Hubbard, S. P., Chabner, B. A., Cannelos, G. P., et al.,** High-dose intravenous bleomycin in treatment of advanced lymphomas, *Eur. J. Cancer,* 11, 623, 1975.
83. **McCullough, B., Collins, J. F., Johanson, W. G., Jr., and Grover, F. L.,** Bleomycin induced diffuse interstitial pulmonary fibrosis in baboons, *J. Clin. Invest.,* 61, 79, 1978.
84. **Adamson, I. Y. and Bowden, D. H.,** The pathogenesis of bleomycin induced pulmonary fibrosis in mice, *Am. J. Pathol.,* 77, 185, 1974.
85. **Phan, S. H., Thrall, R. S., and Ward, P. A.,** Bleomycin induced pulmonary fibrosis in rats: biochemical demonstration of increased rates of collagen synthesis, *Am. Rev. Respir. Dis.,* 121, 501, 1980.
86. **Kelley, J., Newman, R. A., and Evans, J. N.,** Bleomycin induced pulmonary fibrosis in the rat. Prevention with an inhibitor of collagen synthesis, *J. Lab. Clin. Med.,* 96, 954, 1980.
87. **Chabner, B. A.,** Pyrimidine antagonists, in *Pharmacologic Principles of Cancer Treatment,* Chabner, B. A., Ed., W. B. Saunders, Philadelphia, 1982, 183.
88. **Haidak, D. J., Hurwitz, B. S., and Yeung, K. Y.,** Tear-duct fibrosis (dacryostenosis) due to 5-fluorouracil, *Ann. Intern. Med.,* 88, 657, 1978.
89. **Bradley, W. G., Lassman, L. P., Pearce, G. W., and Walton, J. N.,** The neuropathy of vincristine in man. Clinical, electrophysiological and pathological studies, *J. Neurol. Sci.,* 10, 107, 1970.

Chapter 8

RESEARCH ASPECTS OF ORAL CANCER

Robin E. Howell and Bruce A. Wright

TABLE OF CONTENTS

I. INTRODUCTION

Perhaps the most interesting and exciting area in the field of oral cancer is that of research and future developments. Research is being carried out in a wide variety of areas ranging from the identification of oncogenes to clinical trials of new chemotherapeutic protocols. Given that this is such a broad area carried on by so many different specialists it would be a herculean task to review this topic in comprehensive detail. Of necessity, a chapter such as this can only highlight a few areas and raise some unanswered questions which will, naturally, reflect personal bias.

Because cancer research of any nature covers so many disciplines, it is not easy to present this in a logical manner. Therefore, it was decided, arbitrarily, to divide this chapter into four overlapping areas, i.e., etiology, pathogenesis, diagnosis, and treatment. Time alone will be the judge as to whether any of the areas highlighted will ultimately prove to be of major significance in the field of oral cancer research.

II. ETIOLOGY

Epidemiologic studies have provided much of the evidence for the various factors, e.g., tobacco, alcohol, etc., which have been traditionally implicated in the etiology of oral squamous cell carcinoma.[1-4] The argument is made in Chapter 2 that there is a chance of too simplistic an interpretation of epidemiologic data with regard to common etiologic agents for lip and intraoral cancer. The two diseases are probably not analogous and should be considered independently when causative factors are discussed. The same argument might be made, although perhaps less convincingly, about combining the different intraoral sites when studying etiologic factors.

In spite of the voluminous epidemiologic data available with regard to oral cancer there is still room for more. Studies in the past have often concentrated on head and neck cancer in general or grouped data from various areas. There is a trend now to consider the different anatomic sites separately, not only for etiologic factors, but also for treatment outcomes. Owing to the relative rarity of oral cancer, multicenter cooperative studies would be needed to achieve sufficient numbers of cases to provide meaningful data about etiologic factors with reference to a single intraoral site. If a large sample was available it would be possible to examine not only individual etiologic factors for different anatomic sites, but also to study the interrelationship, by regression analysis, among a number of different facts, e.g., synergism between tobacco use and alcohol consumption, for any particular site. Binnie and Rankin pointed out in Chapter 2 that in some studies, strenuous efforts have been made to avoid overlap between different factors which may in fact not be independent but may act synergistically.

A. Tobacco
There is evidence that smoking may be causally related to the development of intraoral squamous cell carcinoma. Moore[5] examined the effect of stopping or continuing smoking on a group of patients apparently successfully treated for oral, pharyngeal, or laryngeal cancer. He found that 44% of patients who continued to smoke developed second cancers of respiratory or upper digestive tracts compared with 6% of patients who stopped smoking after their initial lesion was treated. His criteria for inclusion in the study were that the second primary neoplasm must have occurred at least 3 years after the primary tumor and that the patient must have had no evidence of any recurrences of the first carcinoma. He was unable to find any meaningful data regarding alcohol intake or liver disease. Other studies have confirmed the high incidence of second malignancies following oral cancer, but failed to demonstrate a relationship with the continuing use of alcohol and tobacco.[6]

This type of study would be worth repeating with larger numbers to examine other parameters, i.e., alcohol intake, dental status, and any immunological abnormalities in the genesis of second malignancies. The following are just some of the questions raised by this data:

1. Is tobacco smoke (or its condensation products) directly carcinogenic for oral epithelium?
2. Are there substances in saliva which alter tobacco smoke to render it more "carcinogenic"?
3. Do microsomal enzymes, i.e., the aryl hydrocarbon hydroxylases, which are known to alter the polycyclic aromatic hydrocarbons in tobacco smoke to carcinogens, play a major role in the development of oral cancer?[7]
4. Could the effect of cigarette smoking be mediated via the immune system?

It is well known, for example, that head and neck cancer patients have defects in their immune systems.[8] However, what is not known is whether these defects lead to the development of oral carcinoma or whether they are a result of the development of the neoplasm. One way to settle this would be through expensive, large-scale prospective studies which may not be practicable.

A recent symposium has concentrated on the permeability of oral mucosa.[9] It is well known from tissue recombination experiments that the connective tissue exerts a major effect on the development and differentiation of the overlying epithelium. Could it be that tobacco smoke products penetrate the thinner oral epithelium of sites such as the floor of the mouth and then exert their effect by altering the underlying connective tissue?

Valentine et al.[10] in a recent cadaver study of oral epithelium, used morphometry to relate lingual epithelial thickness to known levels of alcohol and tobacco use. They found a reduction in the maturation layer due mainly to cell shrinkage. In contrast, the progenitor layer was increased due mainly to cell hypertrophy. The effect was apparently greater when related to alcohol intake rather than tobacco use. They concluded that the observed changes appeared to be nonspecific reactions to local toxic effects of alcohol and tobacco, but speculated that they might indicate an increased vulnerability to carcinogens.

The use of smokeless tobacco among adolescent males has also been the subject of a study into its effects on caries, periodontal status, and mucosal pathology, e.g., ulceration and leukoplakia.[11,12] Offenbacher and Weathers[12] found about a sixfold increase in soft tissue pathology in smokeless tobacco users compared with nonusers. This is an area where more research is needed to identify the various factors, both in the tobacco and in the host, which are responsible for the mucosal changes observed. Prospective studies will yield meaningful data regarding the long-term effect of these products.

In the logical progression of scientific research, once factors are identified epidemiologically, they must be tested in the laboratory. This would include both animal studies and mutagen testing. The classical animal model for oral chemical carcinogenesis has been the hamster cheek pouch,[13,14] which is by no means ideal.[15,16] The use of 4-nitroquinolone-*N*-oxide (4NQO) on the rat palate is a model closer to the human situation.[17] Prime et al.[18] studied the effect of iron deficiency on 4NQO palatal carcinogenesis in the rat and found that tumor development was significantly earlier in the experimental group than the controls. In addition, the experimental animals had a significantly greater incidence of tongue tumors. Eveson[16] reviewed the studies relating to tobacco products and their failure to produce tumors in hamster cheek pouches. Repeating these experiments with modifications such as iron deficiency may prove extremely fruitful. Recently, other studies[19,20] have reported local synergistic effects such as that between herpes simplex virus (HSV) infection and tobacco products, e.g., snuff. Park et al[20] reported that 50% of hamster cheek pouches treated with both HSV and snuff developed dysplasia and invasive squamous cell carcinoma. Other studies using combinations of known risk factors could be informative.

B. Alcohol

Alcohol consumption has long been associated with the development of oral cancer[2,21] or abstinence associated with low risk of cancer.[22] Graham et al.[23] reported a relative risk of 7.7 for the development of oral cancer in males with tobacco use, excessive alcohol consumption, and poor dentition. However, the relative risk was much lower when only two of the three factors were present. The possible synergy between alcohol consumption and tobacco products has previously been noted.[24] Whether alcohol produces its effects topically in the oral cavity to produce epithelial changes[10] or whether it works systemically, e.g., via the immune system, the liver, or via alterations in vitamin A metabolism,[25] is not known. Rothman[24] has suggested that alcohol may dissolve tobacco products and thus affect the epithelium. Vitale and Gottlieb[26] have concluded that alcohol per se is not a carcinogen, but in combination with nutritional deficiencies, may be carcinogenic. The immunosuppressive effect of alcohol and its related nutritional deficiencies cannot be ignored.[26] As previously stated when discussing tobacco products, what is needed are carefully controlled epidemiologic studies to review the potential synergy between alcohol and other factors, such as tobacco use, nutritional and immunologic status, and infectious agents, together with animal and basic science research to examine mechanisms of action.

C. Infectious Agents

There has been a great deal of interest recently in chronic infections with *Candida* species. Clinically[27,28] and experimentally,[29,30] candidosis has been associated with epithelial hyperplasia. Candidosis has been shown to be present in speckled leukoplakias[31] and associated with a certain percentage of leukoplakias, epithelial dysplasias, and carcinomas.[32,33] Also, the development of malignancy in candidal leukoplakia has been reported to be much higher than in other types of leukoplakia.[34] At present, it is not known whether chronic candidosis per se is a premalignant lesion or whether *Candida* species are merely colonizing a preexisting oral lesion. Perhaps the most promising line of research in this area would be experimentally to combine one or two systemic factors, e.g., iron deficiency[35] and local candidosis in an experimental animal model and observe the effects on the epithelium. It has been noted that patients with various forms of chronic mucocutaneous candidosis do have abnormalities of iron metabolism.[35]

HSV type 2 and type 1 have been associated with cervical[35] and oral cancer,[37] respectively, as judged by raised circulating antibody titers. However, recently, Shillitoe et al.[39] were unable to demonstrate the presence of various HSV-1 proteins in 11 cases of oral cancer. However, as alluded to earlier, the synergy between HSV and topical carcinogens may provide exciting new avenues in this area.[19,20]

Human papillomavirus (HPV) infection has been associated with cervical dysplasia and invasive carcinoma. This has recently been reviewed by Brescia et al.[40] It seems that, in part, the lesions are associated with only certain of the nearly 40 HPV types.[40] Of extreme interest in the field of oral cancer are the following obervations. First, HPV structural antigens and Epstein-Barr virus (EBV) have been demonstrated in ''hairy'' leukoplakia. ''Hairy'' leukoplakia is an oral finding in some patients with acquired immunodeficiency syndrome (AIDS).[41] Secondly, Silverman et al.[42] have reported a greater than expected incidence of oral squamous cell carcinoma in patients having AIDS or at risk (i.e., homosexual partners of known AIDS patients) to develop the disease. Also, Eisenberg et al.[43] have observed morphological virus-like changes in a high percentage of oral verrucous carcinomas. In addition, Loning et al.[44] reported the finding of HPV structural antigens in oral papillomas and leukoplakias. What is not known at present is the precise role of these viruses in the development of mucosal lesions. Is a defect in the immune system necessary for the virus to infect the oral mucosa and thus exert its effect? Or do only those patients who have an immune deficiency go on to develop malignancy in their oral lesions (lack of immune surveillance)? Or are other factors operating, such as synergy with tobacco use? Obviously, further carefully controlled clinical data together with animal experimentation are needed in this potentially fascinating field. More detailed discussion of this subject and the possible mechanisms of action(s) of oncogenic viruses are given in Section III.

D. Deficiency States

There are a number of deficiency states of great interest in studies on the etiology of oral cancer. The first of these is iron deficiency. The association of iron deficiency, dysphagia, and an increased incidence of oral and pharyngeal carcinoma has long been known (either as the Paterson-Kelly or Plummer-Vinson syndrome; Chapter 2). Although oral mucosal lesions in iron deficiency anemia have been described[45] there has been recent interest in developing an animal model for iron deficiency.[18] Changes in the oral epithelium in iron-deficient hamsters and mice have been described.[46,47] In addition, as noted previously Prime et al.[18] found that iron-deficient rats developed tumors significantly earlier and developed more tongue tumors when exposed to 4NQO than control animals. It is also of interest that "iron deficiency" has been associated with oral candidosis[35] and that chronic hyperplastic candidosis has an apparently higher incidence of malignant transformation than other forms of oral leukoplakia.[34] Whether these are truly cause-and-effect interrelationships or merely incidental associated findings will require a great deal more research both clinically and in the laboratory.

There has been a great deal of interest both clinically and experimentally in the effect of retinoids on head and neck cancer.[25,48-51] It is known that vitamin A and its analogs are necessary for normal epithelial differentiation.[52] There are at least two distinct intracellular retinoid binding proteins. One is cellular (or cytoplasmic) retinoic acid binding protein (CRABP) and the other, cellular retinol binding protein (CRBP). One study[48] has found that CRABP is almost absent in carcinoma of the esophagus, while adjacent normal esophagus contained significantly higher levels. More recently still, in a series of 37 head and neck cancers, Gates and Rees[49] found a 3-fold increase in CRBP while there was a 2.5-fold decrease in CRABP when compared with adjacent normal tissue. This phenotypic change in malignant epithelium may be related to its failure to "mature" normally. D'Antonio et al.[25] have found relatively normal blood levels of retinol in an alcoholic population. However, they did observe alterations in metabolism of cholesterol and carotene. This, together with the observation of a different cytoplasmic content of CRBP and CRABP from normal epithelium surrounding carcinomas, should prompt clinical and experimental studies into local factors causing these alterations at particularly susceptible sites.

In the experimental situation, retinoids have been found to inhibit transplanted tumor growth in the rat palate,[50] and both retinoic acid and selenium were found to delay the development of leukoplakia and tongue cancer induced by dimethyl-benzanthracene (DMBA) in hamsters.[51] More work remains to determine the precise mode of action of induced-carcinoma inhibition by retinoids and whether this has any application to the human situation.

There are other deficiency states which may be associated with oral mucosal change, e.g., B12. However, whether these and other nutritional deficiencies such as those associated with alcohol ingestion[20] play any role in the etiology of oral cancer remains to be seen.

E. Chronic Trauma

Trauma is another of the quoted potential factors in the etiology of oral cancer.[53] Graham et al.[23] speculated that the increased risk of oral cancer in their group associated with poor dentition (and smoking and heavy alcohol intake) might have been due, in part, to mucosal trauma. Experimentally, Renstrup et al.[54] found that although mechanical irritations alone could not produce carcinoma, they did hasten the onset of DMBA chemical carcinogenesis in the hamster cheek pouch. The precise role of mucosal trauma, i.e., whether it actually promotes carcinogenesis, merely allows the ingress of noxious substances, or is coincidental in the development of oral cancer, is still unclear at this time.

F. Premalignant Lesions

Premalignant lesions of the oral cavity have been extensively discussed in Chapter 3. Whether further studies of the causes of the various known premalignant lesions of the oral cavity, e.g., leukoplakia, erythroplakia, etc., may help to shed some light on the genesis of oral cancer is not clear. There is the potential that prospective studies of keratin staining patterns or the distribution of keratin proteins in both normal and premalignant lesions may help to unravel the mystery of which ones will become malignant.[55-57] As technology advances and different and more sensitive techniques for localizing the various keratin proteins become available, the missing pieces of this puzzle may be found. However, given the limits of morphology these answers may come from the molecular biology of keratins.

G. Mutagens

Mutation is the acquisition of inheritable changes in the genetic material of a cell. Some mutations can lead to cancer, many chemical mutagens are also carcinogens, and many carcinogens are also mutagens. Shorter (48 hr) in vitro tests for mutagens have been developed using specially developed strains of bacteria, and substances which are mutagenic in such tests are also carcinogenic in 85 to 95% of cases.[58] Mutagenesis testing is now widely accepted as making a valid contribution to cancer research, and very extensive literature now exists on this subject.[59,60] Tobacco smoke condensates have been tested extensively and many mutagens have been discovered. However, very little testing has been done on alcoholic drinks. One study has shown that red wine contains mutagens,[61] and it may be relevant that the only study of oral cancer in which the type of alcoholic drink was taken into account did find that patients drank more wine than did control subjects.[20]

Another aspect of mutagenesis testing could be to look for mutagens which are in contact with oral tissue of oral cancer patients and controls. It is known that urine of smokers contains mutagens[62] and that smoking is associated with bladder cancer. If saliva of oral cancer patients contained higher concentrations of mutagens or different types of mutagens than saliva of matched controls, this would provide an extremely important lead in determining the possible etiology of cancer in those patients.

A related aspect concerns the activation of mutagens. Many carcinogens/mutagens are inactive until they have been metabolized to the active form. This can be done by certain tissue enzymes or by bacteria. The intestinal bacteria of many persons make enzymes which convert premutagens into mutagens.[61] The saliva of some persons can convert amines to nitrosamines[63] which are carcinogenic. It might be that oral bacteria, fungi, or salivary enzymes of oral cancer patients are particularly effective at activating carcinogens, and this could be tested in mutagenesis tests. Future research would then be aimed at preventing this activation.

Finally, the need for a representational animal model for oral chemical carcinogenesis should be emphasized. Recently, Eveson,[16] in an excellent review, has discussed the relative merits of the traditional hamster cheek pouch together with other models, i.e., the rat palate and nonhuman primates. With the continued search for different models and various cofactors, i.e., iron deficiency and synergy between potential carcinogens, there are many different models from which to choose. It is only by continuing to apply careful clinical observations to the experimental situation that the various etiologic factors in oral cancer will be discovered.

III. PATHOGENESIS

The etiological agents suspected of causing oral cancer have been fairly well delineated by epidemiological studies. However, the mechanisms by which these agents change normal cells into malignant cells really lie at the heart of the problem. A better understanding of the molecular basis of malignant transformation is essential if there is to be hope of treatment or preventive measures which would be both highly effective and acceptable to the people who have this disease. This sort of detailed understanding of the molecular biology of cancer cells requires complementary basic research into the normal mechanisms of important cellular functions, such as growth and differentiation. While a great deal of oral cancer research has been done in areas such as etiology, diagnosis, and treatment, only relatively recently has more work been done on pathogenesis at the molecular level.

A. Genetic Alterations

Cancer researchers have amassed a great deal of data indicating that changes occur in the genetic control apparatus as cells progress to a malignant state. Almost all carcinogenic agents whether chemical, physical (radiation), or infectious (oncogenic viruses) are mutagens, i.e., they change the structure of genes and chromosomes by producing point mutations, deletions, insertions, or rearrangements.[64-69] The tendency to develop specific types of tumors is inherited in a number of different situations including breast cancer, retinoblastoma, Cowden's syndrome, Gardner's syndrome, and neurofibromatosis.[70-74] Specific chromosomal aberrations have been consistently found in a number of tumors, such as Burkitt's lymphoma, chronic myelogenous leukemia, acute myeloblastic leukemia, and Wilms' tumor in the aniridia-Wilms' tumor syndrome.[75] These aberrations have been translocations and deletions with break points at characteristic locations.[76] Another chromosomal change characteristically found in malignant tumors is that of an abnormal number of chromosomes. Aneuploidy can be found in almost all tumors and tumor cell lines by karyotyping or flow cytometry.[75-77]

Other findings which indicate that genetic alterations are critical events in the pathogenesis of malignant tumors are data from research on oncogenic retroviruses. These viruses carry genes which act in a dominant fashion to transform cells into malignant cells and can rapidly and efficiently produce malignant tumors in the appropriate host animal.[69] These retroviral tumor-causing genes, or oncogenes, have been found to be mutated genes derived from normal eukaryotic cell genes which are termed protooncogenes.[78] A rather large number of protooncogenes have been identified in the human genome, and mutated, amplified, and rearranged oncogenes have been found in a wide variety of malignant tumors including carcinomas of the bladder, lung, breast, gall bladder, pancreas, and colon as well as lymphomas, leukemias, and other sarcomas.[79-81] Many of the chromosome deletions and translocations which are characteristic of certain tumors have breakpoints at or near the locations of known protooncogenes.[76]

Although no one has precisely delineated the pathogenic events in the development of any cancer, the most promising area of investigation likely to lead to a molecular understanding of this process is that of research into genetic changes occurring in malignant transformation. Oral cancer research in this area is just beginning, but some tantalizing results have already been found. Changes in the DNA content and chromosome number in squamous carcinomas of the head and neck have been studied by several investigators.[82-84] Measurements of individual cells by flow cytometry indicate that all tumor cells have an abnormally high DNA content ranging from 1.1 to 3.3 times the normal diploid level.[82] An interesting flow cytometric study of oral leukoplakias found that the benign keratoses and mild to moderate dysplasias had diploid DNA content while two of three lesions of severe dysplasia to carcinoma *in situ* were aneuploid with DNA levels of 1.31 and 2.38 times the diploid value.[83] The number of chromosomes in cells from tumors or derived cell lines varies considerably, but most tend to be near triploid or tetraploid.[84] One study found aberrations of chromosome 1 in nine head and neck carcinoma cell lines examined which mainly involved deletions at 1q21, 1q32, 1q13, or 1p22.[22] Two known protooncogenes map to these areas

As previously mentioned, protooncogenes are normal genes found in eukaryotic cells which when "activated" by a number of different mechanisms can, under the right circumstances, cause malignant transformation of cells.[69,85-87] Protooncogenes have generally been found to code for functions involved in regulating cellular growth and differentiation.[69,88-91] A number of different techniques can be used to study genes in tumors and normal tissues. To obtain the DNA for these studies, tissue samples are obtained at surgery and frozen in liquid nitrogen where they can be stored for at least 5 years.[92] The samples are thawed, digested with proteolytic enzymes, and the DNA isolated by phenol/chloroform extraction.[93] The DNA samples, which contain all the genetic information from the malignant cells or from normal tissues, can then be analyzed in a variety of ways. One technique which has proved valuable in detecting activated oncogenes in tumor DNA is transfection.[94-96] Tumor DNA is co-precipitated with calcium phosphate and placed into the medium of cultured NIH 3T3 cells which are an immortalized, but contact inhibited a mouse fibroblast cell line that will not form tumors when injected into nude mice. These cells take up the precipitated tumor DNA, and a percentage of them will incorporate it into their own genomes. If they incorporate certain activated oncogenes from the tumor DNA, the mouse cells will become transformed and will form masses of cells on the culture dish which, if injected into nude mice, will grow as fibrosarcomas. Several dominantly acting transforming oncogenes have been identified in many human malignant tumors and tumor cell lines in this manner.[85,92,97]

Preliminary experiments of this kind have been performed using DNA from squamous carcinomas of the head and neck. While transfection experiments surveying many different types of solid malignancies have found that 15 to 30% of these tumors contain transforming genes,[85,92,97] studies of head and neck carcinomas indicate that nearly 100% may have transforming genes.[98-100] Transforming genes from head and neck carcinomas have been passed by transfection through four generations of mouse fibroblasts[99] which will then produce fibrosarcomas when injected into nude mice.[98] The Ki-ras oncogene has been tentatively identified in mouse fibroblasts transformed by DNA from a squamous carcinoma of the gingiva.[100] This oncogene is the one most commonly identified in transfection assays,[92] and it is usually activated by a point mutation in the 12th or 61st codon.[101-103] Work is proceeding to identify whether an activated Ki-ras gene is present in the original tumor DNA and what alterations may have activated it.

A recent study of a series of various malignant tumors and normal tissues found that alterations in a limited number of oncogenes were fairly common in tumors, but did not occur in normal tissue.[81] Amplification of the c-myc oncogene was found in 11 to 22% of carcinomas and sarcomas and appeared to correlate with more aggressive primary tumors, tumor progression, and metastasis. Amplification of Ki-ras occurred in a few tumors, and the loss of one allele of c-myb or c-Ha-ras was found in 11 to 15% of solid tumors. Preliminary studies of these genes in head and neck tumors using Southern hybridizations have indicated that 1 of 8 (12.5%) primary squamous carcinomas studied had a deletion of one allele of the c-Ha-ras oncogene.[100] Investigations are continuing into the status of these and other oncogenes in carcinomas of the head and neck.

B. Viruses

Viruses have been known to be the causative agents of certain malignant tumors in animals for many years,[88,104] but recently, a great deal of evidence has accumulated linking a number of types of human cancer with several specific viruses. (Some of the clinical data has been discussed under etiology.) These include HSV and HPV which are associated with genital tumors, hepatitis B virus with hepatocellular carcinoma, EBV with Burkitt's lymphoma and nasopharyngeal carcinoma, and human T-cell lymphotrophic viruses (HTLV) with leukemias, lymphomas, and other tumors.[105,106] Viruses can transform cells through several different mechanisms. The oncogenic retroviruses carry transduced, host-cell-derived oncogenes which, in infected cells, are very efficiently transcribed into proteins which effect cellular transformation.[107] Virally derived transforming genes may encode proteins that interact with the host-cell nucleus, cytoplasm, or cell membrane to cause malignant transformation.[105,108,109] Viral infection has been associated with chromosomal deletions or translocations such as EBV infection in Burkitt's lymphoma. The characteristic translocation that occurs in Burkitt's lymphoma transfers the c-myc oncogene coding sequences to the site of the heavy chain immunoglobulin gene cluster, where inappropriate transcriptional activation of the oncogene occurs in the B lymphocyte.[110,111] When viral DNA integrates into the host genome, it may interrupt host sequences that are important in regulating transcription of protooncogenes thus activating them. Another way in which viral genes can activate host protooncogenes is by insertion of viral promoters, which are regions of viral DNA that greatly increase transcription of adjacent genes, next to host-cell protooncogenes.[108,112] Also viral genes may be integrated into host genes in such a way that a fusion protein, coded for partly by viral and partly by host genes, is generated which may have transforming properties.[113] Oncogenic viruses may also act at the level of the whole organism, i.e., by modulation of the immune system so that tumors of other systems are free to develop. This appears to be important in AIDS patients who have an increased incidence of oral squamous carcinoma as well as other tumors.[114,115]

The HPVs are a group of oncogenic DNA viruses, of which there are around 40 known types each tending to infect stratified squamous epithelium at relatively specific sites.[105,116] Since these viruses only reproduce in terminally differentiating keratinocytes and no satisfactory in vitro method for producing the virus has been established, they have, until recently, been extremely difficult or impossible to study.[116] Molecular biology techniques have allowed researchers to clone HPV DNA in plasmid vectors and to generate a great deal of information about them.[117] Various animal papilloma viruses are associated with benign and malignant tumors in the appropriate host animals, and HPV have been strongly implicated as etiologic agents in carcinomas of the skin arising in patients with epidermodysplasia verruciformis (EV)[118] and in epithelial dysplasia[119] and squamous carcinoma of the uterine cervix.[120,121] Cervical carcinoma has a number of similarities to oral cancer in that it is a carcinoma of squamous cells occurring on a mucous membrane and it goes through a premalignant phase where a progression from mild dysplasia to carcinoma *in situ* is generally thought to occur before the development of invasive squamous carcinoma.[12] Investigations of cervical lesions have found HPV types 6 and 11 in nearly all benign squamous papillomas, i.e., condyloma acuminatum. The viral DNA is not integrated into the host genome, but is maintained episomally in a plasmid-like state.[122] Epithelial dysplasias contain unintegrated HPV DNA as well; however, they usually contain types 16 or 18. The majority of squamous carcinomas also contain HPV types 16 or 18, but the viral DNA is often found integrated into the host DNA where there may be multiple copies of the viral genome or only fragments of incomplete viral DNA.[105,120,121] When HPV viral DNA integrates into a host genome it usually disrupts a specific region of the viral genome which encodes for early viral proteins which may result in loss of control of expression of other viral genes thus leading to cellular transformation.[105] Alternatively, one of the previously mentioned or other mechanisms may be responsible for the association between cervical cancer and HPVs.

Current research also indicates a link between HPVs and benign and malignant squamous proliferations of the oral cavity and other mucous membranes of the upper aerodigestive tract (UADT). Morphologic, epidemiologic, and electron microscopic studies have indicated for some time that papillomaviruses are the major etiologic agents in UADT papillomas, such as laryngeal papillomatosis, condyloma acuminatum, verruca vulgaris, squamous papilloma, and focal epithelial hyperplasia,[123-126] although in some instances convincing evidence for HPV involvement was not consistently found.[125-127] The histological features that are suggestive of an HPV lesion have been listed as hyperkeratosis, dyskeratotic superficial cells, papillomatosis, acanthosis, koilocytosis, multinucleation, single cell dyskeratosis, and a sharp border between the deep and superficial epithelial layers.[128] HPV can be detected in squamous papillomas by immunoperoxidase or immunofluorescence techniques with antibodies to common structural antigens.[129] Staining occurs within a limited number of the nuclei of superficial keratinocytes and koilocytes in the stratum granulosum.[130-132] Paraffin sections of tracheal and laryngeal papillomatosis have been found to be positive for HPV antigens in 40 to 50% of cases, and an esophageal papilloma which contained HPV antigens within the nuclei of koilocytes has been reported.

If serial biopsies of several tumors in a patient with laryngeal papillomatosis are examined, nearly all of them will stain positively,[133] but usually, as with other lesions, HPV antigens will be found only in a few isolated groups of cells. This indicates that even though a lesion may be induced by HPV and is producing infectious viral particles, it may be very difficult to demonstrate viral antigens in any individual tissue sections, and even though a squamous cell proliferation is caused by the presence of HPV DNA, it may only periodically and focally produce complete viral particles detectable by immunohistochemical techniques. Conclusions about the etiological relationship between HPV and proliferative squamous lesions are very insecure when based on a failure to demonstrate viral proteins within specific tissue sections.

Studies of HPV antigens in oral papillomas have yielded variable results. Immunoperoxidase studies of formalin fixed paraffin embedded material have found that about 60% of oral lesions histologically diagnosed as verruca vulgaris or condyloma acuminatum contain HPV antigens as do 40% of multiple oral papillomas.[130] Some studies of solitary oral papillomas found very few that contain HPV antigens.[127] However, using frozen sections of six solitary oral squamous papillomas, one group found HPV antigens in 83% of them.[44]

Studies of oral leukoplakias and carcinomas have also found HPV antigens. One found that four of seven homogenous leukoplakias which were nondysplastic histologically contained HPV antigens and two of two nodular leukoplakias were also positive for HPV.[44] One of the nodular leukoplakias was nondysplastic, and the other was a severe epithelial dysplasia adjacent to a squamous carcinoma. Another study found histological features of HPV infection in 44% of 40 oral squamous carcinomas, but only half of these morphologially suggestive lesions were positive for HPV antigens by immunoperoxidase on paraffin sections.[128]

With Southern hybridization techniques, it is possible to detect very small amounts of HPV DNA in head and neck papillomas and to determine the HPV type. About 50% of laryngeal papillomas can be shown to contain HPV 11 DNA which is also found in cervical condylomata.[122] In oral squamous papillomas and lesions of focal epithelial hyperplasia, DNA from HPV types 2, 6, 11, 13, 16, and 32 has been found.[44,116,117,134,135] HPV DNA has also been demonstrated in oral leukoplakias, dysplasias, and carcinomas.[44,136] A study of seven squamous carcinomas of the tongue using limited amounts of DNA found three that contained detectable HPV DNA.[136] Two of these were poorly differentiated carcinomas and contained HPV 16 which is commonly found in cervical carcinomas. The other, a well-differentiated squamous carcinoma contained HPV 2 which is an uncommon finding in malignant tumors, but commonly causes verruca vulgaris on the skin.

HSV are also associated in some way with squamous carcinoma of the cervix and the oral cavity. Cervical cancer patients have been found to have elevated serum titers of antibodies to HSV-2,[137] and there is evidence that HSV-2 genes are transcribed and translated in cervical cancer cells.[138,139] Increased serum levels of antibodies to HSV-1 of the IgM and IgA class have been demonstrated in patients with oral cancer,[38,140] and transcription of HSV-1 genes has been found in some oral cancers.[141] An immunohistochemical examination of oral cancer tissue for specific HSV-1 proteins, some of which are thought to possibly have transforming functions, failed to detect any HSV-1 antigens.[39]

Studies of viruses and cancer of the head and neck have shown a clear association between them; however, the demonstration of any cause-and-effect relationships will be very difficult. Viruses may be associated with tumors without necessarily causing the tumor, e.g., HPVs could possibly be found in oral dysplasias and carcinomas because they preferentially infect already premalignant or malignant epithelial cells. It is important, though, to first establish associations that occur between viruses and tumors before any etiological relationship can be proven. A virus may be etiologically important in the development of a tumor without being present in the tumor cells as in some experimental systems where the virus produces changes in the cells which lead to transformation but the virus is not then necessary for maintenance of the malignant phenotype.[142] Classical-type experiments using Koch's postulates to prove causation in the case of human oncogenic viruses are, of course, ethically impossible and in addition would be practically very difficult. Research which establishes a precise molecular mechanism producing malignant transformation and which if modified will inhibit tumor formation is needed in the field of oral cancer. This kind of information is obviously pivotal in the effort to develop truly effective treatment and prevention of oral cancer.

C. Immunology

Studies into the immunology of oral cancer promise to yield information regarding pathogenesis, treatment, and prevention as well as providing help with simplified and more accurate techniques for diagnosis, follow-up, and prognostication. Research to date has been mainly concerned with the inflammatory cells involved and to some extent with humoral immunity and chemical mediators of inflammation. Investigations of the inflammatory infiltrate in oral carcinomas have shown most of the cells to be T-lymphocytes, and the intensity of the T-cell infiltrate appears to be positively correlated with a better prognosis.[143] A tendency for suppressor/cytotoxic T-cell-dominated infiltrates has been found in stage I and II tumors and for helper/inducer T-cell infiltrates in stage IV tumors.[144] Circulating T-lymphocytes have also been evaluated in patients with oral cancer, and a reduction in a subset of T-helper cells which produces interleukin-2 was found in a group of head and neck cancer patients.[145] A lowered amount of interleukin-2 would result in diminished cell-mediated and humoral immunity, and head and neck squamous carcinoma patients are known to have impaired T-cell function and poor tumor-specific responses.[146-152] Reduction of another T-cell subset defined as high affinity rosette-forming cells has also been reported in oral cancer patients.[153] Decreased levels of these cells were more pronounced in advanced clinical stages, returned to normal in patients who were cured, but remained low in patients with residual disease. A recent study found an increase in circulating suppressor T-cells in oral cancer patients which did not change following treatment[154] and also found suboptimal phytohemagglutinin and mixed lymphocyte culture responses in the oral cancer patient. Similar findings have been reported previously.[155]

Natural killer (NK) cells are thought to be important in the control of tumor cells.[156] Studies have found NK activity to be decreased in some groups of cancer patients,[157,158] but unchanged or increased in others.[159] Recent studies on patients with squamous carcinoma of the head and neck have shown no changes in activity of circulating NK cells.[154,156] A significant reduction in NK activity was found in cells from lymph nodes as compared to peripheral blood cells. This difference was markedly greater in tumor-draining lymph nodes from head and neck cancer patients than controls.[156] Another study showed a significant decrease in NK activity in head and neck cancer patients following tumor surgery[160] which was not seen in noncancer surgical patients. The decreased activity could be reversed by removal of monocytes from the lymphocyte cultures or by incubation of the cultures with the naturally occurring immunopotentiator tuftsin.[161] Similarly, NK activity in lymph node cell cultures could be increased by incubation with β-interferon.[156] These findings suggest that a population of suppressor cells may be found in tumor-draining lymph nodes and postoperatively in peripheral blood of head and neck squamous carcinoma patients which reversibly induce NK activity and that these suppressor cells would likely be monocytes or macrophages.

Peripheral monocytes from head and neck cancer patients have impaired chemotactic responsiveness.[152] Recently a low molecular weight factor derived from head and neck carcinomas was found to depress macrophage accumulation.[162] This effect was more pronouned when filtrates of more poorly differentiated tumors were used. In a study of patients with lip cancer, a significant increase in expression of Fc-IgG receptors on circulating monocytes was seen, but only in patients with metastatic disease.[163]

Changes in humoral immunity have been reported in oral cancer patients. Serum levels of IgA and IgE were found to be elevated whereas IgG, IgM, and IgD levels are similar to control values.[164] The percentage and number of circulating B-cells was shown to be increased in oral cancer patients, and they had an increased number of circulating immune complexes which correlated positively with tumor load.[154] Addition of aggregated IgG and Fc fragments to monocyte cultures enhanced the production of prostaglandin (PG) E[165] which may be an important modulator of immune function in patients with oral cancer. PGE2 acts to suppress a number of immune responses including T-cell functions, NK cell activity, and antibody-dependent cytotoxicity against tumor cells.[166,167] Excessive production of PGE2 has been reported in head and neck cancer patients.[168] Current studies of squamous carcinomas of the head and neck have found that the concentration of PGE2 is increased to levels about four times that of adjacent normal tissue[169] and that when given radiolabeled arachidonic acid, tumor tissue homogenates could synthesize a variety of metabolites of the cyclooxygenase and lipoxygenase pathways.[169,170]

There is obviously a great deal of scope for further research in all of these areas to elucidate the various mechanisms possibly involved in the pathogenesis of oral squamous cell carcinoma.

IV. DIAGNOSIS

Much of the current research in oral cancer is devoted to improving methods of detection, diagnosis, and prognostication. There have been some interesting recent discoveries with regard to tumor thickness and prognosis. This is along similar lines as that found for malignant melanoma, and it has been presented in Chapter 4.

Several substances have been investigated as possible biochemical serum markers of oral cancer which would be useful for screening and early detection as well as for following patients after treatment. The biochemical markers which have been studied and show some potential include carcinoembryonic antigen (CEA), ferritin, β2-microglobulin, thymidine kinase, alkaline deoxyribonuclease, IgA, and IgE. Serum CEA levels have been found to be elevated in head and neck cancer patients and to correlate with tumor burden; however, they were not predictive of survival and are also elevated in smokers without tumors.[171] Elevated CEA levels have also been detected in the saliva of oral cancer patients. Serum ferritin may be a useful marker as it was found at elevated levels in head and neck cancer patients. These levels were higher in more advanced stages of disease, returned to normal within 5 months after successful treatment, but remained at high levels in patients with a poor prognosis.[172] Elevated plasma levels of β2-microglobulin have been reported in patients with a number of different malignant tumors.[173-176] While only 8.5 to 12% of head and neck cancer patients had elevated β2-microglobulin levels, there is evidence that the tumor volume doubling time is inversely correlated with the β2-microglobulin concentration in tumor tissues.[177] Serum thymidine kinase activity has been found to be elevated in oral cancer patients[178] as has serum alkaline deoxyribonuclease.[179] Serum IgA and IgE levels were shown to be elevated in head and neck cancer patients[164,180] and have been suggested as useful markers.

Although a number of different biochemical markers show significant changes in oral cancer patients, there are problems which limit their usefulness, especially in individual cases. The ranges for tumor patient values and controls generally overlap to some extent. Abnormal values for particular markers are often seen in a variety of non-neoplastic conditions and in users of tobacco or alcohol. Clearly, more research is needed if we are to discover reliable biochemical serum markers of oral cancer.

There is currently a great deal of interest in finding histochemical markers that may distinguish premalignant or malignant epithelium from nonmalignant mucosal lesions. One area of active research which shows some promise is that of cell surface glycoconjugates, which specifically bind to plant lectins. A number of different lectins are available which bind to different terminal sugar residues that are generally located on the cell surface.[181] The lectins can be conjugated with markers such as fluorescein or biotin to allow visualization by standard immunohistochemical methods.[181-183] Normal and hyperplastic oral epithelia bound a variety of lectins mainly on cell surfaces, intercellularly in the spinous layer, and in the cytoplasm of the basal layer.[181] Squamous carcinomas showed variable lectin binding with loss of cell surface binding, and patchy cytoplasmic staining especially with Con A.[121] Binding of the lectin RCA-1 was found to be absent or greatly decreased in invading nests of squamous carcinoma cells.[182] Lesions diagnosed as carcinoma *in situ* bound lectins in the cytoplasm similarly to normal basal cells.[121] Blood group antigens A, B, and H, and the intercellular substance antigen of pemphigus (ICS) are also cell membrane or intercellular glycoconjugates. These have been studied by immunohistochemical methods which have yielded results similar to those of lectin binding studies.[184-186] Nearly all oral squamous carcinomas have been found to have undetectable or reduced levels of the normally occurring blood group antigens on cell surfaces as have the vast majority of epithelial dysplasias.[186] Epithelial ICS antigens were generally diminished or absent in almost all squamous carcinomas and epithelial dysplasias, but present on mature, more differentiated cells even in carcinomas.[185] Although many of these cell surface changes were quite consistently seen in epithelial dysplasia and squamous carcinoma, they appear to be nonspecific, as reactive lesions may show similar changes.[182,185] It is likely that these are nonspecific cell surface alterations which may be seen at times when cells are less differentiated, i.e., in benign and malignant neoplasms, wound healing, and hyperplasias.

Studies of other possible histochemical markers have not identified an ideal marker for oral squamous carcinoma or premalignant lesions, but some interesting results have emerged. The distribution of fibronectin and laminin in leukoplakia and squamous carcinoma of the oral cavity was found to be essentially the same as that in normal oral mucosa, with the exception that laminin was lost around islands of deeply invasive carcinoma.[187] Hexokinase, an important enzyme in glucose metabolism, was found by histochemical studies to have the same distribution in oral squamous carcinoma as in leukoplakia or normal oral mucosa; however, the intensity of staining was greater in the carcinomas than in adjacent normal-appearing epithelium.[188]

The development of antibodies which specifically recognize antigens exclusively in head and neck squamous carcinomas or premalignant epithelial dysplasias is the goal of a number of investigators. A monoclonal antibody, SQM1, has been produced which recognizes a surface membrane antigen in squamous carcinomas of the head and neck and in cell lines derived from them.[189] It did not bind to normal oral or upper airway mucosal epithelium or to the majority of tumors and normal tissues tested. It is not, however, absolutely specific as it did bind to some carcinomas of the lung and breast as well as bronchial epithelial cells and epidermal keratinocytes. This antibody could still have important applications in diagnostic immunohistochemistry and other techniques, i.e., radioimmunodetection of tumors as has been accomplished using radiolabeled antibodies to CEA in head and neck carcinomas.[190] Although the oncofetal protein CEA is not produced solely by head and neck squamous carcinoma cells, it has often been found on tumor cell surfaces.[171,191] Radiolabeled anti-CEA antibodies when injected into head and neck cancer patients were found to bind to primary and metastatic tumor masses and could be detected by gamma camera imaging.[190]

Other research into the clinical detection of premalignant and malignant oral disease also shows promise. Evaluations of the usefulness of tolonium (toluidine blue) rinses for screening of patients for oral cancer have been recently published.[192,193] The considerable amount of research that has been done in the field of colposcopy of premalignant and malignant neoplasms of the cervix may have applicability to oral cancers. The colposcope is essentially a stereoscopic operating-type microscope which is used to visualize epithelial and vascular patterns of cervical lesions in vivo. Characteristic patterns have been identified which can differentiate between benign lesions, varying degrees of dysplasia, and squamous carcinoma with great accuracy.[194,195] Similar patterns have recently been reported in dysplasias and carcinomas experimentally induced in the hamster cheek pouch, and observations of human oral lesions are currently in progress.[196]

The ability to predict which patients are at highest risk for developing oral cancers would have important patient management implications. One test that may generate predictive information is the determination of aryl hydrocarbon hydroxylase (AHH) inducibility in users of tobacco products.[7,197] Polycyclic aromatic hydrocarbons are hydroxylated to epoxides, which are probably the active or ultimate carcinogens, by AHH. The ability for the AHH enzyme system to be induced in a patient's lymphocytes can be determined and categorized as high, intermediate, or low and may be a useful measure of the patient's ability to activate carcinogens. An overrepresentation of high AHH inducibility has been found in patients with smoking-related cancers, i.e., laryngeal[198] and lung carcinomas,[199] and was also found in a study of oral cancer patients.[7] Further, AHH inducibility has been shown to be unaffected by age or smoking history.[197]

Obviously, there is further research to be done in the area of diagnosis. As discussed briefly under etiology, the potential for identifying different keratins in premalignant lesions may hold some promise.

V. TREATMENT

The traditional methods of treatment for oral cancer have been surgery and/or radiation therapy. Probably the main area in surgical treatment of oral squamous cell carcinoma, apart from the development of specific new surgical techniques, which requires further study is the question of elective neck dissection. This refers to the performing of a radical neck dissection in the absence of clinically suspicious lymph nodes. The trend with regard to elective neck dissection has varied over the years.[200-202] Although there have been limited numbers of controlled clinical trials, a number of authors are reporting a high incidence of false negative neck nodes and a high rate of clinically negative lymph nodes subsequently becoming clinically positive.[203-205] Because there is still controversy and because most centers have only small numbers of patients, what is needed is a multicenter prospective controlled clinical trial.

Radiation therapy has long been a mainstay in the treatment of oral cancer.[205-207] In many instances, it provides a viable alternative to surgical treatment. The advent of more sophisticated equipment and the use of combined modalities have been discussed elsewhere in this book. Obviously, there is room for further investigation.

In addition, changing dose fractionation schemes may lead to further improvement in the effectiveness of radiotherapy. Two such changes are hyperfractionation, where the daily dose remains the same but is given in two or three fractions, and accelerated fractionation, with a twice daily dose given for a total of 180 to 220 rad. Hyperthermia, either with external or interstitial radiation, is another physical change which could improve the overall outcome with radiation therapy.

There has been a great deal of interest in so-called radiation sensitizers, e.g., metronidazole. These agents render the tissues more sensitive to radiation therapy. There is also work being done on the more conventional chemotherapeutic agents, e.g., *cis*-platinum and 5-fluorouracil, as radiation sensitizers. A detailed discussion of these agents is outside the scope of this chapter. However, they may prove to be an exciting new avenue in the treatment of oral cancer.

One of the more interesting developments in recent years in the treatment of oral cancer has been the use of chemotherapy as adjunctive therapy. Initially, it was used for advanced lesions.[208-219] O'Brien et al.[220] do not advocate its use for early stage carcinoma. Mead and Jacobs[212] have reviewed many of the chemotherapy regimens and discussed the disadvantages of preoperative chemotherapy. One criticism of these trials is that they, for the most part, have put all head and neck cancer into one group assuming homogeneity. The reason for this is that because of the relative rarity of oral cancer, numbers of cases from any one anatomic location are too small in most centers to achieve statistical significance in prospective trials. In Chapter 6, Wright et al. have discussed some of the trials now underway as well as emphasized the need for future multicenter cooperative studies. Once the present round of trials is completed, trends and future directions will be clearer.

There have been other "advances" in treatment of oral cancer which represent new techniques rather than improvement upon traditional methods. One of these has been the carbon dioxide laser. Rhys Evans et al.[221] have recently reviewed their experience with this technique for oral cavity and pharyngeal lesions. They conclude that in certain instances, e.g., leukoplakia, it may offer some advantages over conventional methods. However, one disadvantage is the lack of tissue to examine microscopically. Whether laser treatment gains an established role for treating oral lesions remains to be seen.

Another advance which is worthy of mention is the subject of hematoporphyrin derivative and photochemotherapy.[222] The use of hematoporphyrin derivative and long-wave UV light has been reported to localize experimentally induced hamster cheek pouch carcinomas. Those tumors additionally receiving photochemotherapy showed tumor cell necrosis. Whether these exciting developments will have application to the human situation for oral cancer, time alone will tell.

VI. SUMMARY

It is only by carefully, properly, and adequately controlled research, clinical and experimental, that advances will be made against oral cancer. There is voluminous literature on the subject. However, sometimes the picture has been obscured because of use of inappropriate animal models or the combining of different anatomic sites of head and neck cancers. The experimental approach has become more rational in recent years. Clinically, because of small numbers of cases, a plea is made for more multicenter cooperative trials.

ACKNOWLEDGMENT

This work was supported, in part, by grant no. MT-9612 from the Medical Research Council of Canada.

REFERENCES

1. **Dorn, H. F. and Cutler, S. J.,** Morbidity from Cancer in the United States, Public Health Monogr. No. 56, U.S. Department of Health, Education, and Welfare, Washington, D.C., 1959.
2. **Keller, A. Z. and Terris, M.,** The association of alcohol and tobacco with cancer of the mouth and pharynx, *Am. J. Public Health,* 55, 1578, 1965.
3. **Wynder, E. L., Bross, I. J., and Feldman, R. M.,** A study of the etiological factors in cancer of the mouth, *Cancer,* 10, 1300, 1957.
4. **Wynder, E. L., Mushinski, M. H., and Spivak, J. C.,** Tobacco and alcohol consumption in relation to the development of multiple primary cancers, *Cancer,* 40, 1872, 1977.
5. **Moore, C.,** Cigarette smoking and cancer of the mouth, pharynx, and larynx, a continuing study, *JAMA,* 218, 553, 1971.
6. **Tepperman, B. S. and Fitzpatrick, P. J.,** Second respiratory and upper digestive tract cancers after oral cancer, *Lancet,* 2, 547, 1981.
7. **Trell, E., Bjorlin, G., Andreasson, L., Korsgaard, R., and Mattiasson, I.,** Carcinoma of the oral cavity in relation to aryl hydrocarbon hydroxylase inducibility, smoking and dental status, *Int. J. Oral Surg.,* 10, 93, 1981.
8. **Wanebo, H. J., Jun, M. Y., Strong, E. W., and Oettgen, H.,** T-cell deficiency in patients with squamous cell carcinoma of the head and neck, *Am. J. Surg.,* 130, 445, 1975.
9. **Schlegel, D., Kilian, M., and Dabelsteen, E.,** Penetration of potentially noxious compounds through oral mucosal surfaces, synopsis of a conference held at Eibsee, Bavaria, West Germany, *J. Oral Pathol.,* 15, 234, 1986.
10. **Valentine, J. A., Scott, J., West, C. R., and St. Hill, C. A.,** A histologic analysis of the early effects of alcohol and tobacco usage on human lingual epithelium, *J. Oral Pathol.,* 14, 654, 1985.
11. **Conolly, G. N., Winn, D. M., Hecht, S. S., Henningfield, J. E., Walker, B., Jr., and Hoffman, D.,** The reemergence of smokeless tobacco, *N. Engl. J. Med.,* 314, 1020, 1986.
12. **Offenbacher, S. and Weathers, D. R.,** Effects of smokeless tobacco on the periodontal, mucosal and caries status of adolescent males, *J. Oral Pathol.,* 14, 169, 1985.
13. **Salley, J. J.,** Experimental carcinogenesis in the cheek pouch of the Syrian hamster, *J. Dent. Res.,* 33, 253, 1954.
14. **MacDonald, D. G.,** A technique for localization of tumors in hamster cheek-pouch carcinogenesis, *Arch. Oral Biol.,* 23, 573, 1978.
15. **Smith, C. J.,** Experimental animal models for oral premalignancy, in *Oral Premalignancy,* MacKenzie, I. C., Dabelsteen, E., and Squier, C. A., Eds., University of Iowa Press, Iowa City, 1980, chap. 7.
16. **Eveson, J. W.,** Animal models of intra-oral chemical carcinogenesis: a review, *J. Oral Pathol.,* 10, 129, 1981.
17. **Wallenius, K. and Lekholm, U.,** Oral cancer in rats induced by the water-soluble carcinogen 4-nitroquinoline *N*-oxide, *Odontol. Rev.,* 24, 39, 1973.
18. **Prime, S. S., MacDonald, D. G., and Rennie, J. S.,** The effect of iron deficiency on experimental oral carcinogenesis in the rat, *Br. J. Cancer,* 47, 413, 1983.
19. **Hirsch, J.M., Johansson, S. L., and Vahlne, A.,** Effect of snuff and herpes simplex virus-1 on rat oral mucosa: possible associations with the development of squamous cell carcinoma, *J. Oral Pathol.,* 13, 52, 1984.
20. **Park, N.-H., Sapp, J. P., and Herbosa, E. G.,** Oral cancer induced in hamsters with herpes simplex infection and simulated snuff dipping, *Oral Surg. Oral Med. Oral Pathol.,* 62, 164, 1986.
21. **Mashberg, A., Garfinkel, L., and Harris, S.,** Alcohol as a primary risk factor in oral squamous carcinoma, *CA,* 31, 146, 1981.
22. **Lyon, J. L., Gardner, J. W., Klauber, M. R., and Smart, C. R.,** Low cancer incidence and mortality in Utah, *Cancer,* 39, 2608, 1977.
23. **Graham, S., Dayal, H., Rohrer, T., Swanson, M., Sultz, H., Shedd, D., and Fischman, S.,** Dentition, diet, tobacco, and alcohol in the epidemiology of oral cancer, *JNCI,* 59, 1611, 1977.
24. **Rothman, K. J.,** The effect of alcohol consumption on risk of cancer of the head and neck, *Laryngoscope,* 88(Suppl. 8), 52, 1978.
25. **D'Antonio, J. A., LaPorte, R. E., Dai, W. S., Hom, D. L., Wozniczak, M., and Kuller, L. H.,** Lipoprotein cholesterol, vitamin A and vitamin E in an alcoholic population, *Cancer,* 57, 1798, 1986.
26. **Vitale, J. J. and Gottlieb, L. S.,** Alcohol and alcohol-related deficiencies as carcinogens, *Cancer Res.,* 35, 3336, 1975.
27. **Cawson, R. A. and Lehner, T.,** Chronic hyperplastic candidiasis-candidal leukoplakia, *Br. J. Dermatol.,* 80, 9, 1968.
28. **Wright, B. A.,** Median rhomboid glossitis, not a misnomer, *Oral Surg. Oral Med. Oral Pathol.,* 46, 806, 1978.

29. **Cawson, R. A.,** Induction of epithelial hyperplasia by *Candida albicans, Br. J. Dermatol.,* 89, 497, 1973.
30. **Russell, C. and Jones, J. H.,** The histology of prolonged candidal infection of the rat's tongue, *J. Oral Pathol.,* 4, 330, 1975.
31. **Pindborg, J. J., Renstrup, G., Poulsen, H. E., and Silverman, S., Jr.,** Studies in oral leukoplakias. V. Clinical and histologic signs of malignancy, *Acta Odontol. Scand.,* 21, 407, 1963.
32. **Wright, B. A.,** Candidosis in Oral Leukoplakia and Epithelial Dysplasia, M.Sc. thesis, Indiana University, Bloomington, 1978.
33. **Hornstein, O. P., Grassel, R., and Schioner, E.,** Prevalence rates of candidosis in leukoplakia and carcinomas of the oral cavity, *Arch. Dermatol. Res.,* 266, 99, 1979.
34. **Cawson, R. A. and Binnie, W. H.,** Candida, leukoplakia and carcinoma: a possible relationship, in *Oral Premalignancy,* MacKenzie, I. C., Dabelsteen, E., and Squier, C. A., Eds., University of Iowa Press, Iowa City, 1980, chap. 5.
35. **Higgs, J. M. and Wells, R. S.,** Chronic muco-cutaneous candidiasis: associated abnormalities of iron metabolism, *Br. J. Dermatol.,* 86(Suppl. 8), 88, 1972.
36. **Melnick, J. L. and Adam, E.,** Epidemiological approaches to determining whether herpes virus is the etiological agent of cervical cancer, *Prog. Exp. Tumor Res.,* 21, 49, 1978.
37. **Shillitoe, E. J., Greenspan, D., Greenspan, J. S., Hansen, L. S., and Silverman, S., Jr.,** Neutralizing antibody to herpes simplex virus type 1 in patients with oral cancer, *Cancer,* 49, 2315, 1982.
38. **Shillitoe, E. J., Greenspan, D., Greenspan, J. S., and Silverman, S., Jr.,** Antibody to early and late antigens of herpes simplex virus type 1 in patients with oral cancer, *Cancer,* 54, 266, 1984.
39. **Shillitoe, E. J., Hwang, C. B. C., Silverman, S., Jr., and Greenspan, J. S.,** Examination of oral cancer tissue for the presence of the proteins 1CP4, 1CP5, 1CP6, 1CP8, and gB of herpes simplex virus type 1, *JNCI,* 76, 371, 1986.
40. **Brescia, R. J., Jenson, A. B., Lancaster, W. D., and Kurman, R. J.,** The role of human papillomaviruses in the pathogenesis and histologic classification of precancerous lesions of the cervix, *Hum. Pathol.,* 17, 552, 1986.
41. **Greenspan, J. S., Greenspan, D., Lennette, E. T., Abrams, D. I., Conant, M. A., Petersen, V., and Freese, U. K.,** Replication of Epstein-Barr virus within the epithelial cells of oral "hairy" leukoplakia, an AIDS-associated lesion, *N. Engl. J. Med.,* 313, 1564, 1985.
42. **Silverman, S., Jr., Migliorati, C. A., Lozada-Nur, F., Greenspan, D., and Conant, M. A.,** Oral findings in people with or at high risk for AIDS: a study of 375 homosexual males, *J. Am. Dent. Assoc.,* 112, 187, 1986.
43. **Eisenberg, E., Rosenberg, B., and Krutchkoff, D.,** Verrucous carcinoma: a possible viral pathogenesis, *Oral Surg. Oral Med. Oral Pathol.,* 59, 52, 1985.
44. **Loning, Th., Reichart, P., Staquet, M. J., Becker, J., and Thivolet, J.,** Occurrence of papillomavirus structural antigens in oral papillomas and leukoplakias, *J. Oral Pathol.,* 13, 155, 1984.
45. **Jacobs, A.,** The buccal mucosa in anaemia, *J. Clin. Pathol.,* 13, 463, 1960.
46. **Steele, B., Sofaer, J. A., and Southam, J. C.,** Lingual epithelial thickness in mice with inherited iron-deficiency anaemia (sla), *Arch. Oral Biol.,* 26, 343, 1981.
47. **Rennie, J. S. and MacDonald, D. G.,** Quantitative histological analysis of the epithelium of the ventral surface of hamster tongue in experimental iron deficiency, *Arch. Oral Biol.,* 27, 393, 1982.
48. **Dowlatshahi, K., Mehta, R. G., Levin, B., Cerny, W. L., Skinner, D. B., and Moon, R. C.,** Retinoic-acid-binding protein in normal and neoplastic human esophagus, *Cancer,* 54, 308, 1984.
49. **Gates, R. E. and Rees, R. S.,** Altered vitamin A-binding proteins in carcinoma of the head and neck, *Cancer,* 56, 2598, 1985.
50. **Huang, C.-C.,** Effect of retinoids on the growth of squamous cell carcinoma of the palate in rats, *Am. J. Otolaryngol.,* 7, 55, 1986.
51. **Goodwin, W. J., Huijing, F., Bordash, G. D., and Altman, N.,** Inhibition of hamster tongue carcinogenesis by selenium and retinoic acid, *Ann. Otol. Rhinol. Laryngol.,* 95, 162, 1986.
52. **Robbins, S. L., Cotran, R. S., and Kumar, V.,** *Pathologic Basis of Disease,* W. B. Saunders, Philadelphia, 1984, chap. 9.
53. **Thumfart, W., Weidenbecher, M., Waller, G., and Pesch, H.-J.,** Chronic mechanical trauma in the aetiology of oro-pharyngeal carcinoma, *J. Maxillofac. Surg.,* 6, 217, 1978.
54. **Renstrup, G., Smulow, J. B., and Glickman, I.,** Effect of chronic mechanical irritation on chemically induced carcinogenesis in the hamster cheek pouch, *J. Am. Dent. Assoc.,* 64, 770, 1962.
55. **Clausen, H., Moe, D., Buschard, K., and Dabelsteen, E.,** Keratin proteins in human oral mucosa, *J. Oral Pathol.,* 15, 36, 1985.
56. **Reibel, J., Clausen, H., and Dabelsteen, E.,** Staining patterns of human pre-malignant oral epithelium and squamous cell carcinomas by monoclonal anti-keratin antibodies, *Acta Pathol. Microbiol. Immunol. Scand. (A),* 93, 323, 1985.

57. **Mori, M., Nakai, M., Hyun, K.-H., Noda, Y., and Kawamura, K.,** Distribution of keratin proteins in neoplastic and tumorlike lesions of squamous epithelium, an immunohistochemical study, *Oral Surg. Oral Med. Oral Pathol.,* 59, 63, 1985.
58. **Ames, B. N.,** Identifying environmental chemicals causing mutations and cancer, *Science,* 204, 587, 1979.
59. **Rinkus, S. J. and Legator, M. S.,** Chemical characterization of 465 known or suspected carcinogens and their correlation with mutagenic activity in the *Salmonella typhimurium* system, *Cancer Res.,* 39, 3289, 1979.
60. **Devoret, R.,** Bacterial tests for potential carcinogens, *Sci. Am.,* 241, 40, 1979.
61. **Tamura, G., Gold, C., Ferro-Luzzi, A., and Ames, B. N.,** Fecalase: a model for activation of dietary glycosides to mutagens by intestinal flora, *Proc. Natl. Acad. Sci. U.S.A.,* 77, 4961, 1980.
62. **Yamasaki, E. and Ames, B. N.,** Concentration of mutagens from urine by absorption with the nonpolar resin XAD-2; cigarette smokers have mutagenic urine, *Proc. Natl. Acad. Sci. U.S.A.,* 74, 3555, 1977.
63. **Tannenbaum, S. R., Archer, M. C., Wishnok, J. W., and Bishop, W. W.,** Nitrosamine formation in human saliva, *JNCI,* 60, 251, 1978.
64. **Ames, B. N., Dunston, W. E., Yamasaki, E., and Lee, F. D.,** Carcinogens are mutagens. A simple test system combining liver homogenates for activation and bacteria for detection, *Proc. Natl. Acad. Sci. U.S.A.,* 70, 2281, 1973.
65. **McCann, J., Choi, E., Yamasaki, E., and Ames, B. N.,** Detection of carcinogens as mutagens in the salmonella/microsome tests. Assay of 300 chemicals, *Proc. Natl. Acad. Sci. U.S.A.,* 72, 5135, 1975.
66. **McCann, J. and Ames, B. N.,** Detection of carcinogens as mutagens in the salmonella/microsome test. Assay of 300 chemicals: discussion, *Proc. Natl. Acad. Sci. U.S.A.,* 73, 950, 1976.
67. **White, S. C.,** Effects of low-level X radiation on chromosomes, *J. Dent. Res.,* 46(Suppl. 6), 1177, 1967.
68. **Hayward, W. S., Neel, B. G., and Astrin, S. N.,** Activation of cellular onc gene by promoter insertion of ALV-induced lymphoid leukosis, *Nature (London),* 290, 475, 1981.
69. **Bishop, J. N.,** Cellular oncogenes and retroviruses, *Ann. Rev. Biochem.,* 52, 301, 1983.
70. **Haagensen, C. D., Lane, N., Lattes, R., and Bodian, C.,** Lobular neoplasia (so-called lobular carcinoma in situ) of the breast, *Cancer,* 42, 737, 1978.
71. **Cavenee, W. K., Hansen, N. F., Nordenskjold, M., Kock, E., Maumenee, I., Squire, J. A., Phillips, R. A., and Gallie, B. L.,** Genetic origin of mutations predisposing to retinoblastoma, *Science,* 228, 501, 1985.
72. **Swart, J. G. N., Lekkas, C., and Allard, R. H. B.,** Oral manifestations in Cowden's syndrome, *Oral Surg. Oral Med. Oral Pathol.,* 59, 264, 1985.
73. **Fader, M., Kline, S. N., Spatz, S. S., and Zubrow, H. J.,** Gardner's syndrome (intestinal polyposis, osteomas, sebaceous cysts) and a new dental discovery, *Oral Surg. Oral Med. Oral Pathol.,* 15, 153, 1962.
74. **Hope, D. G. and Mulvihill, J. J.,** Malignancy in neurofibromatosis, in *Advances in Neurology,* Vol. 29, Riccardi, V. M. and Mulvihill, J. J., Eds., Raven Press, New York, 1981, 33.
75. **Yunis, J. J.,** The chromosomal basis of human neoplasia, *Science,* 221, 227, 1983.
76. **Yunis, J. J. and Soreng, A. L.,** Constitutive fragile sites and cancer, *Science,* 2216.
77. **Greenebaum, E., Koss, L. G., Elequin, F., and Silver, C. E.,** The diagnostic value of flow cytometric DNA measurements in follicular tumors of the thyroid gland, *Cancer,* 56, 2011, 1985.
78. **Temin, H. M., Chen, I. S. Y., Watanabe, S., and Wilhemsen, K.,** Evolution of retroviruses, in *Perspectives on Genes and the Molecular Biology of Cancer,* Robberson, D. L. and Saunders, G. F., Eds., Raven Press, New York, 1983, 243.
79. **Pulciani, S., Santos, E., Lauver, A. V., Long, L. K., and Barbacid, M.,** Transforming genes in human tumors, *J. Cell. Biochem.,* 20, 51, 1982.
80. **Willecke, K. and Schafer, R.,** Human oncogenes, *Hum. Genet.,* 66, 132, 1984.
81. **Yokota, J., Tsunetsugu-Yokota, Y., Battifora, H., LeFevre, C., and Cline, M. J.,** Alterations of myc, myb and ras^{Ha} proto-oncogenes in cancers are frequent and show clinical correlation, *Science,* 231, 261, 1986.
82. **Roa, R. A., Carey, T. E., Passamani, P. P., Greenwood, J. H., Hsu, S., Ridings, E. O., Swartz, D. R., Wolf, G. T., and Hudson, J. L.,** DNA content of human squamous cell carcinoma cell lines: analysis by flow cytometry and chromosome enumeration, *Arch. Otolaryngol.,* 111, 565, 1985.
83. **Grassel-Pietrusky, R., Deinlein, E., and Hornstein, O. P.,** DNA-ploidy rates in oral leukoplakias determined by flow cytometry, *J. Oral Pathol.,* 11, 434, 1982.
84. **Hauser-Urfer, I. H. and Stauffer, J.,** Comparitive chromosome analysis of nine squamous cell carcinoma lines from tumors of the head and neck, *Cytogenet. Cell Genet.,* 39, 35, 1985.
85. **Cooper, G. M. and Lane, M.-A.,** Cellular transforming genes and oncogenesis, *Biochim. Biophys. Acta,* 738, 9, 1984.
86. **Andersson, P., Goldfarb, M. P., and Weinberg, R. A.,** A defined subgenomic fragment of in vitro synthesized Moloney sarcoma virus DNA can induce cell transformation upon transfection, *Cell,* 16, 63, 1979.

87. **Coffin, J. M., Varmus, H. E., Bishop, J. M., Essex, M., Hardy, W. D., Jr., Martin, G. S., Rosenberg, N. E., Scolnick, E. M., Weinberg, R. W., and Vogt, P. K.,** Proposal for naming host cell-derived inserts in retrovirus genomes, *J. Virol.,* 40, 953, 1981.

88. **Erikson, R. L.,** Towards a biochemical description of malignant transformation, *Cancer,* 53, 2041, 1984.

89. **Cohen, P.,** The role of protein phosphorylation in neural and humoral control of cellular activity, *Nature (London),* 296, 613, 1982.

90. **Devare, S. G., Shatzman, A., Robbins, K. C., Rosenberg, M., and Aaronson, S. A.,** Expression of the PDGF-related transforming protein of simian sarcoma virus in *E. coli, Cell,* 36, 43, 1984.

91. **Dmitrovsky, E., Kuehl, W. M., Hollis, G. F., Kirsh, I. R., Bender, T. P., and Segal, S.,** Expression of a transfected human c-myc oncogene inhibits differentiation of a mouse erythroleukaemia cell line, *Nature (London),* 322, 748, 1986.

92. **Pulciani, S., Santos, E., Lauver, A. V., Long, L. K., Aaronson, S. A., and Barbacid, M.,** Oncogenes in solid human tumors, *Nature (London),* 300, 539, 1982.

93. **Stafford, D. W. and Blin, N.,** A general method for isolation of high molecular weight DNA from eukaryots, *Nucleic Acids Res.,* 3, 2303, 1976.

94. **Shih, C., Shilo, B.-Z., Goldfarb, M. P., Dannenberg, A., and Weinberg, R. A.,** Passage of phenotypes of chemically transformed cells via transfection of DNA and chromatin, *Proc. Natl. Acad. Sci. U.S.A.,* 76, 5714, 1979.

95. **Perucho, M., Goldfarb, M., Shimizu, K., Lama, C., Fogh, J., and Wigler, M.,** Human-tumor-derived cell lines contain common and different transforming genes, *Cell,* 27, 467, 1981.

96. **Shih, C. and Weinberg, R. A.,** Isolation of a transforming sequence from a human bladder carcinoma cell line, *Cell,* 29, 161, 1982.

97. **Krontiris, T. G. and Cooper, G. M.,** Transforming activity of human tumor DNA, *Proc. Natl. Acad. Sci. U.S.A.,* 78, 1181, 1981.

98. **Friedman, W. H., Rosenblum, B., Loewenstein, P., Thornton, H., Katsantonis, G., and Green, M.,** Oncogenes: preliminary studies in head and neck cancer, *Laryngoscope,* 93, 1441, 1983.

99. **Friedman, W. H., Rosenblum, B., Loewenstein, P., Thornton, H., Katsantonis, G., and Green, M.,** Oncogenes in laryngeal cancer: serial passage of transformed cellular DNA, *Otolaryngol. Head Neck Surg.,* 93, 346, 1985.

100. **Howell, R. E., Fenwick, R. G., and Wong, F. S. H.,** unpublished data.

101. **Capon, D. J., Seeburg, P. H., McGrath, J. P., Hayflick, J. S., Edman, U., Levinson, A. D., and Goeddel, D. V.,** Activation of Ki-ras 2 gene in human colon and lung carcinomas by two different point mutations, *Nature (London),* 304, 507, 1983.

102. **Santos, E., Martin-Zanca, D., Reddy, E. P., Pierotti, M. A., Della Porta, G., and Barbacid, M.,** Malignant activation of a K-ras oncogene in lung carcinoma but not in normal tissue of the same patient, *Science,* 223, 661, 1984.

103. **McCoy, M. S., Bargmann, C. I., and Weinberg, R. A.,** Human colon carcinoma Ki-ras 2 oncogene and its corresponding proto-oncogene, *Mol. Cell. Biol.,* 4, 1577, 1984.

104. **Shope, R. E.,** Infectious papillomatosis of rabbits, *J. Exp. Med.,* 58, 607, 1933.

105. **Marks, J. L.,** Viruses and cancers, *Science,* 231, 919, 1986.

106. **Marks, J. L.,** The slow, insidious natures of the HTLV's, *Science,* 231, 450, 1986.

107. **Bishop, J. M. and Varmus, H. E.,** Functions and origins of retroviral transforming genes, in *Molecular Biology of Tumor Viruses, Part III, RNA Tumor Viruses,* Weiss, R., Teich, N., Varmus, H. E., and Coffin, J., Eds., Cold Spring Harbor Press, Cold Spring Harbor, N.Y., 1982, 199.

108. **Varmus, H. E., Payne, G. S., Nusse, R., Luciw, P., Westaway, D., and Bishop, J. M.,** Insertional mechanisms in oncogenesis by retroviruses, in *Perspectives on Genes and the Molecular Biology of Cancer,* Robberson, D. L. and Saunders, G. F., Eds., Raven Press, New York, 1983, 233.

109. **Howley, P. M., Yang, Y.-C., Spalholz, B. A., and Rabson, M. S.,** Papillomavirus transforming functions, in *Papillomaviruses (Ciba Foundation Symposium 120),* John Wiley & Sons, Toronto, 1986, 39.

110. **Aerikson, J., Ar-Rushid, A., Drwinga, H. L., Noel, P. C., and Croce, C. M.,** Transcriptional activation of the translated c-myc oncogene in Burkitt lymphoma, *Proc. Natl. Acad. Sci. U.S.A.,* 80, 820, 1983.

111. **Adams, J. M., Gerondakis, S., Webb, E., Corcoran, L., and Corey, S.,** Cellular c-myc oncogene is altered by chromosomal translocation to an immunoglobulin locus in murine plasmacytomas and is rearranged similarly in human Burkitt lymphomas, *Proc. Natl. Acad. Sci. U.S.A.,* 80, 1982, 1984.

112. **Cullen, B. R., Lomedico, P. T., and Ju, G.,** Transcriptional interference in avian retroviruses — implications for the promoter insertion model of leukemogenesis, *Nature (London),* 307, 241, 1984.

113. **Stephenson, J. R. and Todaro, G. J.,** Viral-encoded transforming proteins and transforming growth factors, in *Advances in Viral Oncology,* Vol. 1, Klein, G., Ed., Raven Press, New York, 1982, 59.

114. **Silverman, S., Jr.,** Epidemiology, in *Oral Cancer,* 2nd ed., Silverman, S., Jr., Ed., American Cancer Society, New York, 1985, 6.

115. **Lozada, F., Silverman, S., Jr., Migliorati, C. A., Conant, M. A., and Volberding, P. A.,** Oral manifestations of tumor and opportunistic infections in the acquired immunodeficiency syndrome (AIDS): findings in 53 homosexual men with Kaposi sarcoma, *Oral Surg. Oral Med. Oral Pathol.,* 56, 491, 1983.

116. **Pfister, H., Krubke, J., Deitrich, W., Iftner, T., and Fuchs, P. G.,** Classification of the papillomaviruses — mapping the genome, in *Papillomaviruses (Ciba Foundation Symposium 120),* John Wiley & Sons, New York, 1986, 3.

117. **Pfister, H.,** Biology and biochemistry of papillomaviruses, *Rev. Physiol. Biochem. Pharmacol.,* 99, 111, 1984.

118. **Orth, G.,** Epidermodysplasia verruciformis: a model for understanding the oncogenicity of human papillomaviruses, in *Papillomaviruses (Ciba Foundation Symposium 120),* John Wiley & Sons, New York, 1986, 157.

119. **Crum, C. P., Mitao, M., Levine, R. U., and Silverstein, S.,** Cervical papillomaviruses segregate within morphologically distinct precancerous lesions, *J. Virol.,* 54, 675, 1985.

120. **Lancaster, W. D., Castellano, C., Santos, C., Delgado, G., Kurman, R. J., and Jensen, A. B.,** Human papillomavirus deoxyribonucleic acid in cervical carcinoma from primary and metastatic sites, *Am. J. Obstet. Gynecol.,* 154, 115, 1986.

121. **Coleman, D. V., Wickenden, C., and Malcolm, A. D. B.,** Association of human papillomavirus with squamous carcinoma of the uterine cervix, in *Papillomaviruses (Ciba Foundation Symposium 120),* John Wiley & Sons, New York, 1986, 175.

122. **Gissman, L., Wolnik, L., Ikenberg, H., Koldovsky, U., Schrurch, H. G., and zur Hausen, H.,** Human papillomavirus types 6 and 11 DNA sequences in genital and laryngeal papillomas and in some cervical cancers, *Proc. Natl. Acad. Sci. U.S.A.,* 80, 560, 1983.

123. **Boyle, W. F., Riggs, J. L., Oshiro, L. H., and Lennett, E. H.,** Electron microscope identification of papovavirus in laryngeal papilloma, *Laryngoscope,* 83, 1102, 1973.

124. **Praetorius-Clausen, F.,** Rare oral viral disorders (molluscum contagiosum, localized keratoacanthoma, verrucae, condyloma acuminatum and focal epithelial hyperplasia), *Oral Surg. Oral Med. Oral Pathol.,* 34, 604, 1972.

125. **Wysocki, G. P. and Hardie, J.,** Ultrastructural studies of intraoral verruca vulgaris, *Oral Surg. Oral Med. Oral Pathol.,* 47, 58, 1979.

126. **Praetorius-Clausen, F. and Willis, J. M.,** Papovavirus-like particles in focal epithelial hyperplasia, *Scand. J. Dent. Res.,* 79, 362, 1971.

127. **Welch, T. B., Barker, B. F., and Williams, C.,** Peroxidase-antiperoxidase evaluation of human oral squamous cell papillomas, *Oral Surg. Oral Med. Oral Pathol.,* 61, 603, 1986.

128. **Syrjanen, K., Syrjanen, S., Lamberg, M., Pyrhonen, S., and Nuutinen, J.,** Morphological and immunohistochemical evidence suggesting human papilloma virus (HPV) involvement in oral squamous cell carcinogenesis, *Int. J. Oral Surg.,* 12, 418, 1983.

129. **Jenson, A. B., Rosenthal, J. D., Olsen, C., Pass, F., Lancaster, W. D., and Shah, K.,** Immunological relatedness of papillomaviruses from different species, *JNCI,* 64, 495, 1980.

130. **Jenson, A. B., Lancaster, W. D., Heartmann, D.-P., and Shaffer, E. L., Jr.,** Frequency and distribution of papillomavirus structural antigens in verrucae, multiple papillomas, and condylomata of the oral cavity, *Am. J. Pathol.,* 107, 212, 1982.

131. **Strauss, M. and Bennett, J. A.,** Human papillomavirus in various lesions of the head and neck, *Otolaryngol. Head Neck Surg.,* 93, 342, 1985.

132. **Syrjanen, K., Pyrhonen, S., Aukee, S., and Koskela, E.,** Squamous cell papilloma of the oesophagus: a tumor probably caused by human papillomavirus (HPV), *Diag. Histopathol.,* 5, 291, 1982.

133. **Lack, E. E., Jenson, A. B., Smith, H. G., Healy, G. B., Pass, F., and Vawter, G. F.,** Immunoperoxidase localization of human papilloma-virus in laryngeal papillomas, *Intervirology,* 14, 148, 1980.

134. **Nagashfar, Z., Sawanda, E., Kutcher, M. J., Swancar, J., Gupta, J., Daniel, R., Kashima, H., Woodruff, J. D., and Shah, K.,** Identification of genital tract papillomaviruses HPV-6 and HPV-16 in warts of the oral cavity, *J. Med. Virol.,* 17, 313, 1985.

135. General discussion. II: sites, types and transmission of infection, in *Papillomaviruses (Ciba Foundation Symposium 120),* John Wiley & Sons, New York, 1986, 257.

136. **DeVilliers, E.-M., Weidaur, H., Otto, H., and zur Hausen, H.,** Papillomavirus DNA in human tongue carcinomas, *Int. J. Cancer,* 36, 575, 1985.

137. **Melnick, J. L. and Adam, E.,** Epidemiological approaches to determining whether herpes virus is the etiological agent of cervical cancer, *Prog. Exp. Tumor Res.,* 21, 49, 1978.

138. **Dreesman, G. R., Burek, J., Adam, E., Kaufman, R. H., Melnick, J. L., Powell, K. L., and Purifoy, D. J. M.,** Expression of herpes virus-induced antigens in human cervical cancer, *Nature (London),* 283, 591, 1980.

139. **McDougall, J. K., Galloway, D. A., and Fenoglio, C. M.,** Cervical carcinoma: detection of herpes simplex virus RNA in cells undergoing neoplastic change, *Int. J. Cancer,* 25, 1, 1980.

140. **Shillitoe, E. J., Greenspan, D., Greenspan, J. S., and Silverman, S., Jr.**, Immunoglobulin class of antibody to herpes simplex virus in patients with oral cancer, *Cancer,* 51, 65, 1983.

141. **Eglin, R. P., Scully, C., Lehner, T., Ward-Booth, P., and McGregor, I. M.**, Detection of RNA complementary to herpes simplex virus in human oral squamous cell carcinoma, *Lancet,* 2, 766, 1983.

142. **Crawford, L.**, Criteria for establishing that a virus is oncogenic, in *Papillomaviruses (Ciba Foundation Symposium 120)*, John Wiley & Sons, New York, 1986, 238.

143. **Hiratsuka, H., Imamura, M., Ishii, Y., Kohama, G.-I., and Kikuchi, K.**, Immunohistologic detection of lymphocyte subpopulations infiltrating in human oral cancer with special reference to its clinical significance, *Cancer,* 53, 2456, 1984.

144. **Hiratsuka, H., Imamura, M., Kasai, K., Kamiya, H., Ishii, Y., Kohama, G.-I., and Kikuchi, K.**, Lymphocyte subpopulations and T-cell subsets in human oral cancer tissues: immunohistologic analysis by monoclonal antibodies, *Am. J. Clin. Pathol.,* 81, 464, 1984.

145. **Dawson, D. E., Everts, E. C., Vetto, R. M., and Burger, D. R.**, Assessment of immunocompetent cells in patients with head and neck squamous cell carcinoma, *Ann. Otol. Rhinol. Laryngol.,* 94, 342, 1985.

146. **Burger, D., Vandenbark, A., and Finke, P.**, Assessment of reactivity to tumor extracts by leukocyte adherence inhibition and dermal testing, *JNCI,* 59, 317, 1977.

147. **Kragina, F. and Bolanca, S.**, Recent theoretical and practical problems in cell mediated immunological reactions in cases of laryngeal cancer, *Acta Otolaryngol. (Stockholm),* 89, 195, 1980.

148. **Krause, C.**, Characteristics of tumor associated antigens in squamous cell carcinoma, *Laryngoscope,* 89, 1105, 1979.

149. **Kragina, F., Koskivic, F., and Bolanca, S.**, Immunological investigations in laryngeal cancer, *Acta Otolaryngol. (Stockholm),* 87, 388, 1979.

150. **Gustafson, R., Neel, H., and Reaisch, G.**, Immunologic studies on cancer of the upper aerodigestive tract, *Otolaryngol. Head Neck Surg.,* 90, 52, 1982.

151. **Tong, A., Vandenbark, A., Kraybill, W., Vetto, R. M., and Burger, D. R.**, Flow cytofluorometric detection of tumor specific rosette-forming cells in patients with squamous cell carcinoma of the head and neck, *Cancer Res.,* 42, 2949, 1982.

152. **Balm, F., Drexhage, H., von Bromberg, M., and Snow, G.**, Mononuclear phagocyte function in head and neck cancer: NBT dye reduction, maturation and migration of peripheral blood monocytes, *Laryngoscope,* 92, 810, 1982.

153. **Vijayakumar, T. and Vasudevan, D. M.**, High affinity rosette forming cells in carcinoma of the oral cavity, uterine cervix and breast, *Cancer Lett.,* 27, 339, 1985.

154. **Saranath, D., Mukhopadhyaya, R., Rao, R., Fakiah, A. R., Naik, S. L., and Gangal, S. G.**, Cell-mediated immune status in patients with squamous carcinoma of the oral cavity, *Cancer,* 56, 1062, 1985.

155. **Angelini, G., Vena, G. A., D'Ovidio, R., Lospalluti, M., and Meneghini, C. L.**, T-cell subsets and soluble immune responses suppressor (SIRS) factor in skin squamous cell carcinoma, *Acta Derm. Venereol. (Stockholm),* 63, 109, 1983.

156. **Wustrow, T. P. U. and Zenner, H.-P.**, Natural killer cell activity in patients with carcinoma of the larynx and hypopharynx, *Laryngoscope,* 95, 1391, 1985.

157. **Poss, H. F. and Baines, M. G.**, Spontaneous human lymphocyte-mediated cytotoxicity against tumor target cells. I. The effect of malignant disease, *Int. J. Cancer,* 18, 593, 1986.

158. **Takasuji, M., Ramseyer, A., and Takasuji, J.**, Decline of natural nonselective cell-mediated cytotoxicity in patients with tumor progression, *Cancer Res.,* 37, 413, 1977.

159. **Hersey, P., Edwards, A,. and McCarthy, W. H.**, Tumor-related changes in natural killer cell activity in melanoma patients. Influence of stage of disease, tumor thickness, and age of patients, *Int. J. Cancer,* 25, 187, 1980.

160. **Schantz, S. P., Romsdahl, M. M., Babcock, G. F., Nishioka, K., and Goepfert, H.**, The effect of surgery on natural killer and cell activity in head and neck cancer patients: in vitro reversal of a postoperatively suppressed immunosurveillance system, *Laryngoscope,* 95, 588, 1985.

161. **Phillips, J. H., Nishioka, K., and Babcock, G. F.**, Tufsin-induced enhancement of murine and human natural cell-mediated cytotoxicity, *Ann. N.Y. Acad. Sci.,* 419, 192, 1983.

162. **Balm, F. J. M., von Blomberg-van de Flier, B. M. E., Drexhage, H. A., de Haan-Meulman, M., and Snow, G. B.**, Mononuclear phagocyte function in head and neck cancer: depression of murine macrophage accumulation by low molecular weight factors derived from head and neck carcinomas, *Laryngoscope,* 94, 223, 1984.

163. **Vena, G. A., Angelini, G., D'Ovidio, R., Pastore, A., and Meneghini, C. L.**, Monocyte Fc-IgG receptors expression and soluble suppressor factor in skin squamous cell carcinoma, *Acta Derm. Venereol. (Stockholm),* 63, 307, 1983.

164. **Scully, C.**, Immunological abnormalities in oral carcinoma or oral keratosis, *J. Maxillofac. Surg.,* 10, 113, 1982.

165. **Passwel, J., Rosen, F. S., and Merler, E.,** The effect of Fc fragments of IgG on human mononuclear cell responses, *Cell. Immunol.,* 52, 395, 1980.

166. **Droller, M. J., Schneider, M. U., and Perlmann, P.,** A possible role of prostaglandins in the inhibition of natural and antibody-dependent cell-mediated cytotoxicity against tumor cells, *Cell. Immunol.,* 39, 165, 1978.

167. **Goodwin, J. S.,** Prostaglandins and host defense in cancer, *Med. Clin. North Am.,* 65, 829, 1981.

168. **Balch, C. M., Dougherty, M. S., and Tilden, A. B.,** Excessive prostaglandin E2 production by suppressor monocytes in head and neck patients, *Ann. Surg.,* 196, 645, 1982.

169. **Jung, T. T. K., Berlinger, N. T., and Juhn, S. K.,** Prostaglandins in squamous cell carcinoma of the head and neck: a preliminary study, *Laryngoscope,* 95, 307, 1985.

170. **El Attar, T. M. A., Lin, H. S., and Vanderhoek, J. Y.,** Biosynthesis of prostaglandins and hydroxy fatty acids in primary squamous carcinomas of head and neck in humans, *Cancer Lett.,* 27, 255, 1985.

171. **Silverman, N. A., Alexander, J. C., and Chretien, P. B.,** CEA levels in head and neck cancer, *Cancer,* 37, 2204, 1976.

172. **Maxum, P. E. and Veltri, R. W.,** Serum ferritin as a tumor marker in patients with squamous cell carcinoma in the head and neck, *Cancer,* 57, 305, 1986.

173. **Shuster, J., Gold, P., and Poulik, M. D.,** Beta 2-microglobulin levels in cancerous and other diseases, *Clin. Chim. Acta,* 67, 307, 1976.

174. **Cassuto, J. P., Krebs, B. P., Viot, G., Dujardin, P., and Masseyeff, R.,** Beta 2-microglobulin, a tumor marker of lymphoproliferative disorders, *Lancet,* 2, 108, 1978.

175. **Teasdale, C., Mander, A. M., Fifeld, R., Keyser, J. W., Newcombe, R. G., and Hughes, L. E.,** Serum beta 2-microglobulins in controls and cancer patients, *Clin. Chim. Acta,* 78, 135, 1977.

176. **Trope, C. G., Logdberg, L., and Johnsson, J. E.,** Beta 2-microglobulin: a tumor marker of gynecologic cancer, *Am. J. Obstet. Gynecol.,* 137, 743, 1980.

177. **Wennerberg, J., Alm, P., Logdberg, L., and Trope, C.,** Beta 2-microglobulin in squamous cell carcinomas of the head and neck and in tumors heterotransplanted in nude athymic mice, *Acta Otolaryngol. (Stockholm),* 98, 335, 1984.

178. **Scully, C.,** Thymidine kinase activity in oral squamous cell carcinoma, *J. Oral Pathol.,* 11, 210, 1982.

179. **Scully, C., Spandidos, D. A., Ward-Booth, P., McGreggor, I. A., and Boyle, P.,** Serum alkaline deoxyribonuclease in oral cancer and premalignant lesions, *Biomedicine,* 35, 179, 1981.

180. **Katz, A. E., Nysather, J., and Harker, L.,** Major immunoglobulin ratios in carcinoma of the head and neck, *Ann. Otol. Rhinol. Laryngol.,* 87, 412, 1978.

181. **Toto, P. D. and Gargiulo, A. W.,** Lectin binding to oral squamous carcinoma, *Cancer Detect. Prev.,* 8, 161, 1985.

182. **Dabelsteen, E. and MacKenzie, I. C.,** Expression of *Ricinus communis* receptors on epithelial cells on oral carcinomas and oral wounds, *Cancer Res.,* 38, 4676, 1978.

183. **Prime, S. S., Rosser, T. J., Malamos, D., Shepard, J. P., and Scully, C.,** The use of the lectin *Ulex europeus* to study epithelial cell differentiation in neoplastic and non-neoplastic oral white lesions, *J. Pathol.,* 147, 173, 1985.

184. **Dabelsteen, E. and Pindborg, J. J.,** Loss of epithelial blood group substance A in oral carcinomas, *Acta Pathol. Microbiol. Scand.,* 81, 435, 1973.

185. **Bovopoulou, O., Sklavounou, A., and Laskaris, G.,** Loss of intercellular substance antigens in oral hyperkeratosis, epithelial dysplasia, and squamous cell carcinoma, *Oral Surg. Oral Med. Oral Pathol.,* 60, 648, 1985.

186. **Gupta, Y. N., Gupta, S., Singh, I. J., Khanna, N. N., and Agarwal, M. K.,** Epithelial isoantigens A, B and H in oral carcinomas, *Ear Nose Throat J.,* 64, 239, 1985.

187. **Meyer, J. R., Silverman, S., Jr., Daniels, T. E., Kramer, R. H., and Greenspan, J. S.,** Distribution of fibronectin and laminin in oral leukoplakia and carcinoma, *J. Oral Pathol.,* 14, 247, 1985.

188. **Matsumura, T., Kobayashi, S., Ishihara, Y., Sugahara, T., Yui, S., and Nakamura, M.,** Histochemical observations of hexokinase in leukoplakias and squamous cell carcinomas of oral cavity and maxillary sinus, *J. Osaka Dent. Univ.,* 23, 133, 1983.

189. **Boeheim, K., Speek, J. A., Frei, E., III, and Bernal, S. D.,** SQM1 antibody defines a surface membrane antigen in squamous carcinoma of the head and neck, *Int. J. Cancer,* 36, 137, 1985.

190. **Tranter, R. M. D., Fairweather, D. S., Bradwell, A. R., Dykes, P. W., Watson-James, S., and Chandler, S.,** The detection of squamous cell tumors of the head and neck using radiolabelled antibodies, *J. Laryngol. Otol.,* 98, 71, 1984.

191. **Toto, P. D.,** Fluorescent antibody detection of CEA in oral cancer, *J. Oral Med.,* 34, 45, 1979.

192. **Mashberg, A.,** Tolinum (toluidine blue) rinse — a screening method for recognition of squamous carcinoma. Continuing study of oral cancer. IV., *JAMA,* 245, 2408, 1981.

193. **Mashberg, A.,** Final evaluation of tolinum chloride rinse for screening of high risk patients with asymptomatic squamous carcinoma, *J. Am. Dent. Assoc.,* 106, 319, 1983.

194. **Kolstad, P.,** Vascular changes in cervical intraepithelial neoplasia and invasive cervical carcinoma, *Clin. Obstet. Gynecol.,* 26, 1938, 1983.

195. **Javaheri, G. and Fegjin, M. D.,** Diagnostic value of colposcopy in the investigation of cervical neoplasia, *Am. J. Obstet. Gynecol.,* 137, 588, 1980.

196. **Howell, R. E., Danforth, R. A., Bray, B. A., and Mathews, F. R.,** Human cervical and hamster oral epithelial neoplasia — colposcopic similarities, *Gynecol. Oncol.,* 24, 17, 1986.

197. **Trell, L., Korsgaard, R., Janzon, L., and Trell, E.,** Distribution and reproducibility of aryl hydrocarbon hydroxylase inducibility in a prospective population study of middle-aged male smokers and non-smokers, *Cancer,* 56, 1988, 1985.

198. **Trell, L., Korsgaard, R., Hood, B., Kitzing, P., Norden, G., and Simonsson, B. G.,** Aryl hydrocarbon hydroxylase inducibility and laryngeal carcinomas, *Lancet,* 2, 140, 1976.

199. **Kellerman, G., Shaw, C. R., and Luyten-Kellerman, M.,** Aryl hydrocarbon hydroxylase inducibility and bronchogenic carcinoma, *N. Engl. J. Med.,* 289, 934, 1973.

200. **Jesse, R. H.,** Cancer of the oral cavity: is elective neck dissection beneficial?, *Am. J. Surg.,* 120, 505, 1970.

201. **Spiro, R. H. and Strong, E. W.,** Surgical treatment of cancer of the tongue, *Surg. Clin. North Am.,* 54, 759, 1974.

202. **Vandenbrouck, C., Sancho-Garnier, H., Chassagne, D., Saravane, D., Cachin, Y., and Micheau, C.,** Elective versus therapeutic radical neck dissection in epidermoid carcinoma of the oral cavity, *Cancer,* 46, 386, 1980.

203. **Teichgraeber, J. F. and Clairmont, A. A.,** The incidence of occult metastases for cancer of the oral tongue and floor of mouth: treatment rationale, *Head Neck Surg.,* 7, 15, 1984.

204. **Ali, S., Tiwari, R. M., and Snow, G. B.,** False-positive and false-negative neck nodes, *Head Neck Surg.,* 8, 78, 1985.

205. **Grandi, C., Alloisio, M., Moglia, D., Podrecca, S., Sala, L., Salvatoni, P., and Molinari, R.,** Prognostic significance of lymphatic spread in head and neck carcinomas: therapeutic implications, *Head Neck Surg.,* 8, 67, 1985.

206. **Gilbert, E. H., Goffinet, D. R., and Bagshaw, M. A.,** Carcinoma of the oral tongue and floor of mouth: fifteen years' experience with linear accelerator therapy, *Cancer,* 35, 1517, 1975.

207. **Fu, K. K., Ray, J. W., Chan, E. K., and Phillips, T. L.,** External and interstitial radiation therapy of carcinoma of the oral tongue. A review of 32 years experience, *Am. J. Roentgenol.,* 126, 107, 1976.

208. **Bertino, J. R., Boston, B., and Capizzi, R. L.,** The role of chemotherapy in the management of cancer of the head and neck: a review, *Cancer,* 36, 752, 1975.

209. **Elias, E. G., Chretien, P. B., Monnard, E., Khan, T., Bouchelle, W. H., Wiernik, P. H., Lipson, S. D., Hande, K. R., and Zentai, T.,** Chemotherapy prior to local therapy in advanced squamous cell carcinoma of the head and neck. Preliminary assessment of an intensive drug regimen, *Cancer,* 43, 1025, 1979.

210. **Stephens, F. O., Harker, G. J. S., and Hambly, C. K.,** Treatment of advanced cancer of the lower lip — the use of intraarterial or intravenous chemotherapy as basal treatment, *Cancer,* 48, 1309, 1981.

211. **Weaver, A., Fleming, S., Vandenberg, H., Drelichman, A., Jacobs, J., Kinzie, J., Loh, J. J.-K., and Al-Sarraf, M.,** cis-Platinum and 5-fluorouracil as initial therapy in advanced epidermoid cancers of the head and neck, *Head Neck Surg.,* 4, 370, 1982.

212. **Mead, G. M. and Jacobs, C.,** Changing role of chemotherapy in treatment of head and neck cancer, *Am. J. Med.,* 73, 582, 1982.

213. **Penacchio, J. L., Hong, W. K., Shapshay, S., Gillis, T., Vaughan, C., Bhutani, R., Ucmakli, A., Katz, A. E., Bromer, R., Willet, B., and Strong, S. M.,** Combination of cis-platinum and bleomycin prior to surgery and/or radiotherapy compared with radiotherapy alone for the treatment of advanced squamous cell carcinoma of the head and neck, *Cancer,* 50, 2795, 1982.

214. **Decker, D. A., Drelichman, A., Jacobs, J., Hoschner, J., Kinzie, J., Loh, J. J.-K., Weaver, A., and Al-Sarraf, M.,** Adjuvant chemotherapy with cis-diamminodichloroplatinum II and 120 hour infusion 5-fluorouracil in stage III and IV squamous cell carcinoma of the head and neck, *Cancer,* 51, 1353, 1983.

215. **Hong, W. K., Schaeter, S., Issell, B., Cummings, C., Luedke, D., Bromer, R., Fofonoff, S., D'Aoust, J., Shapshay, S., Welch, J., Levin, E., Vincent, M., Vaughan, C., and Strong, S.,** A prospective randomized trial of methotrexate versus cisplatin in the treatment of recurrent squamous cell carcinoma of the head and neck, *Cancer,* 52, 206, 1983.

216. **Ringborg, U., Ewert, G., Kinnman, J., Lundqvist, P.-G., and Strander, H.,** Sequential methotrexate-5-fluorouracil treatment of squamous cell carcinoma of the head and neck, *Cancer,* 52, 971, 1983.

217. **Mohit-Tabatabai, M. A., Rush, B. F., Hill, G. J., Ohanian, M., Raina, S., Dasmahapatra, K. S., and Cheung, N. K.,** Multimodality preoperative treatment for advanced cancer of the head and neck, *Am. J. Surg.,* 148, 521, 1984.

218. **Ensley, J. F., Jacobs, J. R., Weaver, A., Kinzie, J., Crissman, J., Kish, J. A., Cummings, G., and Al-Sarraf, M.,** Correlation between response to cisplatinum-combination chemotherapy and subsequent radiotherapy in previously untreated patients with advanced squamous cell cancers of the head and neck, *Cancer,* 54, 811, 1984.

219. **Cobleigh, M. A., Hill, J. H., Gallagher, P. A., Kukla, L. J., Lad, T. E., Shevrin, D. H., Applebaum, E. L., and McQuire, W. P.,** A phase II study of adriamycin in previously untreated squamous cell carcinoma of the head and neck, *Cancer,* 56, 2573, 1985.

220. **O'Brien, C. J., Lahr, C. J., Soong, S.-J., Gandour, M. J., Jones, J. M., Urist, M. M., and Maddox, W. A.,** Surgical treatment of early-stage carcinoma of the oral tongue — would adjuvant treatment be beneficial?, *Head Neck Surg.,* 8, 401, 1986.

221. **Rhys Evans, P. H., Frame, J. W., and Brandrick, J.,** A review of carbon dioxide laser surgery in the oral cavity and pharynx, *J. Laryngol. Otol.,* 100, 69, 1986.

222. **Burns, R. A., Klannig, J. E., Shulok, J. R., Davis, W. J., and Goldblatt, P. J.,** Tumor-localizing and photosensitivity properties of hematoporphyrin derivative in hamster buccal pouch carcinoma, *Oral Surg. Oral Med. Oral Pathol.,* 61, 368, 1986.

INDEX